29 Update in Intensive Care and Emergency Medicine

Edited by J.-L. Vincent

Springer
Berlin
Heidelberg
New York
Barcelona
Budapest
Hong Kong
London
Milan
Paris
Santa Clara
Singapore
Tokyo

D. Reis Miranda D. W. Ryan
W. B. Schaufeli V. Fidler (Eds.)

Organisation and Management of Intensive Care

A Prospective Study in 12 European Countries

With 46 Figures and 133 Tables

Springer

Series Editor

Prof. Dr. Jean-Louis Vincent
Clinical Director, Department of Intensive Care
Erasme University Hospital
Route de Lennik 808, B-1070 Brussels, Belgium

Volume Editor

Dr. Dinis Reis Miranda
University Hospital Groningen, Health Services Research Unit
F.O. Box 30.001, NL-9700 RB Groningen, The Netherlands

Dr. David W. Ryan
Freeman Hospital, ICU, NE7 7DN Newcastle upon Tyne,
United Kingdom

Dr. Wilmar B. Schaufeli
University of Utrecht, Department of Social and Organisational Psychology, P.O. Box 80140, NL-3508 TC Utrecht, The Netherlands

Dr. Václav Fidler
University of Groningen, Faculty of Medicine, A. Deusinglaan 1,
NL-9713 AV Groningen, The Netherlands

ISSN 0933-6788
ISBN-13:978-642-64328-6 e-ISBN-13:978-3-642-60270-2
DOI: 10.1007/978-3-642-60270-2

Library of Congress Cataloging-in-Publication Data
Organisation and management of intensive care : a prospective study in 12 European countries / (eds.) D. Reis Miranda ... [et al.].
(Update in intensive care and emergency medicine ; 29)
Includes bibliographical references and index. ISBN-13:978-642-64328-6 (alk. paper) 1. Intensive care units – Administration. 2. Intensive care units – Europe. I. Miranda, D. Reis (Dinis Reis) II. Series. RA975.5.I56074 1997 362.1'74–DC21 97-13204 CIP

Softcover reprint of the hardcover 1st edition 1998

Typesetting (Data conversion) and printing: Zechnersche Buchdruckerei, Speyer
Bookbinding: J. Schäffer, Grünstadt

SPIN: 10566781 19/3133-5 4 3 2 1 0 – Printed on acid-free paper

Foreword

From the viewpoint of a health economist, the intensive care unit (ICU) is a particularly fascinating phenomenon. It is the epitome of "high-tech" medicine and frequently portrayed as the place where life-saving miracles are routinely wrought. But the popular imagination is also caught up in the darker side, when agonizing decisions have to be made to avoid futile and inhuman continuation of expensive treatments.

My analytical interests led me to approach these issues by asking what the evidence tells us about which ICU activities are very beneficial in relationship to their costs and which are not. This quickly translates into a slightly different question, namely, which patients are most appropriately treated in an ICU and which not. Unfortunately, it is very hard to answer these questions because it has proved very difficult to investigate these issues in the manner which is now regarded as the "gold standard," namely by conducting randomized clinical trials or alternative courses of action. I think this is a pity, and I am not at all convinced that it would be unethical to do so in many cases, because there is wide variation in practice and genuine doubt as to which practices are best – the two conditions that need to be fulfilled before such a trial is justifiable.

Be that as it may, the next best alternative is to use the variation that exists in practice as a "natural experiment." This too is a difficult task, requiring careful and systematic collection and sifting of evidence for clues as to underlying relationships, which could then become the subject of more detailed investigation. Intensive care is a fertile field for this kind of data-hungry investigation, because intensive care is stronger than most medical specialties on computer-based information retrieval from well-maintained databases, which is what such studies require. The conceptual and analytical problems remain formidable, however, as the current discussions about rival scoring and prediction systems testify only too clearly.

A further leap of the imagination is required if we are to assess the overall effectiveness of an ICU and its appropriate role in the whole spectrum of health care. Intensive care is not a simple "hands-on" relationship between an individual practitioner and an individual patient. It is a complex multidisciplinary activity relying on extremely complex logistical support from the technological hardware and software that constitute the physical environment of the ICU. Thus the successful delivery of intensive care requires much more than good clinical practice. It also requires good logistic management and good personnel management. Just as with clinical practice, we know that there are wide variations in practice and genuine doubt as to which practices are best. This nonclinical area should be a fertile field for the same kind of natural experiment, as is becoming increasingly common with respect to clinical practice itself.

Investigating the influence of nonclinical factors upon the performance of ICUs, we are somewhat further back the road and still at the stage of exploring the possibilities of formulating and tackling these problems in a systematic manner. The EURICUS-I project occupies an interesting middle ground between a simple descriptive study and a rigorous evaluative study. It has an analytical thrust which takes it well beyond the former, but it lacks the enormously large and representative database, and the experimental design, that would be necessary for the latter. It is of the nature of an extensive pilot study, testing whether particular analytical and data collection methods can be made to work in quite diverse circumstances and whether any provisional conclusions emerge concerning nonclinical factors that seem likely to be positively or negatively associated with the clinical outcomes for patients treated in ICUs.

As will be seen in what follows, EURICUS-I has been a resounding success in both of these respects. It has demonstrated the feasibility of collecting the nonclinical information required and of relating it systematically to patient outcome. But it has also identified some key factors to do with working arrangements within an ICU which appear to affect those patient outcomes. This places a strong ethical obligation on ICU directors to review their current practices and to assure themselves, their staff, and their colleagues that they have done everything which seems reasonable to ensure that their units are run in a manner that does not endanger their patients' well-being. It also places a strong ethical obligation on those with responsibilities for intensive care medicine outside the units themselves to review the role and function of the units for which they have general responsibility and to ensure that they are neither over-stretched in relation to the tasks placed upon them or over-resourced in relation to their actual workload. Both phenomena appear to be present amongst the units covered in the study, and it would be very surprising if both phenomena were not also widespread if the range of units were made more representative in each country.

Another interesting finding has been the apparent significance for patient outcome of the size of the unit (after controlling for many other variables). This is such an important organizational and logistical factor that it would appear worthwhile to investigate this more closely in its own right. There are so many different features associated with unit size that require quite careful disentangling; thus the conclusion here, that the optimal size is probably about nine beds (or, say, between six and 12?), should be treated as no more than a first approximation but not something to be swept under the carpet. At the level of national and regional planning this is a key variable which deserves close investigation.

As someone outside the field of intensive care, I was impressed with the willingness of all the participants in this study to devote their time and energy to what must have been regarded as a high-risk investigation in two senses. In the first place there was a high risk that the data would not be collectable or analyzable, so that the entire enterprise would prove abortive. In the second place there was a high risk that the results would turn out to be damaging to the participants' own self-esteem (for even with the protection of anonymity, each unit knows where it stands in the order of things!). It shows a commendable willingness to put the interests of patients above one's own personal and professional feelings, and I congratulate all concerned for their altruism and dedication. I hope they feel personally rewarded by what follows in this report.

Alan Williams
Centre for Health Economics, University of York, UK
Chairman of the Steering Group of EURICUS-I

Preface

In 1952 an unusually severe epidemic of poliomyelitis, with many patients experiencing respiratory difficulties, struck Copenhagen. Successful management of patients with respiratory failure initiated the development of more sophisticated mechanical ventilators and monitoring equipment and prompted the foundation of intensive care units (ICUs) in several European countries. The year 1952 is, therefore, generally considered as the beginning of intensive care medicine in Europe. Gradually, care of the critically ill patient became more professional, such that in many European countries intensive care medicine is now recognized as a primary specialty (Spain), subspecialty or secondary specialty.

Recent surveys and studies among European ICUs have demonstrated many similarities but also many differences in the practice of intensive care medicine. In this book the first extensive and in-depth European study on features and performance of ICUs, in which 89 ICUs in 12 countries participated, is presented. The basic goal of this study, conducted by the Foundation for Research on Intensive Care in Europe (FRICE) under the leadership of Dr. D. Reis Miranda, was to explore the effects of organization and management on the effectiveness and efficiency of ICUs. The uniqueness of this study is its emphasis on nonclinical factors. Elaborate methods such as extensive questionnaires and site visits have resulted in a wealth of information and a thorough analysis of various aspects of European intensive care. Among these are case mix, occupancy and mortality rates, professional activities of ICU nurses and physicians, nurses' workload and participation in decision-making, ICU organization and use of facilities, budgetary and cost-accounting procedures, and ICU performance.

This diagnostic journey to a relatively large number of European ICUs has provided us with an extremely comprehensive view and has allowed identification of those factors which influence clinical performance of ICUs. The investigators are to be congratulated with their results. Information and analysis such as presented here are urgently needed as they identify areas in which major improvements can be made. This book is the next step in the tradition of the FRICE, which since 1989 has given organizational support to a core network of more than 30 European research teams of diverse disciplines. It is also a basis for further studies, as already planned by FRICE, which ultimately will result in major improvements of ICU performance in Europe.

Lambert G. Thijs
Past President of the European Society of Intensive Care Medicine

Table of Contents

Part II

How to Read This Book

The Content

This book presents the results of the research developed during a multicenter concerted action involving intensive care units (ICUs) in Europe and a multidisciplinary group of research teams. According to the specificity of the research teams involved, the study was divided into several substudies.

The book is divided into three parts. Part I (Introduction and Chaps. 1–5) describes and briefly presents the results of the research done, focusing on integration of the results of the substudies. In the sequence of the results obtained, the conclusions of the study are presented, and recommendations made to those European policy makers involved with intensive care medicine. Part II (Chaps. 6–8) consists of separate and detailed presentations of the various substudies, focusing on the survey analysis made in each of them concerning the total sample of ICUs in the study. Part III presents the list of ICUs, the individuals and the organizations that participated in EURICUS-I.

The Limitations

It is important that the reader of this book is aware of the limitations of the research reported.

Nonrandomization of ICUs

The criteria for selection of ICUs will be addressed in Chap. 1. It was agreed during the preparation phase of EURICUS-I that nonrandomization of the participating ICUs at the country level would better serve the objectives of the study: to reveal the large variation that is possible across Europe regarding the variables organization and management. In each country the ICUs were therefore selected in an open manner according to a previously defined protocol. The value of the research concerning the influence of organization and management on the effectiveness and efficiency of ICUs, the main objective of the study, was not affected by the nonrandomization of the participating units.

The results of the survey of ICUs concerning the data presented at substudy level do need, however, to be interpreted in light of the non-randomization of the ICUs. In particular, limitations concerning data on substudy *Patients and Facilities*, topics most likely to invite analysis and comparison, should be emphasized.

The data on patients and facilities collected from a large number of ICUs spread across Europe provide an extensive and detailed survey of the most relevant characteristics of the units. The study produced the first reference data-set of its kind in many of the participating countries. The data will also allow for useful comparisons between individual ICUs or between particular and well defined aggregates of ICUs. It is not possible, however, because of the non-randomization methodology followed, to use the data for comparing ICUs when aggregated at country level. Besides not being representative of the ICUs at country level, only in a very limited number of cases (in which all the ICUs of a province or other well-defined region are included) do the participating ICUs represent a specific part of a country. Country and European area were the labels used. It was, however, difficult to label data concerning aggregates of ICUs from particular geographic areas without naming the respective country. It is therefore important to emphasize that the various groups of ICUs in the study are not representative of the countries to which they belong, although the name of their country was used to label them.

Different Research Methodologies

Three different research methodologies were used for the collection of EURICUS-I data:

1. Daily collection of clinical data from patients enrolled in the study. The majority of these data were collected as continuous variables ready for (statistical) analysis.
2. Collection of organization and management data by means of questionnaires administered to the leadership and personnel of the ICUs. The majority of these data needed to be transformed into categorical or continuous variables by the use of specific instruments. The majority of these instruments were previously tested and validated. Concerning one substudy (*Organization*) the instruments used were developed in the EURICUS-I data prior to hypothesis testing.
3. Collection of observational data by one interviewer. This was the case of the data collected during the one-day site visit to the ICUs.

The various types of collected data were analyzed independently at the respective substudy level. Integrative analysis of the substudies, however, used data collected differently and with obvious differences concerning validity and reliability. This is clearly the case for data collected during site visits, although the site visits turned out to be a very valuable undertaking, as they provided the advantages of real-time observation, spontaneity and close contact with the working environment in which the research took place.

The limitations pointed out above need to be kept in mind when interpreting the results of the integration of the EURICUS-I substudies.

Size of Samples

The collected data were subdivided into various samples, mainly at ICU level, to address the analysis of those variables selected by the substudies. The sample sizes were often different, usually because the number of entries varied with the ICU (e.g., number of patients enrolled, number of respondents to questionnaires). The large variation in sample size concerned the number of patients enrolled per ICU. This is of particular importance for evaluating ICU performance, as the analysis requires samples that are larger than those provided by some of the ICUs.

During the study many attempts were made to reduce the number of values missing from the data collected. It must be emphasized that the efforts developed at all levels of management of the study were, to our knowledge, without precedent in multicenter studies of this size and complexity. Yet, these attempts were not completely successful and the size of the final samples varied due to missing values. For example, one important effect of missing values is that, in some of the analyses, the number of ICUs is smaller than the 89 units participating in the study. Consequently, the number of ICUs cited in the various tables may vary according to the variable(s) under analysis.

The Interpretation of Two Important Concepts

Country

One of the most interesting findings in the EURICUS-I study was the consistent importance of the area of Europe (country) on the majority of the analyses performed. This variable was significantly related to performance (defined as risk-adjusted mortality) as well as to many other variables in the substudies *Patients and Facilities*, *Personnel*, *Organization* and *Culture*.

Although it was not possible to find an exact explanation for this variable, some reflections about its meaning are nonetheless due. In the EURICUS-I study analyses, the importance of the variable country was that it appeared as a confounder, in other words, as a factor that might distort the relationship of the study variables of central interest by virtue of being related to the outcome under analysis.- Alternatively, it might be extraneous to the study question and unequally distributed among the groups being compared. This was the reason why this variable was consequently used in the majority of the analyses – a strategy that worked very well but did not provide any clues as to its interpretation. By contrast, analyses done in order to relate this variable to other variables in the study were not successful. So, what does country mean? At least three possibilities have been advanced to explain this effect: individual-based, collectively based and sampling bias.

Individual-Based Characteristics

One of the possibilities is that the variable country represents a surrogate marker for differences between patients in diverse European areas, explained for example by differences in nutritional status, use of tobacco, and prevalence of chronic diseases. In this hypothesis, we assume that these factors are unequally distributed among European areas and that they strongly affect short-term mortality. In other words, country would act as an "effect-modifier," changing the relationship between severity of illness and mortality and affecting clinical performance.

Collective-Based Characteristics

The second hypothesis is that the variable country is a surrogate marker of other characteristics, such as gross national product, percentage of expenses in health care, or the cultural characteristics of the population and health personnel aggregated at a collective level (area of Europe). It would be easy to accept that some of these differences (e.g., different admission policies, different attitudes of health care personnel to their work) could have an impact on clinical and nonclinical variables, since they may affect the process of care and the outcome of patients. The correlation introduced in data derived from the same European area, however, should then affect similarly (in a positive or negative direction) all the individuals/institutions in that area. More research is therefore necessary.

Sampling Bias

As stated above, selection of the ICUs was not random. Within each country, the respective country coordinator selected the ICUs according to predefined criteria, in which the ICUs should belong to hospitals of different types and size and the selection should enable study of the professional interaction between the ICUs. In other words, the ICUs should be clustered in groups of at least four units within a national area. This could have introduced a sort of correlation within all the ICUs chosen from each European area based on the criteria (objective or subjective) used by the country coordinator in the selection process. If true, this phenomenon could explain the observed importance of the variable country in the study or at least contribute to magnifying the real differences between different European areas.

Each of these hypotheses probably has some component of truth and they should thus be the subjects of further research. To what extent this line of investigation lies within the scope of the EURICUS studies may be discussed, but its importance cannot be underestimated.

In light of the above, it should be noted that appropriate interpretation of the variable country was not possible from the collected data. Therefore, and although some of the results of the study are clearly influenced by the aggregates of ICUs at country level, it would be incorrect to interpret the observed effects as conclusive characteristics of the countries involved.

Performance

To perform is to achieve. In managerial terms this entails prior definition of objectives. EURICUS-I did not address the definition of objectives by the participating ICU. Nonetheless, the term "performance" is often used in this study, the most important example being "clinical performance." This term is not new as it is commonly used in the literature in association with the observed mortality compared with the mortality predicted by severity of illness scoring systems.

In this study, a ranking of ICUs was computed from the observed mortality in the units after controlling for severity of illness. According to the obtained ranking, the risk-adjusted mortality in one ICU may be higher or lower than in other units. This ranking has been associated with clinical performance. The ranking of ICUs suggests that clinical performance is higher or lower and hence that it may be better or worse. However, a previous definition of objectives is the necessary end-point for this type of comparison. Furthermore, mortality in the ICU is intimately dependent on the case mix of the patients admitted to the unit. Although severity of illness is probably the most relevant element of case mix, the precise definition of case mix in the ICU is not yet available. The correct evaluation of clinical performance is therefore also dependent on the case mix.

This misconception (jargon) regarding clinical performance has made its way into the medical literature.While we dispute the accuracy of this and other generally accepted terms, we have accommodated their usage in this book, as any acceptable alternative would have made the text less easy to understand and to read. It is therefore necessary to emphasize that, used in this way, clinical performance merely reflects a ranking of ICUs and cannot be interpreted as being indicative of quality.

Finally, the EURICUS-I study will be an important reference for future research on the issues addressed, besides constituting a source of hypotheses in its own right.

Part I

EURICUS-I: Introduction

Intensive care is a development of modern medical practice, with the goal of providing for and treating life threatening illness. Caring for such patients is a most demanding job with unremitting hard work, the skilled use of high technology equipment and, literally, life and death dramas occurring every day.

The evolution of intensive care units (ICUs) has been uncontrolled, haphazard and variable across Europe. There is no evidence of financial control or scrutiny of how money is allocated and spent. This is remarkable as the ICU is, in financial terms, a most expensive hospital "hot spot". The ICU is an employer of a large nursing staff and the purchaser of sophisticated and costly equipment; it has a large pharmacy budget, using an enormous amount of disposable equipment; and it is a constant drain on laboratory resources. There is likewise little published scientific work to question the quality of care given, audit the success of treatment, and determine if the resources are being well spent.

The absence of planning, regulation, training and an overall strategy must influence the way the ICU performs and its contribution overall to patient care.

EURICUS-I, or the First European ICU Study, explores the effect of organization and management on the effectiveness and efficiency of ICUs in the countries of the European Community (EC). The study is an interdisciplinary survey of the relevant characteristics of ICUs from a health service research perspective. EURICUS-I tests the hypothesis that variables refelecting nonclinical organization and management influence the clinical outcome of patients admitted to the ICUs. Therefore, the study collected clinical and nonclinical data on several types of ICUs from the various EC countries in order to maximize the variance of the variables to be addressed. EURICUS-I was divided into five complementary substudies, *Patients and Facilities, Personnel, Organization, Culture,* and *Finances,* because of the multidisciplinarity of the subjects to be studied.

The results presented represent sampled data from selected units across Europe. The participants were prepared to let their work practices and professional views be scrutinized, their staff to be interviewed, and their organization to be evaluated. This inevitably creates a bias, as the participating units may feel they represent a better, more open, type of practice than other units in their country and have nothing to fear by such independent scrutiny. The choice of units may also be unrepresentative in that the country coordinator was responsible for selection.

Differences in clinical practice, hospital funding, whether the hospital is large or small, an academic institution or not and the geographic distribution of illness will cause variations to occur. Nevertheless EURICUS-I does provide a revealing insight, albeit a "snapshot" of ICU practice across Europe.

International scientific authorities have reviewed the EURICUS-I final report. Their comments and suggestions, with a focus on the individual substudies, were presented and discussed during a symposium held in December 1996 in Groningen, The Netherlands.

Acknowledgements. This volume presents the results of a Concerted Action (contract no. BMH1-CT93-1340), included on the program BIOMED 1 of the Commission of the European Communities. The study was performed by the Foundation for Research on Intensive Care in Europe (FRICE) under the auspices of the European Society of Intensive Care Medicine (ESICM).

1 Study Design

Background

The intensive care unit (ICU) is, after the operating theater, the most expensive ward in the modern hospital. Generally speaking, the ICU admits annually 5% of the total hospital admissions and consumes approximately 20% of the hospital budget. In a pilot survey of ICUs in Europe, tremendous and unpredictable diversity has been documented with respect to the organization of ICUs in the countries of the European Community [1]. This diversity has been examined by a European multidisciplinary task force under the auspices and general support of the Foundation for Research on Intensive Care in Europe (FRICE) and the European Society of Intensive Care Medicine (ESICM). A major requirement was found to be the definition and use of a minimal set of data which could indicate the "business" characteristics of each ICU and, at the same time, allow for comparisons of different ICUs. The task force concluded that the reorganization of intensive care in a more rational way (at micro and macro levels) is necessary. It also reviewed and recommended ways and methods of research to achieve these goals [2].

Acting upon the recommendations made by the European task force, FRICE performed, in 1990–1992, a national study of Dutch ICUs, supported by the Dutch Ministry of Health. This multidisciplinary study followed a system theory-based research model and analyzed data pooled during a 6 month observation period involving a representative sample of 36 ICUs and 13000 patients. The Dutch study has shown that the methods proposed by the task force had enabled a business-like analysis of the Dutch ICUs. The study produced recommendations which may lead to the reorganization of ICUs at the local and regional levels in the country and to a better match between supply of and demand for resources in the Dutch health care system [3, 4]. The results of this study can be summarized as follows:

1. The development and implementation of ICUs has followed local views and finances, in the absence of planning at regional or national levels. However, a significant association was observed between the operational characteristics of the ICUs and the type and size of the hospitals in which they were located. Considering the daily nursing care required by each patient (patients/nurse; P/N), the possibility of stratifying the ICUs according to the levels of care proposed by the European Task Force was demonstrated and validated [2]. The mean P/N ratios observed were: level I >2.5, level II 1.6–2.5, and level III <1.6.

2. There is no standard for determining admission or use of ICU facilities. There are also no rules governing admission and discharge policies or the use of the different ICU technologies. Overall, 74% of the admitted patients did not use any specific technology and thus a more objective view of the admission policy might frequently result in an increase in the daily ICU bed availability to above 50%.
3. There is no system for the appraisal and control of quality of care.
4. The organization and management system of the ICU has never been professionally evaluated. The more demanding the intensive care, as measured by severity of illness, use of technology, workload, etc., the lower the job satisfaction and the more frequently burnout occurred [5]. This rather unexpected result was tentatively associated with several weak points of the organization and management: the ICUs did not have a strategic plan; the design of the nursing jobs was not defined; the inputs and the outputs of the ICUs were either not known or evaluated; there were no control mechanisms concerning different policies such as those of personnel, budget or "production process"; and the medical organization was generally considered to be the weakest point of the whole ICU organization, particularly concerning availability and continuity of care. Given these conclusions, FRICE designed a large research project, the EURICUS Project, to study the ICUs in the countries of the European Community from a health services research perspective.

The EURICUS Master Project

To address the ICUs as a health care subsystem in European Community hospitals, the project used a methodology based on general system theory, in which the relationships between inputs, throughputs and outputs come under analysis.

Previous international research addressing inputs and outputs from a medical perspective has provided powerful tools (e.g. severity of illness scoring systems) to characterize the case mix of the ICUs and to predict mortality of the admitted groups of patients, allowing establishment of standard mortality ratios (SMRs) between observed and predicted mortalities [6]. One rationale of the EURICUS project is that knowledge of SMRs has to be complemented with knowledge concerning the process of care of patients (throughputs), thereby transforming inputs (patients' case mix) into outputs (patients' outcomes). Considering the ICU as a health care system in itself, patient care is therefore one of its subsystems. One other rationale supporting the EURICUS project is that the standardization of policies and work processes leading to: (a) the effective functioning of the ICU as a system and (b) the efficient match of demands by the ICUs with resources provided to them can only be achieved when the relevant subsystems have been defined and made controllable and reproducible. Organization and management, for instance, is an important subsystem in the ICU. A further goal of the project is to develop robust auditing systems for the various relevant subsystems in the ICUs.

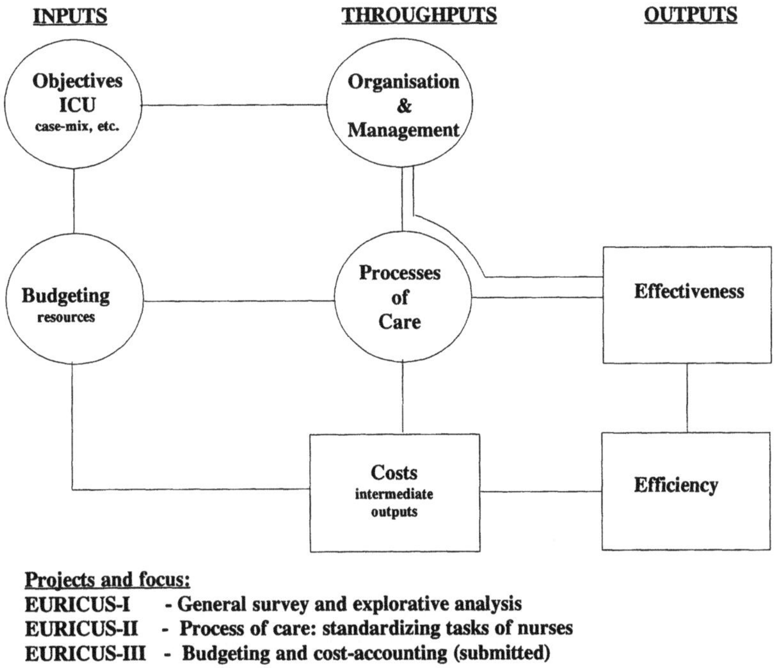

Fig. 1. European ICU studies: project model

The general design for addressing the numerous aspects of the EURICUS project is depicted in the research model of Fig. 1. The complexity of the project led to its division into subprojects, the final design of the EURICUS project is dependent on the results obtained as the research progresses.

The EURICUS-I Project

The aims of the first study of the EURICUS project, EURICUS-I, the results of which are presented and discussed in this book, are a general survey and explorative analysis of ICUs throughout Europe from a health services research perspective, focusing on the organization and management aspects of the ICUs.

Objectives

- To undertake an interdisciplinary inventory of the relevant characteristics of ICUs in Europe from a health service research perspective.
- To define performance indicators for evaluating the effectiveness of organiza-

tion and management (OM) of ICUs.
- To determine the operational aspects of OM which influence the performance, effectiveness and efficiency of ICUs.
- To generate the first database of ICUs in Europe, from a health service research perspective, which may contribute to the effective harmonization of methodologies and protocols of care, management and financing of ICUs.
- The program for achieving these objectives was carried out by a group of researchers from several disciplines. The results should strengthen and improve the existing interdisciplinary networks of researchers in the European Community countries.

Methodology

Setting

The program was developed in the ICUs of one national region in each of 12 participating European countries, with a total of 89 ICUs. Development of the program involved research teams from different disciplines (medicine, health services research, economics, organization and management, occupational psychology, methodology and statistics).

Design

The participating ICUs were selected from university and nonuniversity hospitals of large, medium and small sizes to participate in a prospective study. In each ICU, the patient care and the OM subsystems were studied and quantified by general system theory (inputs/throughputs/outputs) using validated methodologies. At the ICU level, patient care subsystem data were collected over 4 months, OM subsystems data over 6 months (questionnaires, site visits and interviews). The pooled data were studied at four levels of aggregation: (1) individual ICU; (2) global European sample; (3) area samples; (4) requirements of care (ICU levels of care) in previous samples.

Measurements

Patient Care Subsystem

1. Inputs and outputs: The approach to this system has been extensively documented in the medical literature. Characteristics of the consecutively admitted patients at the ICUs included: demographics, location in the hospital before ICU admission, and case mix (diagnosis, severity of illness, surgical status and previous health status). Severity of illness was measured with the Simplified Acute Physiologic Score (SAPS) and the Mortality Prediction Mo-

del (MPM) [6, 7]. Patient characteristics at discharge included: length of stay; destination; mortality in the ICU; mortality in the hospital after discharge from the ICU. Output data, referring to the study group of patients, was collected during two additional months which allowed for registering outcome at hospital discharge of patients admitted towards the end of the field research period.

2. Throughputs: With the exception of patient characteristics, very little research has been done concerning the process of care. The Dutch study that was used as a database collected information regarding therapeutic options; utilization of manpower; and utilization of other resources. Therapeutic options concerned those major interventions meant to support vital functions: mechanical ventilation (respiratory failure); Swan-Ganz catheters and the use of vasoactive drugs (cardiovascular failure); and hemofiltration techniques (renal failure). The utilization of manpower concerned the nursing care consumed daily by each patient. This was measured with a simplified version of the Therapeutic Intervention Scoring System, the so-called NEMS (Nine Equivalents of Nursing Manpower Use Score). The use of other resources was monitored, such as laboratory, pharmacy, radiology and blood bank services. Consumption of these resources, along with those relating to therapeutic options, was related to the duration of use (in days). The use of the facilities, in terms of daily occupancy rate, was derived from the above data.

Organization and Management Subsystem

1. Inputs and outputs were measured by means of various questionnaires administered to the leadership and to the staff of the ICUs. Financial questionnaires were also administered to the financial staff of the hospitals and to the country coordinators concerning the general organization of finances in each national health care system.
2. Throughputs. At each ICU, OM was evaluated by means of site visits, interviews, and questionnaires administered to the ICU staff.

Project Management

Due to its complexity and the specific expertise required for addressing the various parts of the study, EURICUS-I was divided into five substudies. The content of each substudy was addressed, prepared (including selection and/or development of measuring instruments) and analyzed by a specific research team of the FRICE network.

1. *Patients and Facilities*: This substudy focused on the clinical data collected in the study and on the physical environment of care (hospitals, ICUs, equipment, etc).
2. *Personnel*: This substudy focused on the nursing staff of the ICUs, addressing aspects such as leadership, subjective workload, commitment, stress, and subjective evaluation of effectiveness.

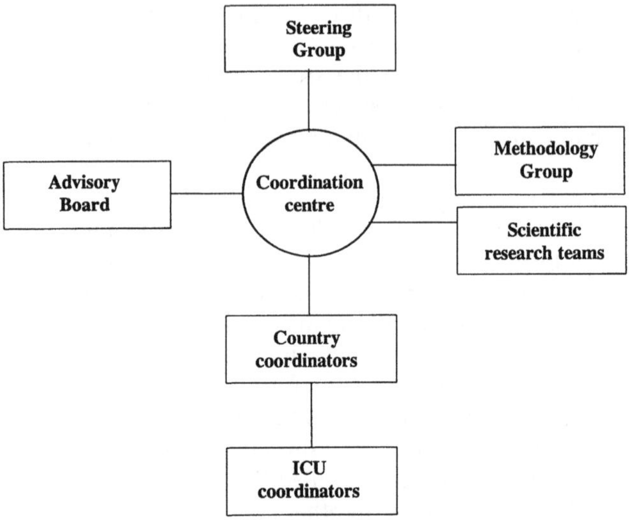

Fig. 2. The structure of the management of the activities developed during the program

3. *Organization*: This substudy focused on organizational aspects of the ICUs such as qualifications of the staff, task differentiation, standardization, work flow, decision making and communication.
4. *Culture*: This substudy explored the "collective mental programming" of the members of the ICUs, related to "values" and "general practices" or "accepted directives" present in each ICU.
5. *Finances*: This substudy explored aspects such as cost calculation, budgeting and budget control at the ICU level and their integration with financial information collected at hospital and at national levels.

The ICU Research Group, at the University Hospital of Groningen, accommodated and staffed the Coordination and Administrative Center (CAC) of the EURICUS-I project. The structure of the management of activities developed during the project is depicted in Fig. 2. All the data were centrally pooled in the EURICUS-I database at the CAC, where the required data handling and control were performed.

Analysis of the data, processed by the various research teams, encompassed two main steps: (1) descriptive and explorative analysis at the substudy level; (2) centralized integration of the results obtained by the substudies and testing of the general hypothesis of EURICUS-I by the CAC together with the involved research teams.

During the development of the project program, communication and interaction between the participants in EURICUS-I were ensured by the organization of various meetings and workshops, by the frequent exchange of research staff and by the regular issuing of newsletters.

A "gentlemen's agreement" was defined among the participants in the project, covering aspects such as circulation of information, use of databank and author's rights. A conflict management committee was put in place in case of need.

Selection of ICUs

The ICUs were selected from particular areas of 12 different European countries. During the preparation phase of the study, it was decided that the selection of the ICUs was not to be randomized. The reasons were: (a) the appropriate randomization at country level would require too large of an effort; (b) a descriptive (actual) survey of the existing ICU facilities does not exist in every European country so that essential information for randomization is lacking; (c) not all of the organizations possessing this information at the national level would accept the need to make this information readily available to the study; (d) in the majority of the European countries involved, the relationship between the ICUs and the national intensive care organizations is often sporadic and not based on a tradition of research designed to solve problems at ICU level. As an alternative to randomization, pooling of data from the selected ICUs would provide the largest possible variance concerning both the clinical effectiveness of patient care and the various modes of OM at the ICUs. It was therefore accepted, given the objectives of the study, that the results would not allow comparative inferences between countries regarding the practice of intensive care.

By virtue of methodology and budget, the selection aimed at obtaining the participation of a minimum of four and a maximum of eight ICUs per country. In each country, the participating ICUs were selected from university and non-university hospitals of large, medium and small size. To explore interactions within their environment, the ICUs belonging to the same geographical region were selected.

The selection of ICUs was done at country level by the respective country coordinator according to the aforementioned criteria. Luxembourg and Spain were exceptional cases; Luxembourg participated with only one ICU, while Spain participated with ICUs of two different regions: Catalonia and Valencia. The additional participation of nine Spanish ICUs was allowed. The data of these ICUs, not included in either of the two regions above, were considered in only some of the analyses performed.

The study started with the participation of 103 ICUs. During the study, 14 ICUs were dropped/withdrew for two reasons: (1) the ICUs did not complete the study and/or (2) the irreliability of the data collected. The list of the 89 ICUs that completed the study is presented in Part III, "The Participants in EURICUS-I". The ICUs completing the study belonged to 86 hospitals: 72 were public and 14 private; 33 were university hospitals. Findings from previous research allowed the hospitals to be divided into four categories: university hospitals and nonuniversity hospitals with <300 beds, with between 300 and 500 beds and with >500 beds. Large differences between the hospital categories were found regarding the size of hospital, clinical services provided, other critical care facilities available in the hospital (e.g. ICU, step-down units), and the availability of a recovery room. In some categories the observed differences were area-related.

Ranging between four and 33 beds, the overall median size of the units was 9.6 ± 5.7 beds. The number of nursing staff of the ICUs varied with the number of nurses/bed (mean 3.6, range 1.3–9.5) and also with the professional education of the nurses. All ICUs had a medical director, but medical coverage of the units varied with the number of physicians appointed to the unit (availability of medical care) and the intensive care education of the professionals involved (continuity of medical care). The availability of ancillary staff to the units (e.g. secretary, technicians) varied between ICUs. All ICUs had the equipment essential for adequate monitoring and treatment of acute conditions threatening vital organ system functions. Important differences were found regarding renal support and equipment required for the transport of patients between units and/or hospitals. The differences in these ICU variables between hospital categories were related to the area of origin. The majority of the ICUs were of the general type (mixed medical and surgical).

References

1. Reis Miranda D (1986) ICUs in Europe. In: Reis Miranda D, Langrehr D (eds) The ICU: a cost-benefit analysis. Excerpta Medica Int. Congr. Series 709, Amsterdam, The Netherlands, pp 207–219
2. Reis Miranda D, Williams A, Loirat Ph (eds) (1990) Management of intensive care: Guidelines for better use of resources. Kluwer Academic, Dordrecht, The Netherlands
3. Reis Miranda D, Spangenberg JFA (eds) (1992) Quality, efficiency and organization of intensive care units in The Netherlands. Van Denderen, Groningen, The Netherlands
4. Hilgeman CN, Koopmanschap MA, Rutten FFH (1992) Costs of intensive care in The Netherlands. Institute for Medical Technology Assessment, Rotterdam, The Netherlands
5. Keijsers G, Schaufeli WB, Weterings M (1992) Organization and management. In: Reis Miranda D, Spangenberg JFA (eds) Quality, efficiency and organization of intensive care units in The Netherlands. Van Denderen 1992, Groningen, The Netherlands, pp 79–93
6. Le Gall JR, Lemeshow S, Saulnier F (1993) A new simplified acute physiology score (SAPS II) based on an European/North American multicenter study. JAMA 270:2957–2963
7. Lemeshow S, Teres D, Klar J et al (1993). Mortality probability models (MPM II) based on an international cohort of intensive care unit patients. JAMA 270:2478–2486

2 Study Results

Patients

A total of 16059 consecutive admissions to the ICUs were enrolled in the study. The number of admissions to the ICU varied from 14 to 1048 (median 130) with an aggregate of 494–3050 at the area level. Some 43% of the total patients were admitted to university hospitals. The nonuniversity hospital patients included 31% enrolled from hospitals with >500 beds, 14% in hospitals with 300–500 beds and 12% in hospitals with <300 beds; 84% of the patients were admitted to general ICUs (Table 1).

Table 1. Number of patients from each European area

	Type of ICU			Type of hospital				Overall
	Medical	Surgical	General	<300 Beds	300–500 Beds	>500 Beds	University	
European area								
Poland	364	71	190	56	300	63	206	625
Germany			1459			1177	282	1459
Denmark			1251	246		477	528	1251
Finland			1349	228		346	775	1349
Netherlands		129	1402		595	807	129	1531
Belgium	332	603	1327	319		935	1008	2262
France	480	110	214	214			590	804
United Kingdom			833			343	490	833
Italy			777		124	401	252	777
Spain	483		1527	387	992	272	1399	3050
Spain-Catalonia			2567	464	97		966	1527
Portugal			439		175	84	180	439
Overall	1659	1065	13335	1914	2283	4905	6957	16059

Data on Luxembourg are not presented.

Case Mix

- Age: The mean age of the patients was 59 ± 18 years. Patients admitted to university hospitals were younger (Table 2). The age of the patients enrolled was significantly associated with the variable area of country.
- Origin of patients: Overall, 37% of the patients were admitted from the operating theater, 4% from the recovery room, 30% from the emergency room, 17% from the ward, 2% from another ICU and 6% from another hospital. This admission pattern was associated with the variables hospital category and European area (Table 3).
- Surgical vs medical patients: About 50% of the patients underwent a surgical procedure within 24 h prior to ICU admission. In two thirds of these patients the surgical intervention was scheduled (at least 24 h in advance); in the other third the surgical intervention was of a nonscheduled type. The remaining admissions (54%) were nonsurgical. The incidence of type of admission was associated with hospital category and with European area.
- Diagnoses: A list of 76 diagnoses, grouped into 18 major categories, was used (see Chap. 7, Table 15). Four diagnostic categories were predominant in the study: cardiovascular and respiratory conditions in the nonoperative group of patients, and cardiovascular and gastrointestinal conditions in the postoperative group of patients (see Chap. 7, Table 15). The incidence of these diagnostic categories was associated with hospital category and with European area.

Table 2. Mean age (years) of the studied patients

	Type of ICU			Type of hospital				Overall
	Medical	Surgical	General	< 300 Beds	300–500 Beds	> 500 Beds	University	
European area								
Poland	60	59	52	62	59	52	55	57
Germany			59			62	49	59
Denmark			58	55		60	58	58
Finland		59	58	59		58	57	58
Netherlands		62	61		60	62	59	61
Belgium	64	42	61	65		62	60	62
France	54		59	59			52	54
United Kingdom			59			58	60	59
Italy			58		60	61	52	58
Spain-Catalonia			60	62	63		59	60
Spain-Valencia	62		60	64	61	62	59	60
Portugal			58		62	61	53	58
Overall	60	58	59	61	60	61	57	59

Table 3. Location in the hospital before ICU admission (number of patients)

	Admitted from [a]:							Overall
	1	2	3	4	5	6	7	
European area								
Poland	76	–	379	141	–	24	4	624
Germany	796	31	109	72	26	55	133	1222
Denmark	436	60	303	302	13	59	31	1204
Finland	788	6	271	227	19	13	5	1329
Netherlands	754	190	254	189	25	71	28	1511
Belgium	1084	86	614	295	10	110	29	2228
France	63	10	207	154	34	115	215	798
United Kingdom	330	39	163	205	14	30	30	811
Italy	265	9	154	198	33	97	18	774
Spain	533	19	1559	576	25	226	25	3003
Spain-Catalonia	378	57	549	209	99	158	63	1513
Portugal	164	24	89	66	48	23	17	431
Type of hospital								
<300 Beds	562	13	669	318	15	150	151	1878
300–500 Beds	486	168	1013	357	20	165	34	2243
>500 Beds	2277	129	914	717	94	293	188	4612
University	2383	263	2128	1254	217	385	228	6858
Type of ICU								
Medical	32	7	916	417	37	167	69	1645
Surgical	679	64	86	63	17	63	72	1044
General	4997	502	3722	2166	292	763	460	12902
Overall *n*	5708	573	4724	2646	346	993	601	15591
(%)	(36.6)	(3.7)	(30.3)	(17.0)	(2.2)	(6.4)	(3.8)	

[a] Admitted from: *1* operating theatre; *2* recovery room ; *3* emergency room; *4* ward; *5* other ICU; *6* other hospital; *7* none of the above.

- Severity of illness: Two severity of illness scoring systems were used: the Simplified Acute Physiology Score (SAPS-II) and the Mortality Prediction Model (MPM_0). SAPS-II was used in the analysis presented in the study because MPM_0 was not scored by four ICUs. With an overall value of 33.5 the mean SAPS-II score varied between 20.9 and 47.0 at ICU level and between 28.3 and 38.5 at area level. The mean SAPS-II score increased with the size of the nonuniversity hospitals and was higher on the ICUs of the university hospitals. In general, medical patients had a higher SAPS-II score than surgical patients (Table 4).

Table 4. Mean SAPS II scores

	Type of ICU			Type of hospital				Overall
	Medical	Surgical	General	<300 Beds	300–500 Beds	>500 Beds	University	
European area								
Poland	35.7	36.4	39.3	37.4	38.9	40.3	33.9	37.1
Germany			28.5			30.2	24.1	28.5
Denmark			29.6	20.9		32.0	32.5	29.6
Finland			30.2	31.4		32.1	27.9	30.2
Netherlands		31.8	29.4		25.8	34.3	31.8	29.7
Belgium	31.5	26.4	30.2	25.0		28.7	32.6	29.8
France	34.7	30.0	38.9	38.9			33.8	35.2
United Kingdom			38.5			38.5	38.6	38.5
Italy			37.3		37.5	35.7	39.9	37.3
Spain-Catalonia			35.4	33.1	32.0		37.0	35.4
Spain-Valencia	36.4		37.5	38.5	36.7	36.5	37.7	37.4
Portugal			37.5		34.4	47.0	35.8	37.5
Overall	34.8	29.4	33.6	31.4	33.1	33.4	34.3	33.5

SAPS, Simplified Acute Physiology Score.

Outcome

Mortality at discharge from the hospital (18%) was the outcome measure used. Overall, 13% of the admitted patients died in the ICU and an additional 6% of patients died in the hospital after discharge from the ICU (Tables 5, 6). It is of note that post-ICU deaths ranged between 0% and 18%. Mortality was also associated with the hospital category and with European area when data were controlled for severity of illness.

Organization and Management Data Results

Field Work

A qualitative survey of ICUs in Europe was made with the goal of providing a global view of the practices and problems of the organization and management of intensive care medicine in Europe. With the focus on the opinions, feelings and wishes of the intensive care professionals, the aim of the qualitative survey was an empirical assessment of ICUs in Europe such that interpretation of the data collected by the substudies might be enhanced. The field work consisted of site visits to all participating ICUs as well as recording of comments that were made by the area coordinators of EURICUS-I regarding the existing national intensive care medical systems.

Table 5. ICU mortality rate (%)

	Type of ICU			Type of hospital				Overall
	Medical	Surgical	General	<300 Beds	300–500 Beds	>500 Beds	Uni-versity	
European area								
Poland	14	30	25	14	21	25	15	19
Germany			6			6	5	6
Denmark			13	6		13	17	13
Finland			8	9		10	7	8
Netherlands		22	9		9	8	22	10
Belgium	11	4	8	5		6	9	7
France	14	29	14	14			17	16
United Kingdom			20			21	20	20
Italy			18		14	19	19	18
Spain-Catalonia			15	10	13		18	15
Spain-Valencia	18		15	12	15	12	18	16
Portugal			14		9	26	14	14
Overall	15	11	12	10	14	11	14	13

Table 6. Hospital mortality rate (%)

	Type of ICU			Type of hospital				Overall
	Medical	Surgical	General	<300 Beds	300–500 Beds	>500 Beds	Uni-versity	
European area								
Poland	19	32	25	20	26	27	17	23
Germany			9			10	8	9
Denmark			20	8		21	26	20
Finland			14	19		16	12	14
Netherlands		29	15		16	14	29	16
Belgium	17	6	13	9		9	14	12
France	19	32	21	21			22	22
United Kingdom			31			31	31	31
Italy			26		21	26	27	26
Spain-Catalonia			21	16	19		23	21
Spain-Valencia	23		20	15	20	18	23	21
Portugal			21		19	32	17	21
Overall	20	14	18	15	20	16	20	18

Site Visits

Site visits were made by the project leader, often accompanied by researchers from nonmedical disciplines, to all participating ICUs during the 4 month field research period of EURICUS-I. The results of the site visits can be summarized as follows:

1. The professional activities of the staff of the ICUs, both those of physicians and nurses, are rather similar across Europe. Their clinical contribution is however poorly defined and/or accepted in the remaining areas of the respective hospitals. It was also found that there was poor communication between the staffs of the various ICUs. The clinical activities of the ICU staff were isolated from those of the other hospital staff. As a consequence a high level of professional insecurity was identified in a large number of the ICUs.
2. The level of skill discretion of ICU nurses was found to be insufficiently developed to cope effectively, efficiently and speedily with the multidisciplinary activities involved with the acute care of patients. The nurses' participation in decision-making was poor, despite the fact that they represented 90% of the ICU staff and possessed crucial information about the patients.
3. Communication between nurses and doctors was inadequate as nurses were only committed to their specific nursing tasks and activities and lacked an overall view of the care of the critically ill.
4. A limited interaction of the ICUs with the patients' families and visitors existed in many ICUs across Europe. A "self-protecting" attitude, on the part of both the nursing and the medical staff, rather than workload and high turnover of patients, was at the origin of the imposed ICU visiting limitations. In general, the ICU announced the imposed limitations in an unpersonal manner (signs on doors, leaflets, etc.). This situation often caused inappropriate information to be conveyed to the families of patients and was sometimes a source of conflict between nurses and physicians.
5. On the day of the site visits, the overall occupancy rate of the ICUs was low and usually dependent on the flow of patients from the operating theater. Several ICUs were empty and were not expecting patients on that day. A shortage of nurses to assist the patients on the ICU was rarely found.
6. When in existence protocols were rarely used as instruments for quality control.
7. In the organizational structure of the ICUs, the "strategic apex" of the units, i.e. where the general ICU policies are decided, was most frequently located outside the ICU and therefore run by medical professionals who were not necessarily involved with the professional activities of the units.
8. In some ICUs structured integration of the professional activities of nurses and physicians merited the attention of the ICU leadership. In the majority of the ICUs, however, this essential process of organization and management seemed to be in its infancy.

Notes on Intensive Care Medical Systems in Europe

The country coordinators of EURICUS-I were asked to write a short memorandum describing what, in their opinion, were the relevant aspects (and possible limitations) of the intensive care medical system in their countries. The overriding conclusion of the descriptions made was diversity.

Several of the problems and differences reported during the site visits have been reinforced by the descriptions at area level. The organization of intensive care medicine (ICM) as a medical activity is very different among the European countries, being an independent specialty in Spain, a subspecialty in some countries, or integrated into other (traditional) specialties in other countries. In France, ICM is dependent on two national medical organizations. Structured teaching and training of ICM is found in very few European countries. The existing teaching and training programs show large differences concerning duration, content and the targeted professional groups.

In general, the nurses are better organized as intensive care professionals than the physicians. The reasons for the lack of medical organization of the ICUs are due to:

1. Insufficient recognition of the ICU as a responsibility center in the hospital's organizational and financial structure
2. The lack of consensus among the existing medical specialties concerning the integration of ICM in medical care
3. The rather independent organization of medical care within the hospital structure

Substudy Patients and Facilities

ICU Performance

Standardized mortality ratios (SMRs), or the observed/predicted mortality ratios, were originally chosen as a measure of ICU performance. Performance was to be used as the clinical reference variable for evaluation of the effects of organization and management variables on ICU effectiveness. SAPS-II was used for computing SMRs.

It has been, however, pointed out that the traditional SMR-based approach has certain theoretical drawbacks which can be avoided by using a different method of analysis. This alternative method essentially estimates the relation between SAPS-II and the mortality separately in each ICU. Using the estimated relations, one can directly calculate standardized ICU mortalities corresponding to some standard case mix defined by suitably chosen SAPS-II values (see Chap. 8, Analysis of ICU Performance).

As it turned, the differences between the standardized ICU mortalities depended on the standard set of SAPS-II values. Thus the standardized probabilities were calculated separately for low risk and high risk patients. Low risk was defined as SAPS-II equal to the 20th percentile of the SAPS-II distribution in the

EURICUS-I sample, high risk as a SAPS-II equal to the 80th percentile. Logits of these standardized mortalities, denoted as B20 and B80, were calculated for each ICU and subsequently used in the analysis as the performance measures (see Chap. 8, Analysis of ICU Performance).

Use of the Facilities

Use of Manpower

- Workload: The Nine Equivalents of Nursing Manpower Use Score (NEMS), a simplified version of the Therapeutic Intervention Scoring System, was used for the daily registration of nursing workload at the patient level. The work of one nurse during three daily shifts corresponds to 46 NEMS points. The overall mean NEMS was 27 points/patient per day (Chap. 2, Table 7) meaning that the work of one nurse per shift was "consumed" by 1.67 patients. The score was highest on the day of admission and decreased gradually at the patient level over the period of stay in the ICU (Chap. 2, Fig. 2). The longer the length of stay in the ICU, the higher the NEMS observed on the admission day. Surgical patients had a higher NEMS than their medical counterparts. These differences

Table 7. First day NEMS and mean overall NEMS

	Day 1 NEMS	Average NEMS of ICUs
European area		
Poland	24.9	22.1
Germany	28.0	28.6
Denmark	23.5	26.2
Finland	27.2	28.4
Netherlands	28.0	28.0
Belgium	27.9	27.0
France	26.0	23.8
United Kingdom	29.3	29.2
Italy	28.4	27.1
Spain-Catalonia	27.0	27.3
Spain-Valencia	25.5	25.2
Portugal	28.0	27.7
Type of hospital		
< 300 beds	23.2	24.0
300–500 beds	24.3	24.5
> 500 beds	28.7	28.1
University	27.3	26.8
Overall	26.8	26.5

NEMS, Nine Equivalents of Nursing Manpower Use Score.

Table 8. Work utilitation ratio by type of ICU and type of hospital

	Type of ICU			Type of hospital				Overall
	Medical	Surgical	General	<300 Beds	300–500 Beds	>500 Beds	Uni-versity	
European area								
Poland	0.62	0.47	0.62	0.60	0.73	0.35	0.52	0.59
Germany			1.12			1.51	0.74	1.12
Denmark			0.49	0.52		0.55	0.45	0.49
Finland			0.65	0.67		0.60	0.70	0.65
Netherlands		0.85	0.74		0.77	0.68	0.85	0.76
Belgium	0.88	1.34	0.94	0.88		1.11	0.99	1.00
France	0.72	0.80	1.12	1.12			0.74	0.89
United Kingdom			0.40			0.39	0.40	0.40
Italy			0.86		0.80	0.86	0.88	0.86
Spain-Catalonia			0.91	0.82	0.65		1.04	0.91
Spain-Valencia	1.12		0.59	0.66	0.54	0.37	0.77	0.64
Portugal			0.91		0.90	0.78	1.00	0.91
Overall	0.78	0.80	0.71	0.77	0.68	0.70	0.74	0.72

in scores were caused particularly by the less frequent use of mechanical ventilation and cardiovascular active drugs by medical patients (see Chap. 7, Table 23). At ICU level the mean overall NEMS ranged between 8 and 34 points. The variance of the incidence of the use of the items in NEMS could be explained by the variables European area, hospital category, or by the interaction between these two variables.

- Work Utilization Ratio: The WUR establishes the ratio between the total nursing work produced (actual cumulative NEMS score) in the unit and the possible total NEMS score considering the number of full-time nursing equivalents working in the unit during the same period of time (Chap. 2, Table 8). On average the ICUs used 72% of the available nursing capacity. At ICU level WUR ranged between 30% and 172%, indicating some use of nursing manpower from outside the unit. Eleven ICUs had a WUR greater than 100%; 19 ICUs had a WUR below 50%.

Use of ICU Beds

1. Length of stay: At the patient level the LOS ranged between <1 day and 291 days: mean 5.2 ± 10.1 days (median 2 days; interquartile range between 0.9 and 4.9 days) (see Chap. 7, Table 24). Besides case mix, LOS was also associated with hospital category and European area. LOS increased with age and with severity of illness. It was shorter for scheduled surgical patients and longer for patients coming from the emergency room (2.8 days), the ward (3.1 days) and other ICUs/other hospitals (4.8 days) (see Chap. 7, Table 24). It

Table 9. Occupancy rate by type of ICU and type of hospital

	Type of ICU			Type of hospital				Overall
	Medical	Surgical	General	<300 Beds	300–500 Beds	>500 Beds	Uni-versity	
European area								
Poland	66.4	37.8	60.4	37.3	69.8	57.2	60.4	58.1
Germany			84.7			91.6	71.0	84.7
Denmark			61.3	60.1		63.7	60.2	61.3
Finland			70.4	73.8		67.4	69.7	70.4
Netherlands		90.4	79.0		78.1	80.9	90.4	80.6
Belgium	63.3	76.9	68.2	67.7		70.1	68.7	68.8
France	63.3	80.1	79.9	79.9			68.9	73.3
United Kingdom			58.5			54.3	62.8	58.5
Italy			79.7		78.2	76.7	86.3	79.7
Spain-Catalonia			82.7	76.1	66.5		91.6	82.7
Spain-Valencia	73.8		63.6	64.3	61.3	44.3	70.3	64.7
Portugal			84.7		74.9	109.8	82.1	84.7
Overall	67.0	63.1	71.0	66.6	69.2	70.6	71.7	70.1

appears that the variance of LOS may be dependent on local factors when controlling for severity of illness and workload required on the first admission day.

2. Occupancy rate (OR). The overall OR was 70%, ranging between 56% and 85% at area level and between 19% and 110% at ICU level (Table 2.9). Eleven ICUs had an OR lower than 50%.
3. Turnover of patients. Turnover was measured by the volume of admissions indexed by the number of beds in the ICU: number of admissions/bed per year (ABY). The overall ABY was 57, ranging between 34 and 87 at area level and between 11 and 117 at ICU level (see Chap. 7, Table 27). High turnover of patients (ABY > 75) was associated with the number of scheduled surgical admissions.

Substudy Organization

The ICU is defined as an "uncertainty reducing" unit. The ICU variables selected as being related to uncertainty were: the percentage of scheduled admissions; the number of unexpected admissions; the incidence of sudden deterioration of the clinical condition of the patients; the occurrence of organ system failure. A variable was constructed from the product of the number of admissions and the mean length of stay in the ICU, indexed by the number of beds in the unit, for indicating the "input" of patients to each ICU. Based on a detailed questionnaire administered to the leadership of the ICUs, the substudy produced a descriptive analysis of the organizational background of the units, especially concerning characteristics, such as staffing and available technology, associated with the hospital category (university and nonuniversity) as used in other substudies. A variable, advanced medical technologies, was constructed and defined as a set of technologies existing in less than 75% of the ICUs.

The aim of the organization and management of the ICU is defined as the reduction of uncertainty at the level of individual tasks and of the workflow at the level of the group of workers in the unit. Predictability, as opposed to uncertainty, is indicated concerning tasks and workflow. In theoretical organizational terms, task predictability is associated with standardization of the tasks (positive effect), the professional qualification of the staff (negative effect) and with the differentiation between the involved professional groups (positive effect). In turn, the predictability of workflow is associated positively with the centralization of decision-making.

In the study, task predictability was influenced by two variables: sudden deterioration of the clinical condition of the patients and the occurrence of organ system failure. Workflow predictability was also determined by two variables: input, as described above, and the percentage of scheduled admissions to the ICU.

The substudy discussed the differences between ICUs and other nonmedical units regarding the effect of technology upon the predictability of tasks and workflow. The technology used in the ICUs, as opposed to in other, nonmedical enterprises, is associated with the diversity and severity of the clinical conditions in the ICU, and its increase is therefore associated with a reduction of the predictability of tasks and workflow in the ICU. The increase of technology use in the ICU results therefore in the need for a more highly qualified ICU staff and, consequently, a lower level of task differentiation. High qualifications and low task differentiation imply simultaneously a lower level of standardization.

Based on the above, the substudy developed the following hypotheses for analysis of the EURICUS-I data:

1. Task differentiation is negatively related to the performance of the ICUs.
2. Professional qualification (only nurses were considered) is positively related to the performance of the ICUs.
3. Centralization of decision-making is negatively related to performance of the ICUs.
4. Standardization of tasks is positively related to the performance of ICUs.

The task differentiation variable was derived from the data collected indicating to what extent tasks assigned to various types of staff were in fact done by other staff members. The professional qualification of the nurses variable was derived from the percentage of nurses with special ICU training and education. The centralization variable was designed to reflect the professional level at which some specific medical decisions were made. The standardization variable was constructed from data regarding the existence of written descriptions of the jobs of physicians and nurses, together with the regular written evaluation of the performance of the involved professionals.

The four hypotheses proposed by the substudy were tested using multiple regression analysis, considering separately ICU performance regarding low risk and high risk patients. For low risk patients, there was a significant negative association between clinical performance of the ICU and both task differentiation and centralization. Clinical performance was positively associated with standardization. In this analysis the best model explained 31% of the variance in performance. For high risk patients, there was a negative, but not significant, association between clinical performance of the ICU and both task differentiation and centralization. In this analysis the best model explained only 19% of the variance in performance.

The substudy concluded by emphasizing the need to organize the ICUs within a team-like structure: low task differentiation and low level of centralization. The existence of such a structure was associated with better clinical performance by the ICUs in EURICUS-I.

Substudy Personnel

In this substudy the focus is on the work of the nursing staff. The descriptive part of the substudy gives a detailed description of the working situation of the nurses participating in this research, based on the results of two survey questionnaires ("Well-Being of ICU Nurses" and "Work and Well-Being") answered by approximately 2000 nurses (77% female; mean age 32.5 years). A research model exploring the relationship between job demands/workload (inputs), levels of job stress (throughputs) and the medical performance of the ICU (outputs) was tested both on the subjective (individual) level and at the objective (ICU) level.

The working situation of nurses is described in terms of: (a) nursing staff characteristics, including sex, part-time vs full-time employment, age and experience; (b) job characteristics, as measured by the "Well-Being of ICU Nurses" questionnaire, including the characteristics of about 40 tasks and activities performed by nurses. These are divided into four categories: operational tasks (nursing and medical care of patients), organizing tasks (job-related cooperation/meetings with others), preparatory tasks and supportive tasks; (c) stress-related characteristics, assessed by the 15 scales of the "Work and Well-Being" questionnaire, including workload, burnout, perceived performance, coping resources and involvement.

The results of the descriptive analyses show that operational tasks are 56% of the tasks performed by nurses; organizing tasks make up 23% of the daily tasks. Preparatory tasks and supportive tasks together constitute 22% of the tasks performed by nurses. Evaluation of the tasks shows that the operational tasks are perceived as the most demanding, as well as the most satisfying. Organizing tasks are perceived as the least demanding and supportive tasks are seen as the least satisfying. A rather unexpectedly strong correlation was found between the demands that tasks pose to the nurses and the satisfaction derived from a task, ranging from $R = 0.41$ for operational tasks to $R = 0.71$ for supportive tasks.

Analysis of 30 potential problem situations indicates that the frequency of occurrence of problem situations is quite low and the autonomy to solve the problems is quite high. The highest frequency is found for problem situations related to the lack of clear "norms" (e.g. unclear instructions). The opinions of nurses indicate that most of the complaints about feedback deal with completeness. Complaints about the work environment are principally related to lack of space, climate, and noise and bustle. It was concluded that the stressfulness of ICU nurses' jobs in this sample due to problem situations is low.

An analysis of risk factors and risk groups was performed. Risk factors were identified as high task demands, low task satisfaction, high frequency of problem situations and low autonomy in solving them. Results indicate that the number of risk factors is higher in the worst performing ICUs than in the best performing ICUs. In particular, problems with respect to lack of resources occur more frequently in the worst performing ICUs. It is found that a lack of autonomy in solving problem situations is associated with a poorer (objective) performance.

Risk groups were identified by comparing the scores of different groups using various scales of the work and well-being questionnaire. Results indicate that women and men were almost equally at risk: women were more at risk in some work-related aspects, whereas men were more at risk on others. Part-time workers were less at risk than full-time workers. Two age groups (corresponding to years of work experience at ICUs) were especially at risk with respect to workload and burnout symptoms: <27 years of age (with ≤ 2 or less years of experience) and in the group of 31–37 years of age (with 5–9 years of experience). It is suggested that the first group probably has to develop a repertoire to cope adequately with the stresses of intensive care nursing, whereas the second group is likely to be depleted by the prolonged exposure to demanding work situations.

The basic research model fitted the data well at the individual level as well as at the unit level. The relationship between workload, burnout, emotional exhaustion and depersonalization was significant and in the expected direction. The relationship between burnout and unit performance was weak at the individual level and not significant at the unit level, suggesting a low impact of burnout on perceived and actual performance of the ICU.

In an extended research model the moderating roles of coping resources and involvement in the relationship between workload and burnout, and burnout and performance were tested. Although little support for such moderating effects was found, significant and important effects of coping resources on burnout are found. The results of the analysis of the extended research model indicate that burnout is significantly lowered by almost all coping resources. Moreover, perceived performance is impaired by poor job involvement and poor organizational commitment.

With respect to the results of the job analysis it can be concluded that, in general, having to work hard is rewarding for ICU nurses, a result that was also found by De Rijk, Le Blanc, Schaufeli and De Jonge (submitted) among Dutch ICU nurses. This applies in particular to operational tasks (nursing and medical care of patients).

Looking at the demands and satisfaction scores within each of the different categories of tasks makes clear that special attention has to be paid to psychosocial aspects of patient care (including contact with relatives) and to (interdisciplinary and external) communication, as these tasks are perceived as either quite demanding or fairly dissatisfying. These results can probably be attributed to the fact that most training programs for ICU nurses are more strongly oriented to technical nursing skills than to psychological or communicative ones. Despite the (emotional) demands associated with it, nurses do enjoy psychosocial care of patients, which is clearly not the case for administrative tasks (e.g. making time tables). Contacts with ICU team colleagues is perceived as very satisfying, probably because they are an important source of work-related social support. Finally, ICU nurses like to maintain their expertise, as training and following courses are perceived as fairly satisfying.

Substudy Culture

In this section a comparative description of ICU culture is presented. The substudy builds on previous research [1], whereby the methodology employed allows mutual comparison of different types of organizational units such as marketing units, production units, research units, head offices and, in this case, ICUs. Two main aspects of culture are distinguished: values and practices. Values are defined as broad, nonspecific feelings about good and evil, normal and abnormal, rational and irrational. Practices are defined as observable manifestations of culture. The analysed data were collected by a survey questionnaire answered by approximately 2500 respondents (79% nurses, 4% ancillary staff, 17% physicians; 74% female).

Four dimensions emerged as significant for the description of ICU culture: process vs results orientation, employee vs job orientation, open vs closed system, and need for security. Comparing the ICUs with a database containing culture analyses of 20 organizational units in Denmark and the Netherlands showed that ICUs can be characterized as having a culture with a relatively high results orientation and a very low need for security. It is suggested that the low need for security is related to the character of the work in ICUs and the ambiguities and uncertainties involved. It may be difficult for people with a high need for security to maintain themselves in the working environment of the ICU. The relatively high results orientation places the ICUs among organizations with direct contact with clients and research departments. Identification of effective ICUs shows that mortality corrected for severity of illness is lower in ICUs that are more results-oriented than process-oriented (corrected for regional differences). This result supports those of Shortell et al. [2] regarding organizational practices and outcomes within ICUs.

Results orientation was further related to morale and satisfaction. This indicates the importance of results orientation as an explanatory variable for medical as well as for human resource management. On the level of the organizational structure, indications are found that positioning of the strategic apex outside the ICU is associated with a higher need for security in the ICU.

Substudy Finances

Here, the cost structure of the sampled ICUs is estimated and budgeting and cost-accounting in European ICUs are described. As far as the cost estimation is concerned, and notwithstanding material differences between the sampled ICUs, some clear conclusions emerge: labor is the most important component of total cost, almost always between 50% and 80% of total cost. Tangibles (if not too old), like equipment and pharmaceuticals, are next in line. The other components are mostly marginal, with the exception of the cost of disposables and, sometimes, blood products and laboratory tests. Probably more importantly, we show that it is possible to develop a standardized cost model for ICUs.

Data collected in 88 ICUs are used to give a systematic description of budgeting and cost-accounting practices. The information about budgetary practices indicates that in a relatively large number of ICUs no specific ICU budget existed. If present, the budget mostly consisted of at least one of the following components: current wage expenses, other current expenses, and investments. Specific investment budgets were found in approximately one third of the ICUs.

Formal procedures for budgetary control at ICU level, required by the hospital, were found in 42% of the ICUs. Some ICUs needed authorization for all expenses and investments, others only for investments, still others for expenses exceeding a certain value. Few ICUs had their own budget control system (16%).

The information about cost-accounting indicates that in 84% of the ICUs no method is present by which the ICU calculates the costs of its activities, globally (for the unit) or per unit of activity, e.g. days, treatment, patient, Therapeutic Intervention Scoring System (TISS) points. Costing systems used, when at all, are very diverse, varying from a detailed system developed by Edbrooke et al. in Sheffield [3] to a system relating cost to TISS points. Some 43% of the ICUs indicate that they do not know the costs/bed per year. The other ICUs use various cost definitions, ranging from the "cost/bed per day" to the amount paid by health insurers. Overall, the budgetary and cost-accounting procedures in ICUs show a nonsystematic diversity. Hospital managers can initiate more or less sophisticated budgetary control systems, but this seems not to be an obligation in most countries. Cost-calculating procedures in a majority of ICUs are rather undeveloped. In general, cost-accounting systems are nonexistent or are so diverse that comparison of costs/bed between ICUs is difficult.

Special Subjects

Levels of Care

Levels of care (LOCs) were defined for the first time by the Bethesda Consensus Conference in 1981 [4]. The aim of defining LOCs was the high costs generated by the intensive care facilities and the consequent need for a better match between the provision and use of resources. The Bethesda task force defined four LOCs based on the number of patients that can be assisted by one nurse. The rationale behind the criterium used is easy to understand.

The resources made available to the ICU are readily measured. The major part of these resources is fixed and is comprised of the permanent staff and the technological environment of the unit. The nursing staff comprises about 90% of the permanent staff. The nurses are the largest part of the fixed resources allocated to the ICU and are the most comparable element of the permanent staff (full-time equivalents) among ICUs.

The use of nursing staff is dependent on the various activities of care required in each unit. The requirements of care are determined by the clinical characteristics of each ICU: the type, volume and severity of patients admitted and the standing practices and policies of care in the unit. These characteristics determine the variable costs in the unit. It is therefore logical that the nursing staff is chosen as a reliable benchmark for evaluating the match between provision and use of resources in the ICU and for independent evaluation of the appropriateness of clinical care in the ICUs.

Following the recommendations of the Bethesda conference, three LOCs are usually described in the ICUs: intensive care unit, high dependency unit (HDU) and medium care unit (MCU). These ICUs are also called step-down units. This type of classification, however, assumes an hierarchy of complexity of care that is related to an hierarchy of severity of illness. Following the step-down care principle, the more severely ill patients are admitted to the ICU, the less severely ill to the MCU. The hierarchy of complexity of care implies that the allocation of nursing staff to these units is also done in a step-down fashion. However, the determining benchmark in this classification of LOCs is the complexity of care rather than allocation of nursing staff.

This classification scheme has two important drawbacks: Firstly, the definition of the various LOCs is not always evident as it is often based on ambiguous terms of complexity of medical care. The Dutch ICU study [5] showed that some MCUs of university hospitals could operate at a higher level of complexity of care, and consequently generated a higher consumption of nursing staff, than the ICUs of some small nonuniversity hospitals. The important implication of this, as was also observed in the same study, is inappropriate allocation of staff to the units and the resulting mismatch of the resources made available compared with those required. Secondly, the classification of LOCs according to complexity of medical care implies that the resulting step-down units are by definition bound to a hierarchy of medical and nursing activities. For example: full critical care on the ICU; artificial mechanical ventilation on the HDU; only monitoring, but no Swan-Ganz catheters on the MCU. The definition of activities pertaining to each LOC is also often bound to time limits, such as artificial mechanical ventilation for only 2 or 3 days.

The use of the classification of LOCs according to complexity of care defines each LOC as an area of medical competence of care. The logical implication of this is that the effective and efficient regionalization of critical care medicine becomes very difficult to realize. One of the aims of EURICUS-I was to explore whether the ICUs were operating at a LOC matching the one planned by the ICU management.

The planned LOC of each ICU was derived from the appointed number of nurses in relation to the number of beds as indicated above. The operating LOC was calculated for each ICU by dividing the number of NEMS points equivalent to the nursing activities of one nurse/shift (46 points) by the mean value of daily NEMS in the ICU during the study. In this way two patients/nurse (P/N) ratios were obtained for comparison: planned and operational. It is noteworthy that these two ratios are calculated differently and measure two different things: the planned P/N ratio is derived from management characteristics at ICU level (numbers of beds and numbers of nurses) and indicates the mean number of nurses available per ICU bed for a given annual rate of occupancy. The operating P/N ratio indicates the annual nursing consumption per average patient-day and is computed by aggregating at ICU level the actual use of nursing resources at patient level.

An important property of the P/N ratios is that they measure the average nursing manpower capacity/use at the ICU level and not at the individual patient level. In other words, two ICUs may have the same P/N ratio and be available to and/or treat groups of patients with different severities of illness, the latter implying requiring care of diverse complexity if other variables such as volume of patients and/or length of stay are also different. This fits the daily practice, as it may be generally anticipated that the severity of illness and the complexity of each patient decreases over time. Therefore, any ICU operating at a low LOC may be able to admit and treat patients requiring much more nursing care than is the average on that particular ICU. Frequency, volume and LOS are the limiting factors to consider.

The two P/N ratios (planned and operational) were calculated for the ICUs participating in EURICUS-I. A ranking of continuous values for the two variables at ICU level was obtained. The following step was to select intervals of P/N ratios which could define three levels of care based on the average P/N ratio of each interval.

The NEMS score data of EURICUS-I were analyzed and two cut-off points were chosen in such a way that the data were divided into three score groups with similar numbers of records. Table 10 shows that there is a large variation in the distribution of NEMS scores stratified at *country* level. In the ICUs of Poland, for example 49% of the records score on group I and only 15% on group III, whereas the inverse score pattern was found for ICUs of the United Kingdom.

Table 11 presents the cut-off points of NEMS scores (second column), the mean value of the NEMS scores in each group and the adjusted average operating P/N ratio corresponding to each group. The adjusted P/N ratios describe the three LOCs defined in the EURICUS-I database. Analysis of the data has shown that an ICU operating at LOC III, for instance, does not mean that all patient-days were performed at a P/N ratio of 1. Conversely, an ICU operating at LOC I does not mean that some patient-days were not performed at a P/N ratio of 1.

Table 12 analyzes the match of LOCs, planned vs operating, of the ICUs in EURICUS-I. The match of LOCs was observed in 21 ICUs (24%). Upgrading of

Table 10. Levels of care (74383 patient days)

		Group I		Group II		Group III	
	ICUs (*n*)	*n*	%	*n*	%	*n*	%
European area							
Poland	9	1929	49	1400	36	606	15
Germany	3	1411	26	1764	33	2238	41
Denmark	6	1459	40	898	25	1290	35
Finland	5	1033	24	1446	34	1784	42
Netherlands	7	1555	29	1627	30	2191	41
Belgium	6	1967	31	2056	32	2312	37
France	5	2128	41	1790	34	1287	25
United Kingdom	8	758	24	923	30	1418	46
Italy	7	1396	29	1702	36	1646	35
Spain	19	6292	36	6612	38	4404	25
Spain-Catalonia	8	2962	29	3408	34	3732	37
Portugal	5	1030	26	1511	38	1460	36
Overall	89	24234	33	25589	34	24560	33

LOC (from I to II) was registered in three ICUs (3%). Upgrading of LOC was observed in ICUs with a low occupancy rate. A larger LOC mismatch was observed in the group of ICUs which had planned to operate at LOC III; these amounted to about 70% of the units in EURICUS-I.

One conclusion of this survey is that there is a very large mismatch between planned and operating LOCs in 74% of the ICUs in the study. This result is not different from that found in the Dutch National ICU Study in which a similar mismatch was found on 40% (12) of the Dutch ICUs. A possible consequence of the current policies of planning ICU facilities in Europe is the inappropriate use of nursing staff as expressed by the WUR of <70% observed in 34 of the units in the EURICUS-I study.

Another conclusion of the survey is that "resources" are a much more suitable describer of LOCs than "complexity of care". First of all resources address the goal of classifying ICUs into LOCs. Secondly, being quantifiable, resources enable the evaluation of planning and management of ICUs. Lastly, and above all, classifying ICUs according to the provision/use of resources separates two important concepts which are unduly mixed up in the current classification of ICUs: medical competence (a rather yes/no issue) and operational capacity (a more/less question).

Using the proposed resource classification, medical competence has to be assured on every ICU regardless of the planned LOC. Progress in almost all European countries concerning the education and training of intensive care personnel and the accreditation of the practice of critical care medicine (CCM) at hospital level will ensure, in parallel with other medical specialties, that CCM can be appropriately practiced where necessary [6]. The definition of various levels of opera-

Table 11. Levels of care according to NEMS

	NEMS score	Mean NEMS	Adjusted P/N ratio
Level of care			
I	<21	16	3
II	21–30	26	2
III	>30	37	1

NEMS, Nine Equivalents of Nursing Manpower Use Score; P/N, patients/nurse.

Table 12. Matching planned with operating level of care

	Operating level of care			
	I	II	III	Overall
Planned level of care				
I	3	3	–	6
II	6	16	–	22
III	14	45	2	61
Overall	23	64	2	89

tional capacity, allowing for the effective match of resources provided and required, will enable the effective and efficient regionalization of CCM at country level.

High Turnover of Patients in the ICU

Nearly 10000 patients, or about 60% of the total number of patients enrolled in EURICUS-I, stayed in the ICUs for a period shorter than 3 days. This large group of patients consumed a total of 13500 nursing days in the ICUs (16% of the total amount of nursing days in the study), or the equivalent of 112 ICU beds (13% of the total number of beds).

Figure 1 presents the decay of the percentage of these patients during the 3 days of stay: 50% of the patients are discharged before the first 24 h of stay, and only 20% of the patients in this group will use the ICU during the third day. The patients who stayed less than 3 days in the ICU had a lower severity of illness, required a lower use of nursing manpower and had a better outcome. A large number of these patients were surgical patients and came directly from the operating theater (Table 12). One of the features of the ICUs receiving a large contingent of patients from the operating theater is that the planned number of beds must be rather large to be able to always match the variable surgical output of the operating theater. It can be seen in Table 12 that the number of patients originating from the recovery room is indeed very small, suggesting that a policy of direct admission to the ICU was agreed upon by the surgical departments involved.

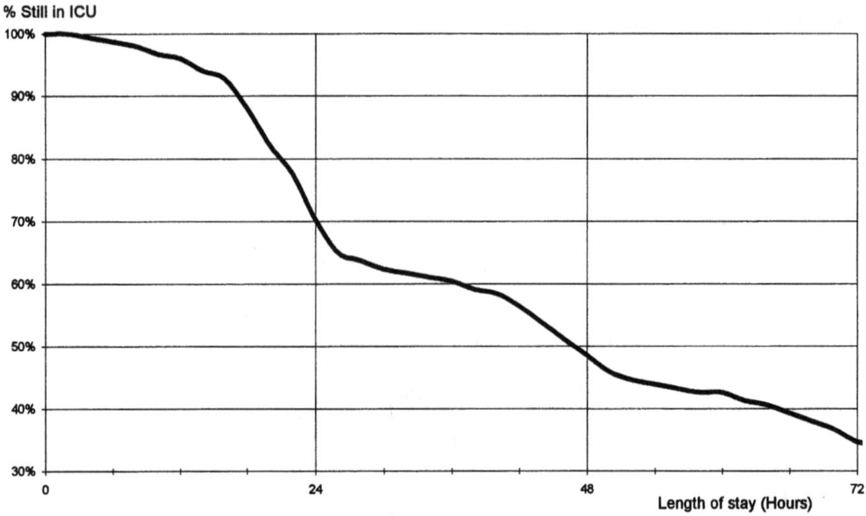

Fig. 1. Percentual decrease of 13006 survivors during the first 3 days of stay

This policy of admission was confirmed on several ICUs during the site visits. One important consequence of this policy is that the admission of scheduled surgical patients necessitates reservation of ICU beds (empty occupation) for a period of time longer than the factual LOS registered during the study. Although impossible to verify in the collected data, this empty occupation might be responsible for the low occupancy rate observed on some ICUs. In addition to this problem of empty occupancy, one has to keep in mind that every new patient entails fixed costs related to his/her admission and discharge [7]. These costs are usually proportional to the LOC of the ICU.

As can be seen in Fig. 2, the weekly admission pattern of patients staying <3 days in the ICU (8000 survivors) is rather peculiar. With 20% of the weekly admissions on Monday, the admission rate falls to 15.8% on Friday and is very reduced during the weekend. The rate of discharges on Friday and Saturday is much higher than the rate of admissions, assuring therefore a low occupancy rate during the weekend and new admissions on the next Monday.

The daily pattern of discharge of this group of patients (stay <3 days) from the ICUs (Fig. 3) suggests that many patients stay in the ICU for a period of time longer than required. As seen in Fig. 3, about 50% of the patients are discharged between 8 a.m. and 12 p.m. in the morning. During this time, staff with responsibility for decision-making regarding patient discharge are on duty. This pattern of discharge is consistent with the admission policy mentioned above: creating room for new short-term admissions. It can be seen by the admission pattern depicted in Fig. 3 that about 50% of the patients in this group are admitted to the ICU between 10 a.m. and 4 p.m. The turnover of 50% of these admissions (about 30% of all admissions) takes therefore about 4 h/day before completion.

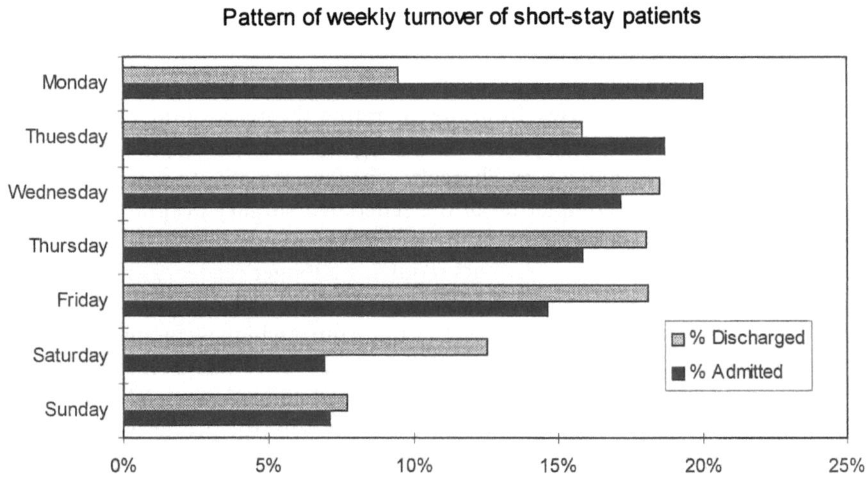

Fig. 2. Pattern of weekly turnover of short-stay patients

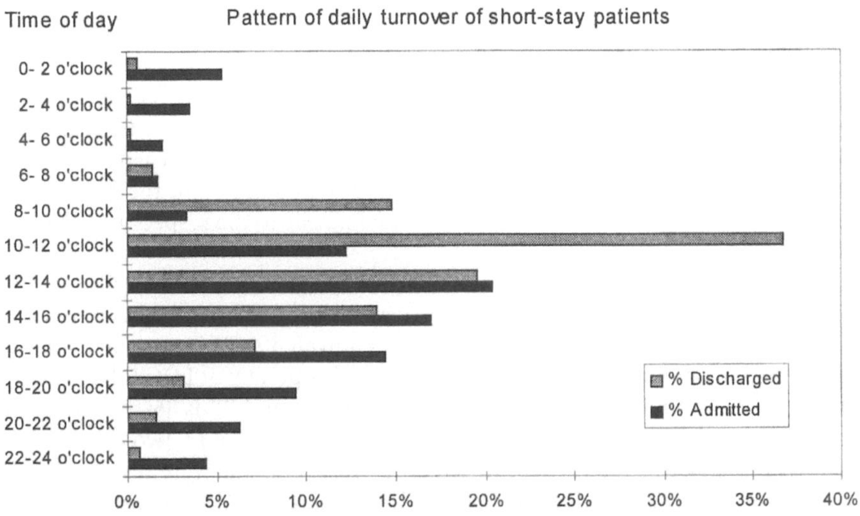

Fig. 3. Pattern of daily turnover of short-stay patients

The Recovery Room

The recovery room (RR) is an essential asset of the surgical activities in the hospital, assuring the appropriate recovery of patients after surgical interventions. Generally speaking, the RR is strictly reserved for admitting new surgical patients. All but 14 hospitals in the EURICUS sample had RR facilities attached to the operating theater. The RR was open around the clock during 5 days of the week in only 30% of the hospitals. The other RRs were operational 8 h/day during 5 days of the week (8 a.m. until 4 p.m.).

The RR is a high turnover unit during working hours. The typical flow pattern is that patients start arriving from the operating theater around 9 a.m. and this flow continues until about 3 p.m., with the highest number of patients being present between 10 a.m. and 2 p.m. Thereafter the flow of patients decreases abruptly in agreement with completion of the scheduled surgery programmed for the day. The typical RR patient stays in the RR between 1 and 3 h before being transferred to the ward of origin. Patients requiring a longer recovery and those arriving later at the RR will be transferred to the ICU around 4 p.m. (Fig. 3).

The P/N ratio at the RR is about 3:1 or more during high occupancy periods of time. Thereafter the P/N ratio decreases to 2:1, 1:1, or less because of the decreased flow of patients. This decreased P/N ratio towards the end of the day is usually very convenient because it may coincide with the presence at the RR of more severely ill patients who therefore require more attention and more complex care. The varying severity of illness and flow of patients in contrast to the same number of nurses staffing the RR leads to a wide range of P/N ratios during working hours.

Two Typical ICUs of EURICUS-I

In order to explore the impact of the recovery function of many European ICUs, two typical units in the sample are described below. The data on the two examples have been slightly adapted so that the respective ICUs cannot be easily identified. It has to be said that more information would be required and the calculations should be more detailed should this be formal advice to the respective ICUs.

ICU-1

This is a general ICU of a nonuniversity hospital with 300–500 beds. With a nursing staff of 25 nurses, or about 3.8 full-time equivalents (FTEs) per bed, the ICU is planned to operate at LOC III. However the ICU operates at LOC I. The WUR is 0.65. The ICU admits a volume of 600 patients/year; the ABY is 86; the mean LOS is 3.6; the occupancy rate (OR) is 70%. As depicted in Table 13, two thirds of the admissions stay less than 3 days in the unit. These patients were responsible for about 24% of the cumulative stay in the ICU. The mean NEMS of the patients with LOS <3 days was 14 points and those who stayed ≥3 days had a mean NEMS of 22 points.

Table 13. ICU-1

LOS	No. of admissions	Mean LOS (days)	Cumulative stay (days)	No. of ICU beds used
<3 days	400	1.2	500	1.4
≥3 days	200	8.7	1600	4.4

LOS, length of stay

A recovery room open 24 h/day would imply the redesign of this ICU both concerning the level of care and the provision of human resources.

If this ICU would not receive those patients with LOS <3 days and if its occupancy rate were improved to around 80%–85%, the size of the ICU could be reduced by two beds. This would result in the saving of 7.2 FTEs. Moreover, considering that the unit should operate at LOC II, for the patients with LOS >3 days this would represent an additional saving of about six nurses. If the 400 patients with LOS <3 days are admitted at the RR, the nursing staff of this unit should be augmented with four to five nurses who would staff the late and night shifts at the RR.

ICU-2

This is a medical ICU of an university hospital. With a nursing staff of 28 nurses, or about 2.5 FTEs/bed, the ICU is planned as a LOC II and is operating at the planned LOC. The ICU has an annual volume of 1000 patients: ABY is 77, mean LOS is 3.2 and OR is 60% (Table 14). The mean NEMS of the patients with LOS <3 days was 22 points and those who stayed ≥3 days had a mean NEMS of 26 points.

A recovery room open 24/day would imply the redesign of this ICU concerning the provision of human resources.

If this ICU would not receive those patients with LOS <3 days and if its occupancy rate were improved to around 80%–85%, the size of the ICU could be reduced by at least four beds. This would therefore result in the saving of 10 FTEs. The unit would keep operating at LOC II for the patients with LOS >3 days. If the 700 patients with LOS <3 days are admitted at the RR, the nursing staff of this unit should be augmented by six to eight nurses who would staff the RR late and night shifts.

The Recovery Room as an ICU of LOC-I

From the examples above we may conclude that the nursing staff of ICU-1 could be reduced substantially if the patients with LOS <3 days were treated in the RR. The proposed reduction of the nursing staff of ICU-2 was less important. For both cases, however, the expanded use of RR beds would allow a marked reduction of the more expensive beds on the ICU without endangering the adequate care of the variable flow of surgical patients. As explained above, the flow characteristics of patients through the RR would allow this unit to operate at

Table 14. ICU-2

LOS	No. of admissions	Mean LOS (days)	Cumulative stay (days)	No. of ICU beds used
<3 days	700	1.5	800	2.2
≥3 days	300	7.5	1600	5.2

LOC I as usual during the morning shift and at LOC II or III during the evening and night shifts without demanding more nursing staff than a typical ICU LOC I.

The ICU Profile of Hospital Categories

The type and size of hospital in which the ICUs were operating took a central position in the analysis performed in this substudy. The rationale behind this decision was the significant association of of hospital and ICUs characteristics found by the Dutch National ICU Study [5]. These associations concerned almost exclusively the medical characteristics of the patients admitted to ICUs of the different hospital categories.

It seemed therefore important to explore whether the same pattern was found in other European countries. In the survey of this issue using the EURICUS-I data, the ICU variables analyzed were clustered into the categories: planning, case mix, intermediate outputs and final output (Table 15). The results of this analysis, most of it included in the above descriptive presentation of the concerned variables, will be summarized in this section. Table 15 indicates whether the variance of the studied variables can be significantly explained by hospital category.

- ICU planning: None of the ICU variables, type, number of beds, nursing staffing and planned LOC, were associated with hospital category.
- Case mix: The variance of the ICU variables concerning case mix of the admitted patients, i.e. age, SAPS-II score, origin of patients, and medical or (un)scheduled surgical type of admission, was related to the hospital category in which the ICUs were located.

Table 15. ICU characteristics associated with hospital categories[a]

	Not significant	Significant
Characteristics		
ICU planning	Number of ICU beds Number of nurses/bed Planned level of care Type of ICU	
Case mix		Age SAPS-II Origin Type of admission
Intermediate outputs	Occupancy rate Work utilisation ratio	Operating level of care Admissions per bed per year Length of stay NEMS
Final output		Mortality

SAPS, Simplified Acute Physiology Score; NEMS, Nine Equiavalents of Nursing Manpower Use Score.

[a] Presented are variables with values that are significantly different between the hospital categories

- Intermediate outputs: The variance of the occupancy rate and of the WUR of the ICUs did not correlate with the hospital category. Conversely, significant correlations between ICU characteristics and hospital category were found for the variables operational LOC, turnover of patients, LOS and NEMS.
- Final output: The mortality at hospital discharge of ICU patients (Tables 5, 6) correlated with hospital category.

The conclusions of the above may be summarized as follows:
1. The variance of case mix of the patients admitted to the ICUs is intimately associated with the type and size of the hospitals in which the ICUs are located. Consequently, and in accordance with these differences, the mortality of these patients varies also with the hospital category.
2. The planning of ICUs in the various hospital categories does not seem tailored to match the volume and type of patients admitted to the respective ICUs. It seems fair to conclude that the rather uniformly planned LOC (number of beds and number of nurses) has to be readjusted to fit the significant differences of operating LOC observed at ICU level.

References

1. Hofstede G, Neuijen J, Ohayv D, Sanders GJEM (1990) measuring organizational cultures: a qualitative and quantitative study across twenty cases. Admin Sci Q 35:286–316
2. Shortell SM, Zimmerman JE, Rousseau DM, Gillies RR, Wagner DP, Draper EA, Knaus, WA, Duffy J (1994) The performance of intensive care units: does good management make a difference? Med Care 32:508–524
3. Edbrooke DL, Wilson AJ, Gerrish SP, Mann AJ (1994) The Sheffield costing system for intensive care. Working paper, Central Sheffield University Hospital
4. Consensus Conference. Critical care medicine (1983). JAMA 250:798–804
5. Reis Miranda D and Gimbrére J (1994) The Netherlands. New Horizons 2:357–363
6. Thijs LG and the Working Group on Guidelines for Training Programmes in Intensive Care Medicine (1996) Guidelines for a training programme in Intensive Care Medicine. Intens Care Med 22:166–172
7. Spangenberg J, Van de Poel JHR, Iapichino G (1990) Management control in the ICU. In: Management of intensive care – guidelines for better resource use. In: Reis Miranda D, Williams A, Loirat Ph (eds). Kluwer Academic, Dordrecht, The Netherlands, pp 103–121

3 Integration of Substudies

Introduction

The integration of the substudies followed two strategies: (1) formal statistical hypothesis testing; (2) explorative integration of the substudies.

Hypothesis Testing

In this analysis the main hypothesis of EURICUS-I, that nonclinical management variables do influence the clinical outcome of patients admitted to the ICUs, is formally tested. Using ICU performance as a dependent variable, the most relevant variables of the substudies were included in a multiple linear regression analysis as the independent variables. For each ICU two variables of performance were used: B20, low risk patients; B80, high risk patients (see Chap. 8).

The Independent Variables

It was prospectively decided that each of the five substudies in EURICUS-I should contribute two independent variables to the analysis of hypothesis testing. After analysis of the data and modeling of the relevant variables, those variables judged to most strongly represent the data in each substudy (two per substudy) were included in the analysis.

The inclusion of two variables per substudy, instead of the (stepwise) inclusion of all variables modeled, was based on two methodologic considerations: (1) inclusion of all the variables would make the analysis extremely difficult from a technical point of view; (2) inclusion of all the variables (more and less meaningful) might lead to a kind of "fishing expedition" through which less meaningful associations could unduly dominate the conclusions of the study.

Substudy Patients and Facilities

This substudy delivered three variables to the hypothesis testing, one of which is the dependent variable discussed in Chap. 8. The two independent variables contributed by *Patients and Facilities* were: number of beds and the wealth of the ICU.

Number of Beds

The argument for including this as an independent variable is that the size of the unit alone may be associated in a significant way with the organizational structure, the culture, and the morale of the personnel.

Wealth of the ICUs

ICUs do not look the same. Besides the number of beds and the case mix of the admitted patients, the physical space in which procedures are implemented differs among ICUs regarding both size and utilization. ICUs may look spacious or crowded, organized or chaotic, clean or messy. These differences were apparent during the site visits. Moreover, it often appeared possible to associate the characteristics of the ICUs with expressions of confidence, satisfaction, planning and expectations during interviews with the leadership of the ICUs .

The hospital environment of ICUs is also not the same. The ICU may be unique or have other critical care areas around it. The case mix of the hospital and the array of sevices that can be provided vary. The number of professionals in the hospital, their areas of specialization as well their care objectives may differ among hospitals. These aspects may determine differences among ICUs.

The financial circumstances of the ICUs are not the same. Besides differences in the resources allocated, differences in the identity of the departments and in the distribution of resources are, expectedly, determinants of some of the ICU characteristics.

The policies concerning the organization of ICUs are not the same. Besides those differences pointed out above, the organization of the ICUs may differ based upon human factors at the decision-making level. Such factors include specific knowledge, professional views, and prestige questions. The particular characteristics of the ICUs and their environment determine the type and volume of the resources invested in them. The invested resources may correspond to those demanded by the medical activities in the unit. They may be inferior but they may also be superior to the resources demanded to match those activities. The various degrees of match between provision and use of resources may influence the clinical performance of the ICUs; moreover, there may also have a relevant influence upon organizational issues. Independent of the differences between provision/use of resources, it may be anticipated that the wealth of the ICU, including the absolute volume of resources invested, may influence significantly several ICU characteristics such as confidence, satisfaction, planning and expectations of the ICU professionals.

The wealth of the ICU may be due to and reinforced by particular developments in the ICU such as the technology available and the number of available professionals. These two elements are intimately associated with relevant characteristics such as: (a) the severity and clinical complexity of the patients' conditions; (b) the type and volume of the standing (un)written routines (procedures and diagnostic); (c) the use of expensive modes of care (e.g. medication); (d) the implementation of innovations and results of research activities. These characteristics are the medical equivalent of wealth of the ICUs.

The development of the variable wealth of the ICU aims therefore at selecting markers which describe wealth without using financial data. Besides taking investment in the ICU at its face value, each of the markers selected should reflect investment in one or more of the resources mentioned above. Furthermore, the selected markers should allow discrimination among ICUs. After statistical analysis, the following markers of wealth were selected and included in the variable wealth of the ICU: (a) number of nurses/ICU bed; (b) ICU secretary; (c) hemofiltration capacity; (d) hemodialysis capacity; (e) intra-aortic balloon pump.

Substudy Organization

The variables of this substudy were derived from analysis of the answers to the questionnaire "Organization and Management", administered to all ICUs. In contrast to the other EURICUS-I substudies, the included variables needed to be developed from the study sample, as there were no dimensions/variables available for ICUs regarding the substudy *Organization*. After statistical analysis of the data provided by 91 ICUs, two variables were selected to contribute to hypothesis testing. These are discussed below.

Centralization of ICUs

This variable was constructed from questions exploring the professional level at which policies and/or decisions are made in the ICU: (a) level of policy-making regarding common interventions in the ICU, particularly antibiotic prophylaxis and decubitus prevention; (b) level of decision-making regarding common activities in the ICU, such as admission and discharge of individual patients.

Elementary Organization Framework

Clinical and nonclinical management responsibilities in the ICU are, generally speaking, in the hands of professionals responsible for patient care in the unit: the ICU physicians (including the medical director) and the nurses. As a result, the clinical and nonclinical organization and management (OM) of the ICU is usually guided by medical views and professional needs. Recent developments in the nursing profession and the more frequent interaction of the ICU with nonmedical managers in the hospital has substantially improved the general approach to the OM of the unit. Some of the managerial improvements were introduced as a consequence of experience acquired in the practice of intensive care, such as the need for continuous communication between the involved professionals and their acquaintance with the general policies and practices in use in the units. Other managerial innovations, mainly introduced in the last decade, are intimately associated with medical care and performance (e.g. job descriptions; individual performance evaluation) and were therefore absorbed into the medical organization of many ICUs.

The existing structure of the OM in the ICU, as a small enterprise in the hospital, is usually focused on the clinical activities of the unit. Several other specific aspects of the OM of enterprises, such as centralization, standardization, hierarchy, or integration of the enterprise (in the hospital), are usually not looked upon by the ICUs as variables with influence upon outcome of medical care. The aim of the elementary organization framework (EOF) variable is to represent what could be described as the basic OM of the ICUs from a medical perspective, upon which the specific nonmedical approach to OM could be further analyzed. This variable was constructed from the following indicators of elementary organization of ICUs, from a medical perspective: (a) the existence of written descriptions of jobs and functions; (b) the existence of daily formal meetings of medical staff for clinical decision-making; (c) the use of formally written protocols to guide implementation of ICU care activities; (d) regular evaluation of the professional functioning of physicians and nurses working in the ICU; (e) the existence of regularly scheduled staff meetings concerning OM aspects other than those related specifically to professional daily practice.

Substudy Personnel

The variables were developed from questionnaires administered to about 2000 nurses. A second-order factor analysis on the dependent variables in the research model (i.e. emotional exhaustion, depersonalization, personal accomplishment, job involvement, organizational commitment and perceived unit performance) yielded a clear two-factor structure. The factors were labeled as: (1) stress (emotional exhaustion and depersonalization) and (2) morale (personal accomplishment, job involvement, organizational commitment and perceived unit performance). This dichotomy parallels the distinction between negative vs positive job-related outcomes that is being made in the current literature on job stress. Based on the results of the second-order factor analysis, two variables were chosen to represent each of the two factors in the general research model of the substudy.

The following two variables were selected for the hypothesis testing analysis:

1. With respect to the stress factor, emotional exhaustion (i.e. the draining of emotional resources) was selected. This decision was based on results of the statistical analysis and on the following reasoning. First, leading theorists in the field of burnout have argued that emotional exhaustion is the defining feature of burnout. Second, emotional exhaustion correlates most strongly with global measures of burnout. Third, emotional exhaustion can be considered as the first stage in the process of burning out. Finally, emotional exhaustion is the burnout component that can be best generalized across different occupations.
2. With respect to the morale factor it was decided to select organizational commitment (i.e. the strength of an individual's identification with and involvement in the ICU). This decision was based on the results of the statistical analysis, and the fact that organizational commitment correlates strongly with perceived unit performance. Also, results of earlier studies have demonstrated that organizational commitment is strongly negatively related to turnover.

Substudy Culture

For this substudy culture scales have been selected from studies in Denmark and the Netherlands involving a wide range of work organizations: private manufacturing organizations, private services companies and public institutions. The units themselves were considered culturally homogeneous by organizational management. Appropriateness and content validity of the scales developed were verified in meetings with participating units and organizations. The culture scales were designed to measure differences between organizational units in cultural dimensions. One value scale and four practices scales have been applied to EURICUS-I: V1, need for security; P1, process-oriented vs results-oriented; P2, employee-oriented vs job-oriented; P3, parochial vs professional; P4, open system vs closed system. The term "values" describes what people feel "should be"; the term "practices" describes what people think "is".

Based on the results of the statistical analysis performed on 2848 questionnaires returned, two variables were selected for hypothesis testing analysis:

1. P1 (process-oriented vs results-oriented): On the process-oriented side of this dimension, the daily tasks and work procedures of the ICU are rather standardized. The procedures, rather automatically implemented, often follow exclusively a criterion of avoidance of risks. In these ICUs the nurses have a low level of autonomy for solving problems and feel themselves dependent on the physicians. On the results-oriented side of this dimension, the tasks of nurses and physicians are implemented more in accordance with the objectives of care regarding each medical case. Nurses and physicians are rather interdependent and work as teams. The autonomy of nurses for solving problems is high and they may be responsible for nursing care and some coordination tasks.
2. P4 (open system vs closed system): On the open system side of this dimension people feel at home quickly. The staff of the ICU feel that the ICU is an integrated part of the hospital. It does not take long before new staff members feel at ease. Conversely, on the closed system side of this dimension, the staff of the ICU feel that the unit is a rather isolated ward in the hospital. There are rather rigid selection criteria for the appointment of new staff members (only special people can work here) and it takes a long time before they feel well integrated into the group.

Substudy Finances

On a priori grounds, departmental budgeting and costing elements might affect ICU performance. Two preliminary hypotheses will be tested. These are to be understood as *ceteris paribus* hypotheses. In EURICUS-I they are integrated with other nonclinical variables such as organization, work force well being and organizational culture in order to assess their influence on the ICU's clinical efficiency.

A budget in this context is defined as a decision by hospital authorities concerning allowed expenses and investments for every unit in the hospital during a given period (mostly 1 year), usually split up for several categories of expenses. We do not consider revenue budgets. A costing procedure is defined as a system by which ICU management is allowed to calculate, in one way or another, a cost per unit of activity. As far as budgeting is concerned, two aspects are considered: the ICU manager's perception of its effect on efficiency, and the tightness of budgetary control.

Flexibility

Two questions in the questionnaire pertain to the managerial perception of budgeting procedures. The first one asks whether ICU managers would like to have more flexibility in their budgets. Managers answering "yes" can have different reasons for doing so: from increasing fringe benefits (such as excessively luxurious furniture or useless equipment), status or power (by, e.g. investing in the newest versions of already owned equipment, or hiring as much staff as possible), to the honest convictions that increasing flexibility would increase the ICU's performance. The managerial theory of "selfish" managers has ben widely discussed. More traditional economic thinking assumes that managers are loyal agents of the organization's owners. In the case of a selfish yes we expect no relationship to performance. In the case of a loyal yes one can expect a negative relationship: ICU managers answering yes expect increasing performance when granted more budgetary flexibility, whereas the others do not. As real managers, like everybody else, are characterized by a mixture of selfishness and loyalty, we have *hypothesis 1: There is a weak negative relation between the ICU manager's wish to have more budgetary flexibiliy and ICU performance.*

Perception of Appropriateness of Budgetary Procedures

The second question pertaining to the managerial perception of budgetary procedures asks whether the ICU manager thinks that budgetary procedures allow him/her to manage efficiently the ICU. When the answer is "yes", we might assume the ICU to be more efficient, *ceteris paribus*, than when the answer is "no": Thus, *hypothesis 2: There is a positive relation between the ICU manager's perception of the appropriateness of budgetary procedures and the ICU's efficiency.*

Results

To study the relationship between ICU performance (dependent variable) and the independent variables selected at substudy level (Table 1), two related approaches were used:

1. The fixed effects approach consisted of calculation of an (SAPS-II-corrected) index of ICU performance; the relation of this index to the substudy variables was studied by means of multiple regression analysis.
2. The random effects approach, which examines the relationship between the patient outcome (alive/dead) and the substudy variables, was studied by means of logistic regression analysis with random ICU effect. The interested reader is referred to the presentation of this methodology in Chap. 8.

Table 1. Summary of variables used

Substudy Facilities	
NoBEDS	The number of beds in the ICU
Wealth	An index of wealth of the ICU
Substudy Personnel	
Emothex	Emotional exhaustion
OrgCom	Organizational commitment
Substudy Finances	
Budget	Budget flexibility
Perceive	Perceived appropriateness of budget
Substudy Organisation	
Central	Centralization
EOF	Elementary organizational framework
Substudy Culture	
P1	Process-oriented vs results-oriented
P4	Open system vs closed system

Both approaches led to similar results: The ICU performance (corrected for differences in SAPS-II) is significantly ($p < 0.05$) related to:

- Number of beds: The optimal number of beds is about nine; smaller or larger ICUs tend to have higher mortality.
- Organizational commitment: Higher organizational commitment lowers mortality.
- Results-oriented culture: Results-oriented culture lowers mortality.
- Elementary organizational framework: Higher EOF lowers mortality.
- European area

Explorative Integration of Substudies

After the hypothesis of EURICUS-I was formally tested by using medical performance as the dependent variable and a set of preselected nonclinical management variables as the explanatory variables, it was important to determine whether other variables of nonclinical management existed which had not been included in the previous analysis but which might influence clinical outcome at the ICU level. Following the research model of EURICUS-I, it can be appreciated that the modes of OM may influence ICU performance on at least at two levels: (1) clinical performance, or the relation between case mix of the patients (input) and mortality; (2) nonclinical performance, or the measurable effects of clinical and nonclinical OM strategies upon a set of selected indicators of OM output. Testing of the effects of OM on the clinical performance of the ICUs was described in the section above.

Here, integration of the results of the substudies will be explored with two objectives: (1) to identify the variables of OM which influence the nonclinical performance of ICUs; (2) to analyze some relevant problems related to the practice of intensive care medicine in Europe, identified during the field work in EURICUS-I.

Nonclinical Performance

Personnel is the major asset of every ICU. It seems therefore logical that the nonclinical outcomes of the ICUs be assessed by the effects (outputs) of variables/ strategies of OM (throughputs) that have been applied to the largest professional group (input), i.e. the nurses, working in the ICU.

The indicators of OM performance were sought among the variables of the substudy *Personnel*. Three nonclinical outcomes were chosen: (1) the nurses' level of burnout (i.e. emotional exhaustion and depersonalization); (2) morale (i.e. accomplishment, commitment, involvement); (3) job satisfaction.

A set of possible explanatory (independent) variables was selected among clinical and nonclinical OM variables and introduced in various stepwise regression models. Selection was based on evaluation of the relevance of these variables as judged by the involved research teams (Table 2). Preliminary analysis using successively country, SAPS-II score, and the interaction country*SAPS-II score as only explanatory variables has shown that country explains 35% (adjusted R^2) of the variance of burnout, 20% of morale and 19% of the variance of satisfaction. SAPS-II score had a negligible (between 1% and 4%) and nonsignificant explanatory power of the variance of the performance indicators. The interaction country*SAPS-II did not add to the explanatory power of country alone.

Using regression analysis the entire set of predictors (Table 2) explained 56% of the variance of burnout and 48% of the variance of satisfaction. The selected set of predictors could not explain the variance of morale. After adding SAPS-II score to the set of predictors the analyzed models did not increase in explanatory power. After adding the variable country, the models explained respectively 65% and 58% of the variance of burnout and morale. For satisfaction the addition of the variable country to the model did not lead to an increase in explanatory power.

In the definitive analysis, the predictor sets of variables (Table 2) were used to explain the variance of the performance indicators by stepwise introduction of the indicated variables in regression models. The best models are presented below.

- Burnout: 58% of the variance of burnout could be significantly explained by a model including perceived job demands (positive effect), work utilization ratio (WUR; negative effect) and perceived appropriateness of budgetary procedures (negative effect). The explanatory power of the model was increased to 68% after adding country to the regression model.
- Morale: 59% of the variance of morale could be significantly explained by two dimensions of culture, results-oriented (positive effect) and employee-oriented (positive effect), only after adding the variable country to the model.
- Satisfaction: 55% of the variance of satisfaction could be significantly explained by a regression model including: patient/nurse (P/N) ratios (positive

Table 2. Selected set of potential performance predictors

Performance indicator	Predictor set of variables
Burnout	Mortality
	Imbalance team
	Imbalance patients
	Process- vs result-oriented culture
	Employee- vs job-oriented culture
	Perceived appropriateness of budgetary procedures
	Budget flexibility
	Perceived job demands
	Workflow
	Work utilization ratio
Morale	Imbalance patients
	Imbalance team
	Process- vs results-oriented culture
	Employee- vs job oriented culture
	Perceived job demands
	Task differentiation
	Elementary organizational framework
	Scheduled staff meeting
	Length of stay
	Perceived appropriateness of budgetary procedures
	Budget flexibility
Satisfaction	Mortality
	Imbalance patients
	Imbalance team
	Perceived job demands
	Task differentiation
	Elementary organizational framework
	Scheduled staff meetings
	Nurse performance evaluation
	Workflow
	Patients/nurse ratios
	Length of stay
	Work utilization ratio
	Perceived appropriateness of budgetary procedures
	Budget flexibility
	Wealth of the ICU
	Process- vs results-oriented culture
	Employee- vs job oriented culture
	Open vs closed system culture

effect), results-oriented culture (positive effect), job demands (negative effect) and wealth of the ICU (negative effect). The explanatory power of the model was not increased after adding country to the model.

Remarks

Variance in the nonclinical performance indicators (burnout, morale and satisfaction) appears to be associated, to a large extent, with the European area (country) in which the ICUs are located. This is particularly true for morale and for burnout, suggesting the influence of nation-related OM characteristics of ICUs (or more general health care policies) which were not identified and/or quantified by the EURICUS-I study. This phenomenon might also be associated with undetermined characteristics of the selected ICUs in each European area, as the ICUs in these areas do not have national representation. This explanation seems less probable, however, as the explanatory power of the variable country was less evident, and even absent, regarding variance in the performance indicator satisfaction in the same ICU sample.

The severity of the conditions of the patients who were admitted to the ICUs did not have a measurable impact on the variance of the performance indicators. Although it may be argued that the severity of illness variable used was aggregated at ICU level for the purpose of this analysis, one has to remember that there were significant differences in the SAPS-II scores aggregated at unit level. Mortality, by contrast, which could be expected to influence the performance indicators in a manner similar to severity of illness, also was not associated with them in any of the regression models tested. The results of the stepwise regression analysis described above do conform somehow with what could be expected and require no further explanation. The negative association of WUR and burnout deserves however to be noted. WUR measures the relation between nursing work provided and the amount of nursing work available in each unit. Association of the two variables suggests that nursing workload is not, in itself, a cause of burnout.

Integration of Results of Substudies in the Light of the Field Work Survey

During the site visits by EURICUS-I the leadership of the participating ICUs indicated as relevant matters of concern, among others, the following aspects regarding the OM of the units:

- Poor definition of jobs and tasks
- Insufficient professional autonomy of the nursing staff
- Insufficient participation of the nurses in ICU decision-making processes
- Lack of an overall view by the nurses of patient care

From the notes of the country coordinators on intensive care medicine systems in Europe three areas of concern could be identified: (1) insufficient organization of intensive care medicine as a medical activity at the national level; (2) insufficient organization and implementation of teaching and training of intensive care medicine with respect to both physicians and nurses; (3) insufficient professional organization, particularly of ICU medical activities, resulting in highly diverse qualifications of care providers and continuity of care provided.

All of the above is obviously interrelated. It would therefore be inappropriate to select one of the aspects mentioned and to address the solution of the related insufficiencies without considering the interdependence with (all) other OM variables.

In the following example of integration of EURICUS-I results, we selected four OM aspects of intensive care medicine which appeared to be at an equally high

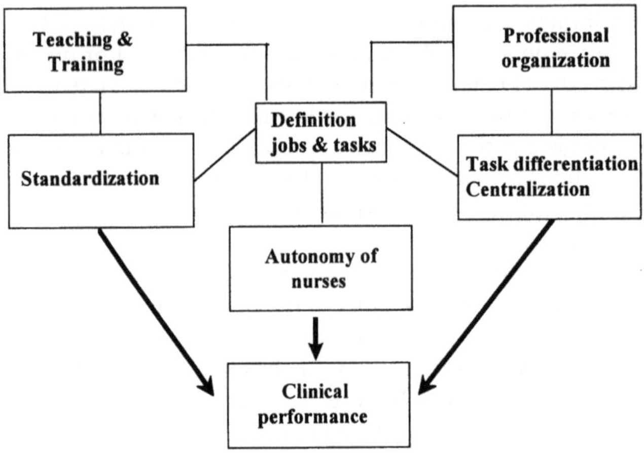

Fig. 1. Integration of results of substudies

level in the hierarchy of interrelations among the variables of OM in the ICUs: (1) professional organization; (2) teaching and training (notes on intensive care medicine systems); (3) definition of jobs; and (4) tasks and autonomy of the nurses (site visits). These aspects were integrated with five OM variables: (1) jobs; (2) tasks and autonomy of nurses (substudy *Personnel*); (3) standardization; (4) task differentiation; and (5) centralization of decision-making (substudy *Organization*). Finally, by means of a "fishing expedition", e.g. multivariable analyses, the existence of meaningful associations between the variables in relation to clinical performance at ICU level was explored. The association with performance varied depending on whether ICU performance concerned high risk or low risk patients. For the sake of simplicity, the differences will not be considered here. The interested reader is therefore referred to the respective substudies. Figure 1 is a guide to the analysis.

Autonomy of the nurses has been shown to correlate positively with performance (more autonomy better performance) and addressed concerns such as norms, materials, information and work planning. In addition, problems regarding the exchange of information (communication) between nurses and other professionals (inside and particularly outside the ICU) were found to be fairly demanding and rather dissatisfying, as opposed to communication within the ICU nurses' professional group. It is interesting to note that problems related to patients were considered to be both demanding and satisfying. In addition, the level of the autonomy which was granted to solve these problems was not significantly associated with performance. This finding seems to reenforce the importance of nonclinical OM variables upon the clinical performance of ICUs. Notwithstanding, the reader should consult the research models used in the substudy *Personnel* in order to better understand how these various aspects can be interconnected.

The substudy *Organization* has shown that standardization was positively correlated with performance. The variables included in standardization concerned written description of the relevant professional jobs in the ICU and structured evaluation of the professional performance of the involved staff members. Furthermore, other aspects of standardization in the ICUs, such as daily formal clinical meetings, written clinical protocols and the existence of scheduled staff meetings for discussing OM issues of the ICU, have been shown to be significantly and positively associated with the clinical performance of the units. It seems therefore clear that better performing ICUs do seek standardization of both clinical and nonclinical OM. The importance of the link between (appropriate) standardization and (well structured) teaching and training is obvious.

The described association of task differentiation and centralization of decision-making with ICU performance (substudy *Organization*) is perhaps one of the most relevant results of EURICUS-I. Although standardization and other OM measures will reduce uncertainty concerning tasks and workflow in the ICU, uncertainty is mainly dependent upon the clinical conditions of the patients and the required care, including the use of technologies.

It was found that better performing ICUs had a lower level of task differentiation (with higher overlap of the tasks comprising the various professional activities) and a lower level of centralization of decision-making with a subsequent increase of professional autonomy at the bedside. Development of a team-like structure for the multidisciplinary staff of the ICU requires comprehensive organization of the various professions involved and detailed descriptions of jobs and tasks, particularly concerning those areas in which the various tasks may overlap. The beneficial reduction of task differentiation implies upgrading of professional knowledge and skills by means of teaching and training.

4 Conclusions

Organization and Planning

EURICUS-I has shown that the organization of intensive care medicine (ICM) in Europe is underdeveloped and that the organization and management (OM) of the intensive care units (ICUs) in Europe shows an immense non-systematic diversity. The European Society of Intensive Care Medicine (ESICM), a society of individual members, was, until now, the only European forum which formally addressed the various aspects relating to developing ICM into a new medical specialty. Understandably, however, ESICM concentrated on clinical research findings and their implications for clinical behavior.

The results of the efforts made by ESICM and the resulting recommendations are not binding and their acknowledgment remains rather limited to ESICM members. Thus the distinctive contribution of the EURICUS projects, and of the Foundation for Research on Intensive Care in Europe (FRICE), is: (1) to broaden the perspective on ICM and (2) to create a research base from which it is possible to offer guidance on how to better organize the nonclinical aspects of the work of an ICU. It should then be possible to use more effectively the skills of those who work within ICUs, to the benefit of the patients treated. The poor organization of ICM in Europe and the observed diversity of OM among the ICUs in Europe appear to be a consequence of the inappropriate focus on these issues at the various levels of European health care policy-making. The importance of ICM in effective and efficient multidisciplinary medical care of the critically ill patient has yet to be recognized.

The following conclusions were made:

1. Apart from Spain, ICM is not recognized as an independent medical specialty in the countries of the European Community (EC). Organizational steps towards the recognition of ICM as a medical subspecialty have been taken or are in progress in some countries. Independently of these developments, however, the ICU remains integrated into the organization of other medical activities in the majority of the hospitals (e.g. anaesthesiology, internal medicine). An important consequence of this organizational set-up is that decision-making and final responsibility (strategic apex) concerning the OM of the ICUs and relevant aspects of patient care are usually entrusted to professionals outside the ICUs and therefore not directly involved with the specific activities performed in the ICUs.

Four major modes of organizational integration of ICUs with other medical activities were identified in the study (see Chap. 6, "Organization Structure"). These were differently associated with variables of OM which, in turn, were associated with the clinical and nonclinical performance of the ICUs. The data collected by the study were not conclusive concerning the position of the strategic apex (inside or outside the ICU) and its effect on the clinical performance of the units. It could however be concluded from the study that the organizational location of the strategic apex inside the ICU had a beneficial effect on the non-clinical performance of the ICU regarding burnout, morale and satisfaction of the nursing staff.

2. There are no written and centrally coordinated guidelines and standards for the planning and the provision of resources for the ICUs in the majority of EC countries. When existent, these guidelines and standards are based upon traditional and/or empirical knowledge. There were significant differences between the ICUs (and the hospitals) in Europe concerning case mix and outcome of patients as well as the majority of the intermediate outputs studied (length of stay, nursing workload, etc). Nonetheless, after considering similar clinical conditions, EURICUS-I has shown that there are no significant differences between the ICUs concerning the provision of important resources to them such as the number of nurses/bed (see Chap. 7, "The Nursing Staff" and Chap. 7, Table 8). It can be therefore concluded that in the EC the actual planning of ICU facilities is not based on precise objectives and forecasted resource requirements.
3. There are no written and centrally coordinated guidelines and standards for the professional organization of ICUs in the EC. EURICUS-I has documented a large degree of diversity among ICUs concerning elementary standards such as medical coverage (both in number and in professional qualification), multdisciplinary evaluation of critically ill patients, professional communication and the use of protocols. The study has shown that these OM variables, among others, do influence the outcome of ICU patients.
4. The rights of patients to receive both information concerning their clinical condition and visits by family and friends are not equally considered in all the countries and in all the ICUs of the EC. EURICUS-I has shown that the different consideration paid to these rights was basically related to the rather insufficient professional education of ICU professionals regarding these ethical issues.

Organization and Performance of ICUs

The EURICUS-I project explores the effects of OM on the effectiveness and efficiency of ICUs in EC countries. The main hypothesis in this research is that nonclinical variables influence performance of the ICUs. EURICUS-I was successful in identifying nonclinical factors related to the performance of ICUs. In the hypothesis testing part of this research, as well as in the substudies, differences in performance were found to be significantly related to OM factors of the ICUs.

On the level of organization, the results indicate the importance of standardization of both job description and evaluation (see Chap. 7, "Standardization") for the medical performance of the ICU . The elementary organizational framework (EOF) should include daily, formal decision-making meetings of medical staff; the use of formal written protocols to guide implementation of ICU care activities; and the existence of regularly scheduled staff meetings concerning OM aspects of the ICU. On the level of organization of work, hypotheses that ICUs with a more team-like structure - characterized by less centralized decision-making and less task differentiation - perform better were confirmed (see Chap. 7, "Task Differentiation"). The positive relationship between performance and less centralized decision-making implies that decisions can be made at lower levels in the organization. Less task differentiation implies that boundaries between functions are relaxed. It appears that ICUs in which people are not strictly confined to their own tasks and functions, but may instead exchange and fill in for each other wherever and whenever required, perform better. Additionally the results indicate that nurses lack of autonomy in solving problems is related to poor performance of the ICU (see Chap. 7, "Problem Situations and Autonomy").

On the level of ICU culture, the hypothesis that better performance is associated with a results-oriented culture was confirmed (see Chap. 8, "Analysis of ICU Performance"). A results-oriented organizational culture corresponds well to a team-like structure. High performance, high commitment work cultures are characterized by delegation, teamwork across boundaries, empowered people, people integrated with technology and a shared sense of purpose (see Chap. 7, "Conclusions and Implications").

On the level of personnel, performance is strongly related to organizational commitment - the strength of an individual's identification with and involvement in the ICU - of the nursing staff. Unexpectedly, no evidence was found for a detrimental influence of burnout in ICUs. This may be explained by the low level of stressfulness of nurses jobs in this research, as indicated by the frequency of problem situations and the quite high level of autonomy.

The results show that the performances of the various ICUs may be different for different categories of severity of illness: some ICUs appear to be good at treating severely ill patients, whereas others appear to be better at treating less severely ill patients. Although not identified in this research, different types of organization may be required for the treatment of patients with different degrees of severity of illness. It was observed that the relationships between non-clinical variables and performance are especially strong for patients who are not severely ill. For more severely ill patients, comparable relations are found, though weaker.

Use of Resources

The results of EURICUS-I have shown the existence of a detrimental mismatch between provision and demands of resources in about 75% of the units in the European sample of ICUs. This results in a rather consistent and very important loss of resources. Though not documented, it is estimated that this loss may be close to 50% of the amount invested. Three aspects deserve mention:

1. The human resources allocated enabled a large number of the ICUs to operate at a level of care which was higher than that required for those units (Chap. 2, Table 12); as a probable consequence of the foregoing it was estimated that an important fraction of the nursing manpower of the ICUs was not being used for patient care tasks(Chap. 7, Table 29). Although the mismatch between human resources provided and required was generally observed across the whole sample of units, the study data have shown that it was more pronounced in the ICUs of particular areas of Europe.
2. It was found, both during the site visits and from the collected data, that the number of beds allocated to the ICUs was frequently substantially larger than the number of beds used (Chap. 6, Table 3). A weekly pattern of use of beds was also found concerning about 50% of the admitted patients: decreasing steadily from Monday through Saturday and Sunday (Chap. 2, Fig. 2).
3. There were clear differences between ICUs concerning the use of nursing manpower and of beds (length of stay) after controlling for severity of illness (see Chap. 7, "Length of Stay"). These differences were already generally anticipated on an empirical basis. EURICUS-I has documented that the (non)-clinical approach to the care of similar clinical conditions may be different among the ICUs in EC countries and that these differences may result in significant differences in the use of resources.

Analysis of the collected data suggests that some aspects of the OM of ICUs may be at the origin of the observed mismatch between provision and demand of resources.

1. Without considering local financial circumstances, the planned level of the nursing staff in the ICUs often followed instructions (recommendations and/or guidelines) existing in the hospital or issued by some authority in the country. These instructions indicate usually a fixed number of nurses per ICU bed (N/B). The recommended N/B ratios varied from two to six, without considering important characteristics of the ICUs such as type and volume of patients, desired occupancy rate, etc. The use of these recommendations, when staffing the ICU of a small peripheral hospital, for example, will expectedly lead to a waste of resources.

   When existent, step-down units were characterized by defining the complexity of the predominant medical activities to be performed in the unit instead of by defining the amount of human resources to be consumed in the performance of those and other activities in the ICU. The EURICUS-I study confirms the results of other studies indicating that the definition of levels of care in terms of nursing staff resources enables a better match of provision and demand of resources than definitions based on terms of complexity of medical care. Use of the latter definition will endanger the effective regionalization of intensive care medicine, as every ICU should be prepared to assist in the treatment of medical conditions of a wide range of complexity even if only sporadically and/or for a short period of time.

2. The surgical activities in the hospital determined to a large extent the patient population on the ICUs and the pattern of admission of patients to the ICUs. Generally speaking, the severity of illness of surgical patients was significantly lower than that of their nonsurgical counterparts: a considerable majority of the surgical patients admitted to the ICUs in the study had a low severity of illness, a short length of stay in the ICU, and were alive at hospital discharge. These patients were predominantly admitted from the operating theater directly after surgery (Chap. 7, Table 12). Admission of these patients to the ICU instead of the recovery rooom (RR) was associated with the limited working hours of the RR (8 h/day) in about 70% of the hospitals in the sample. An important consequence of these organizational policies was the "empty occupancy" of beds, as the planning of admissions to and discharges from the ICU was made dependent on the surgical program (Chap. 2, Figs. 2, 3). Another consequence of these organizational policies is, besides other costs, that the cost associated with the procedures of admission and discharge of these short-stay patients is much higher when using the ICU than when using the RR.
3. Differences in intermediate outputs between ICUs (e.g. workload and length of stay) which cannot be explained by the severity of illness of the involved patients may be caused by social and/or hospital care aspects external to the ICU. It is however important to point out that differences observed in the organizational characteristics of the ICUs, such as availability of care (medical staffing of the ICU), continuity of care (education and training of the medical staff) and the level at which professional decision-making takes place can be at the origin of the observed differences in use of resources.
4. The medical and the nursing staff of the ICUs is in its majority not educated and trained to effectively understand the relevant cost-effectiveness aspects involved in the ICU. This seems to be related to the insufficient financial policies of the ICUs in the EC countries: when existing, ICU budgetary and cost-accounting procedures show a nonsystematic diversity; budgetary control systems are not obligatory in most countries; and cost-calculating procedures are rather underdeveloped in the majority of ICUs.

5 Recommendations*

Summary and Recommendations

On the basis of an in-depth international study involving 86 intensive care units (ICUs) in 12 European countries, a number of conclusions were drawn as to the influence of organization and management on the effectiveness and efficiency of intensive care practice. The Simplified Acute Physiology Score (SAPS-II) was used to describe severity of illness and mortality at time of hospital discharge as the clinical outcome measure.

Very large differences between countries were identified with respect to intensive care practice and outcome. Nonetheless, certain broad conclusions could be reached and tentative recommendations made as to the way forward. The emphasis of the recommendations is on effective communication and consultation, improved research methodology, focused pilot studies/natural experiments, review of internal management processes and revision of education and training goals. Clearly, the manner in which these recommendations might be implemented would be substantially influenced by local factors.

Effective Communication and Consultation

Intensive care is part of a continuum of progressive patient care, and decisions as to the delivery of this component of care involve other health care professionals and managers as well as the patients themselves and their relatives. More generally, society at large is increasingly concerned about the deployment of costly medical resources. EURICUS-I is a unique study, the results of which need to be widely disseminated with a view to sharing knowledge, the wider involvement of interested parties, identifying „good practice", and increasing the likelihood of support for future research.

* The author of this chapter was Professor I. McA. Ledingham, one of the reviewers of the EURCIUS-I final report.

Recommendation 1

The participants of EURICUS-I should undertake to share the results of the study at the European, national and local levels. Government, institutional, professional and community bodies need to be informed and mechanisms devised for continuing consultation.

Improved Research Methodology

Measurement of clinical outcome in relation to severity of illness is clearly an indicator of clinical performance. However, evidence has shown mortality (particularly short-term) to be a relatively insensitive parameter of performance. There is a need to develop other measures of outcome as well as to continue to improve severity of illness scores. The importance of valid and reliable statistical analyses cannot be exaggerated.

Recommendation 2

Measures other than short-term mortality need to be developed to determine standards of performance in relation to intensive care delivery. These might include, in the short-term, restoration of stable or normal organ function, freedom from pain, discomfort and anxiety, or acceptance of professional competence by relatives. In the longer term, out of hospital survival and quality of life assessment are additional parameters. The statistical basis of such measures needs to be sound.

Pilot Studies/Natural Experiments

Data from EURICUS-I implies that certain intensive care organizational and management practices affect clinical outcome. These conclusions need to be confirmed by more specifically focused trials. The perceived importance of progressive patient care and regionalization of ICUs was highlighted. The inherent organizational challenges were appreciated, particularly the need for interdisciplinary consultation and collaboration. The cost implications of resource mismatch was considered to be substantial. In this connection, rigid adherence to conventional subclassification of ICUs, e.g. intensive care, high dependency, etc, may be less cost-effective than creative deployment of locally available resources. Finally, the concept of optimal size for individual ICUs needs further study together with evidence of minimal critical mass, both at institutional and regional levels.

Recommendation 3

Institutions should review the overall (rather than piecemeal) requirement for acute care services and consider ways and means of improving cost-effectiveness. Implementation of a policy of progressive patient care should be prospectively evaluated. Specifically, around the clock utilization of recovery rooms might offer a more effective use of resources for the large number of postoperative patients requiring short-term intensive care.

Recommendation 4

Likewise, regions should review overall (rather than piecemeal) requirement for acute care services and consider ways and means of improving cost-effectiveness. Regionalization of acute care services should be prospectively evaluated. Several examples of good practice exist within the European context and could act as role models for collaborative pilot studies. Linking transport systems are an integral part of such systems.

Recommendation 5

Procedures should be devised at the local level for detailed calculation of acute care costs and systems put in place for budget control.

Review of Internal Management Processes

EURICUS-I revealed serious and widespread deficiencies in intensive care management. These included inadequate leadership, ambiguous lines of responsibility, lack of team ethos and evidence of work-related stress.

Recommendation 6

Institutions should ensure that all aspects of acute care management policy are developed in conjunction with the staff providing the care. A full-time medical director and head nurse should be directly responsible for development and audit of individual unit activities in consultation with other relevant health care professionals.

Recommendation 7

Intensive care unit management should develop an effective system of feedback to all involved staff, particularly concerning individual job performance.

This implies the prior existence of relevant job descriptions. The emphasis should be on support of the staff member as part of a multiprofessional health care team.

Recommendation 8

Intensive care unit management should develop, control and regularly update the operational aspects of the unit (e.g. protocols, duties, meetings, etc.) and ensure that these are known to and accepted by staff inside the unit and available to relevant staff in other departments.

Revision of Education and Training Goals

EURICUS-I has provided evidence that the existence of a team ethos within an ICU is associated with improved performance. The team approach was consistent with low task differentiation and low centralization of clinical decision-making. This approach is only possible when staff have appropriate qualifications and experience and a commitment to continuing professional education. They should have high problem solving skills and be maximally adaptable to change.

Recommendation 9

The health care authorities of the countries of the European Community should: (a) adopt and implement the recommendations of the European Society of Intensive Care Medicine concerning education and training of ICU professionals; (b) develop and implement national programs for the teaching and education of ICU nurses.

Recommendation 10

Institutions should explore the potential for multiprofessional education and training. The concept of learning together to work together is particularly relevant in the context of intensive care. Increased attention should be paid to the topics of ethics, quality assurance, budgeting, rationing etc. Relationships with health care staff outside the unit and with the community at large should also be a focus of discussion.

Part II

6 Field Work

Introduction

During the preparation phase of EURICUS-I it was felt that the meaningfulness of the data collected by the different substudies could be enhanced if interpreted with respect to the daily practices and living circumstances on the participating ICUs. It was therefore decided that the aim of the site visits to the ICUs, originally planned to control and support the field research, should be enlarged to include a qualitative survey of the units. This survey focused on aspects of daily practice in the ICU and on interactions of the staff both within the unit and with their professional environment, paying particular attention to individuals' views, feelings and wishes. This qualitative survey of ICUs is described in the following section. The comments made in "Notes on Intensive Care Medicine in Europe", by the country coordinators of EURICUS-I, address the intensive care medicine systems at the national level and clarify many aspects which were highlighted during the site visits.

Site Visits

D. Reis Miranda

Introduction

During the field research of EURICUS-I (October 3, 1994 through January 31, 1995), site visits were performed by the project leader, who was often accompanied by researchers in nonmedical disciplines involved in the study. The site visits took between four and eight hours per ICU and were essentially composed of four parts:

1. Review of the questionnaire concerning organization and management in the ICU with the ICU leadership (usually the medical director and the head nurse).
2. Photographic documentation of ICU aspects (two standard photographs): (1) one ICU bed (with a nonidentifiable patient) and its surroundings (equipment); (2) the entrance giving access to "outsiders" (e.g. family) to the ICU. These photographs were, whenever possible, shot from an equal distance and made after having received permission from the unit. Other aspects found

during the site visits that were of importance to the study were also documented, in agreement with unit representatives.
3. Direct observation aimed at detecting not previously addressed characteristics of the ICUs; identifying "life aspects" at the level of the functioning ICU. The purpose of the site visit was to observe in detail the work process at the units, paying particular attention to the role of the nursing staff. The various elements of the ongoing field research were also discussed with the staff, in particular those related to collection of the study data. Other aspects such as the physical characteristics of the ICU and the availability of beds as well the estimate of the clinical severity of illness of the patients in the ICU were also observed during the site visit.
4. Interview with the ICU leadership, including questions targeting a fixed list of issues such as: (a) number, type and use of protocols; (b) regulations concerning visitors and attitude towards families of patients; (c) users of the ICU in the hospital and relations with them regarding: structured interdisciplinary decision-making, strengths, weaknesses, opportunities, threats, beliefs and wishes at the ICU level. The main goal of the interviews was however to listen to different points of view and to the description of unexpected cases and problems. This was done by means of open questions and dialogue with the ICU staff.

Quite often, the leadership of the unit had organized a short interview with the leadership of the hospital during which the study program was explained and other issues were raised. The overriding impression from the visits was that of careful organization of the project at the national level. At the ICU level, there was detailed knowledge of the program by the responsible staff and the study was accepted with sympathy and even enthusiasm by doctors and nurses. We felt that the collection of data was done according to the stated protocols in all ICUs. We saw that the Field Research Manual of EURICUS was to be found in places easily accessible to the nursing staff. In some ICUs, instructions regarding administration of the data after collection were also translated into the native language and affixed, together with the protocols, at least in the coffee room.

The collection of individual data for questionnaires of the substudy *Personnel* did not pose any particular problem at the local level. The anonymity protocol had the agreement of the ICUs. Completion of the financial questionnaires presented, however, more difficulties than originally expected: one hospital refused to provide the information; two other hospitals were prepared to provide reduced information after consent from the hospital management; one hospital questioned the confidentiality of the response. The majority of hospitals did not have a particular problem in providing data, apart from the often experienced difficulty related to retrieval.

The description of the site visits, reported in this chapter, addresses only particular aspects observed in the ICUs. The most frequent finding was that conditions which we thought were unique to our own ICU or to the ICUs in our country were also found elsewhere. In general, the report of the site visits focuses on those aspects requiring the attention and reflection of the clinicians involved with practice and decision-making in intensive care. The report is therefore obviously often biased by the individual interpretations of the observers. Above all, the report does not intend to provide a real picture of the ICUs, as the observed aspects of adequate practice of care and of good entrepreneurial functioning were often omitted from the description made.

Expectations of the Study

"*Voir si je suis bien dans le peloton*"

During the site visits one of the questions made to the leadership of the ICUs was: "What do you expect from this study?" This question explores some of the reasons which might have led to participation, and the answers might be of guidance in the analysis and reporting strategies of EURICUS-I.

There were 142 different expectations expressed. Few leaders could not indicate any particular expectation, others indicated more than one (usually two); many of the expressed expectations were coincident. Overall they could be grouped into four major categories:

- *Comparison* was a key expectation of 51 ICUs. This meant detecting unknown/unexpected differences among ICUs, "making an inventory of problems around the world", "to identify the different ways of running the ICU" and "to find our own weak points". The idea behind many of the answers was that of positioning the ICU within the total EURICUS sample (*'voir si je suis bien dans le peloton'*). Some ICUs were more interested in the comparison of their units within the country sample (Denmark, Italy and Spain), whereas others (Poland, UK and Spain) were more interested to know the position of their ICUs within the European sample.
- *Improvement of nonmedical aspects.* Many ICUs (54) agreed to participate in EURICUS-I because they wished to better understand organization and management (OM). This included: (a) ways to improve ICU effectiveness and efficiency; (b) new insights into the policies of personnel; (c) relations between physicians and nurses; (d) rules to regulate functioning of the ICUs; (e) how to define objectives; (f) how to define a new structure; (g) methods for registration and control of OM, including the collection of financial data.

Although not particularly well informed about the nonmedical aspects of OM, the leadership of the ICUs was not indifferent to the currently increasing importance attributed to it. They wished therefore to improve their knowlede of OM techniques and to see these could be helpful to them. Their commitment to using this information was, however, rather unclear ("Macro organization issues have little influence upon the results of the ICU", as one person said). In other words, EURICUS-I would provide them with comparative medical data, ready for their own use, while, at the same time, they would get "not binding information" regarding modern trends of thinking in health care.

The nurses were very interested in the nonclinical management part of the study, as they had the opportunity to express their views and be heard. Those questionnaires concerning nurses' well-being were particularly appreciated ("It is the first time that someone approaches the problem"), and high expectancies were attached to the results. The leadership of some of the ICUs felt that the questionnaires offered them the opportunity of knowing more about their nurses ("to know why do other nurses feel better than our nurses"; "what are the differences in well-being"; "when do they burn out").

- *Improvement of medical aspects* was expected by 20 ICUs. Some leaders found that the project offered material important to the evaluation and registration of patients (see the A- and B-sheets). They hoped that the value of quantifying using the scoring systems would be supported by the study and that standard methods of registration would emerge allowing objective comparison of groups of patients and the related consumption of manpower. Nine respondents expected that the study would reinforce the need for an European consensus concerning the definition and practice of intensive care medicine.
- *Strategic aspects* (17 ICUs) Sometimes the need for recognition was the basis for the expectations: "to obtain recognition of the work done in the ICU"; "to get a better understanding of the unit in the hospital"; "to have data to force the administration of the hospital to give more attention to the ICU"; "to show that the hospital has a good ICU"; "to use the results against the administration"; "to show that we can work with other disciplines". The expectations were often aimed at solving problems experienced as serious and difficult to solve at an individual level: "concentrating all the ICUs in the hospital"; "to increase the number of beds, particularly intermediate beds"; "to support the development of high-dependency units (HDUs) in the UK". There were some that were less hopeful: "There will be good and bad news" and "We know that the results of the study never will change the views of our administration".

The Nurses

Responsibilities of Nurses and Physicians

"*We are not a team; we work together*"

The traditional relationship doctor-patient dominates the medical care at the ICUs. This relation is, to a large extent, a logical consequence of the know-how and the responsibilities involved. However the content and the areas of responsibility of the nursing profession have changed enormously over the last few decades. Clinical knowledge of the nurses has increased radically, as has their responsibility concerning daily evaluation of the patients' clinical condition.

One example may help to clarify the kind of problems raised by these new developments. Of the four important ICU activities (observation, registration, comparison/judgement/decision and intervention), also called "titrated therapy", the nursing staff of the European ICUs performs three of them: observation, registration, and intervention. The task of comparison/judgement/decision, before any further intervention may be performed, belongs to the responsible physicians. Without discussing whether the latter is right, the point we would like to make is that performance of a cycle of titrated therapy, the quality of which is often time-dependent, requires at least two professionals. Consequently, appropriate integration of the responsibilities of nurses and physicians around titration therapy in the ICU becomes a matter of major concern to the nursing staff, as they often recognize the problem at the outset of a relentless process of care.

In the majority of the ICUs, the quality of the medical coverage around the clock is not homogeneous and/or sufficient. Inexperienced medical staff has detrimental consequences regarding at least the prompt and appropriate titrated therapy of patients. A delay before experienced medical help is available may cause a relevant delay in correcting diagnoses and therapy plans. The observed frequent change of medical responsibility (or the existence of more than one responsible physician) may result in conflicting professional views and/or the definition of conflicting policies. It was often reported during the site visits that more experienced nurses are tempted to follow their own clinical opinions by managing existing conflicts and choosing which issues to address to which physician.

Integration of the "new style" of nursing activities into the process of care in the ICU was not openly addressed by the various professionals involved. Over the last few years, the hospital management has reduced the dominating role of the medical professionals by creating independent medical and nursing hierarchy lines. This was the situation in the majority of the ICUs visited. While a new and beneficial culture of professional inter-(in)dependence is perhaps emerging, for now each professional group works on unilateral definition and consolidation of its own tasks and duties. The resultant climate is that of two different worlds without common and clear objectives and without a definition of interdisciplinary responsibilities ("We are not a team; we work together", one head nurse said).

In the sequence of these developments, primary nursing care was found in some ICUs: after admission each patient is allocated to one nurse, who is responsible for delineating the nursing care plan of his/her patient. The written plan is to be followed by the nursing staff during the subsequent shifts. The primary nurse will care for the same patient until discharge and is also responsible for other activities with respect to that patient, such as communication with his/her family. Primary nursing care is thus in contrast to the usual practice of allocating nursing care in each shift according to principles of equity regarding workload and stress: nurses do not frequently care for the same patients. In Finland one head nurse said: "Primary nursing is good for everyone, patients, families and nurses and for the quality of care; burnout occurs from the occurrence of problems which do not receive appropriate solution and which you are not prepared to solve".

However, particularly in ICUs of the UK, we found that primary nursing care could be associated with principles of equity regarding workload and stress: the primary nurse would hold responsibility for the plan of nursing care and all the contacts with the family of one patient without necessarily being responsible for the active care of that patient. This suggests that the practice of primary nurse in these ICUs replicates, to the nurses, the traditional doctor-patient relationship.

In some ICUs attempts were made to involve the nursing staff in the medical activities of diagnosis and treatment planning. Members of the nursing staff attend the ward rounds held formally every day in the presence of all physicians involved in the care of the patients in the ICU and often are present at ad hoc clinical discussions of individual cases. However, the role allocated to the nurses is rather passive and their participation often meets with problems of continuity and motivation.

Professional Power in the Team

"Our work is not appreciated"

In this context, the site visits also explored differences in the professional power of the nurses regarding general policy-making issues at ICU level, such as staffing, choice of equipment, admission and discharge policies. The differences found can be aggregated into three modes of professional power:

1. The ICU has two directors (directorate), the medical and the nursing director. Each director coordinates the issues directly related to his/her profession, but decisions are generally made in consensus and the two directors can replace each other in case of absence (e.g. holidays). This model of organization is more often found in northern European countries (see below).
2. The ICU has a medical director and a head nurse for the coordination of nursing affairs. All the decisions concerning non-nursing issues are made by the medical director without/after consulting with the ICU medical staff. This model of organization is more often found in southern European countries.
3. The ICU has a medical director and a head nurse. The function of the medical director is essentially that of coordinating medical care at the ICU and representing the ICU in the interface of the unit with the other medical departments and the hospital directors. The head nurse exerts extensive control over the internal organization of the ICU, including often the unit's budget. He/she usually receives the full support of the medical director. This model of organization is particularly evident in the UK, where the nursing profession has a high social status. One example of interaction at the leadership level is the effective use of the British concept of "funded beds": the occasional reduction of beds based on the available number of nurses, decided by the nursing staff and implemented by the medical director.

It is of note that an hierarchy of professional power did develop within the nursing staff whenever the nursing leadership was more defined and/or more powerful: older experienced nurses were more powerful than younger staff ("older staff don't like it that doctors transmit orders to the younger nurses; they like to be in charge"), or there were clear differences of professional power between levels of nursing staff ("doctors never ask us nursing aids how the patients are").

Social Atmosphere

"We have staff and line personnel"

During the site visits the climate between doctors and nurses was evaluated by the interviewer and rated as friendly in less than 50% of the ICUs and often experienced as tense. Doctors and nurses seldom socialize outside their work. In many ICUs physicians and nurses have separate coffee rooms. During work time social contacts may be more frequent among nurses and the younger medical staff. It was frequently reported that the nurses felt professionally less happy during the early shifts when more (and senior) medical staff were active in the unit. The nurses experience this lack of social communication as condescension from the medical staff both towards them and their contribution to the successful care of patients. However, physicians were seldom aware of this ("I talk to the nurses everyday and I don't see any problem"). Meetings of nurses and doctors are held in some ICUs for discussing common issues. A medical director reported: "Everything here is a drama: too much work; too little work. There is a meeting with all the nurses once a month. If we don't do it they don't protest, if we do it they come. They do cooperate on research projects, and afterwards they don't care about the results of the research. Nurses do think differently from doctors; they do not have a professional project or a wish to progress".

The lack of professional communication between doctors and nurses at essential moments, such as the prescription of medical orders, was an overriding complaint: "They come, they write something and they go away without talking to the nurses"; "Sometimes it is much later when we discover that therapies were changed"; "If we call them to explain things they come, if we don't they don't notice that we can have major difficulties with performing adequately their orders".

The Visiting System

One important aspect surveyed during the site visits was the approaches of the different ICUs to relationships with relatives of ICU patients. These relationships are known to be difficult to establish and to maintain in an effective and appropriate manner given the characteristics of high turnover and the severity of illness of the admitted patients. Nonetheless, the importance of these relations is not disputed because of the legitimate rights of the patients and their relatives, the valuable clinical information that might be collected, and the role that relatives take when important decisions are to be made. The severity of the clinical conditions being treated in an increasingly complex high-technology environment makes it imperative to understand whether the developments around the ICU are consistent with social principles, particularly those concerning family and the autonomy of the patients under treatment.

This survey addressed three aspects: (1) visits to patients and contact with relatives; (2) background rationale of the various systems; (3) the main entrance door of the ICU and the there-affixed rules for visitors as a formal indicator of the interaction of the ICU with patients' relatives.

Visits to Patients

Each ICU has developed a system to regulate visits by relatives of the patients. We looked at the rules regarding: (a) daily timetable of visits; (b) duration of each visit; (c) number of persons allowed at each time; and (d) discussions between relatives and responsible physicians. Issues such as age of visitors, specific ICU clothing, and hygiene recommendations were also examined.

- *Daily timetable of visits.* Table 1 depicts the various visitation timetables adopted by 86 European ICUs (for reasons of anonymity one ICU in Luxemburg is not included). The system was classified as *open* when there was no visiting time. Instead, the visits were previously agreed upon by the ICU staff or simply organized at the moment of the visitors' arrival at the hospital. The system was considered *liberal* when visits were allowed for more than 2 h/day. A *restrictive* policy regarding visits was considered when the visiting time was reduced to 2 h or less per day.

One important aspect related to visits by relatives was when daily medical information concerning the clinical condition of the patients was provided. In open systems, there are usually no fixed times: the doctors talk to the relatives when the latter are there or when they ask for additional information. In restrictive

Table 1. Visiting system in practice

	Open	Liberal >2 h	Restrictive		Forbidden
			1 h–2 h	≤1 h	
European area					
Poland	5			1	2
Germany	2			1	
Denmark	6				
Finland	5				
Holland		1	4	2	
Belgium				6	
France			4	1	
UK	7				
Italy			3	3	1
Spain		3	15	9	
Portugal			2	3	
Overall	25	4	28	26	3

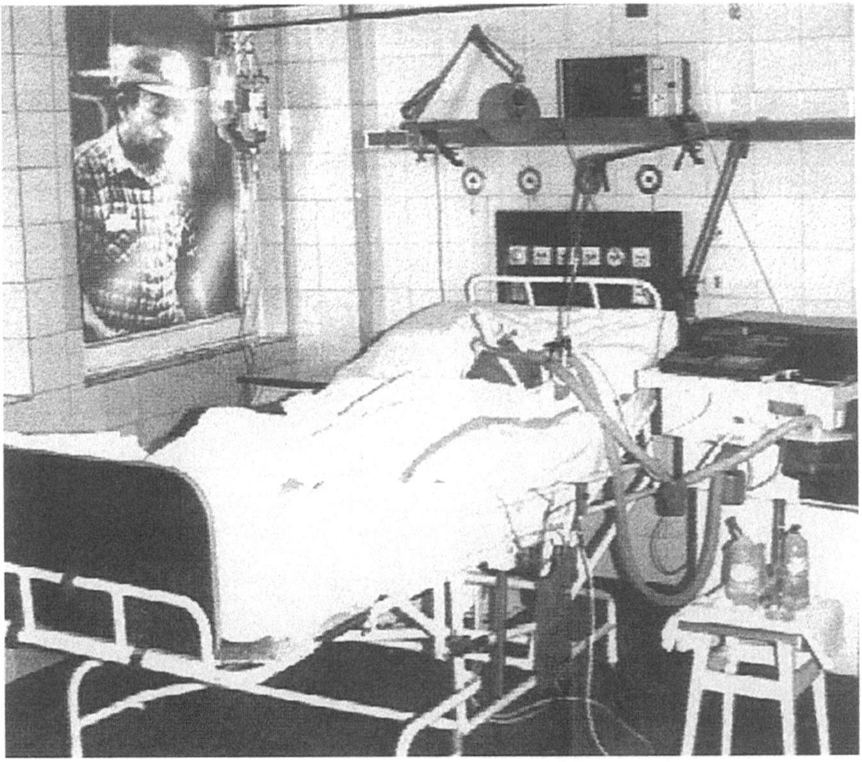

Photograph 1. In ICUs with a restrictive visiting system, window visits were often allowed

systems, there are usually one or two particular times each day when information was provided.

Generally, nurses played an important role in providing information to relatives; it was seldom the case that nurses were not allowed to give information to families.

The consistency of the information given to relatives was often experienced as a major problem, as reported by both nurses and physicians. The providers of information could be different persons, have different knowledge and insights into the clinical conditions of the patients, or express information differently. These differences were often distressing for the nursing personnel and were sometimes at the origin of more or less open interprofessional conflicts in the unit. One head nurse said: "The nurses are kinder with patients and families than doctors; the dialogues are different although they (the doctors) are sometimes even human".

The overriding complaint, particularly from the nurses, concerned the absence of a clear system to indicate which information was appropriate to provide to relatives ("our doctors never find the time to address these issues"). Several ICU leaders reported concern, but no effective system to cope with this difficulty was

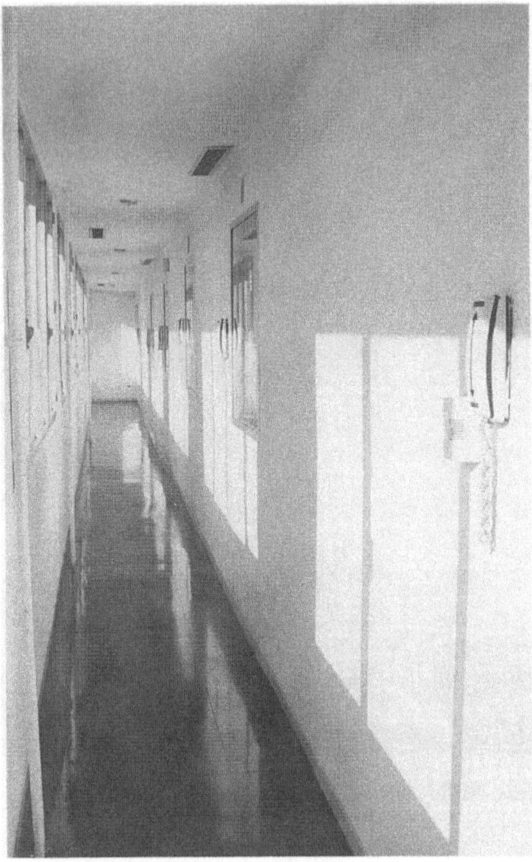

Photograph 2.
Corridor around an ICU

found during the site visits. One ICU, for example, produced a daily informative bulletin with the health state of all patients to be transmitted to relatives: better; worse; stationary; etc.

"Touching" vs Distant Visual Visits

The two Polish ICUs to which visits were not allowed had galleries ("spectatories") in an upper floor from which the family could look at the patients on particular occasions. Such a construction, though not in use as such for many years, was also found in a Portuguese ICU. In this ICU, the gallery was transformed into a large office for staff and staff meetings. In several Spanish and Italian ICUs, particularly those constructed more than 20 years ago, the same spectator principle was achieved by the existence of corridors located externally to the patient rooms. These corridors, of various sizes and forms, could involve the whole ICU area.

An overriding physical consequence of the corridors was that they subtracted a large proportion of the daylight from the patient rooms. Each patient room had one or more windows to the corridor. In general, the glass area of each window

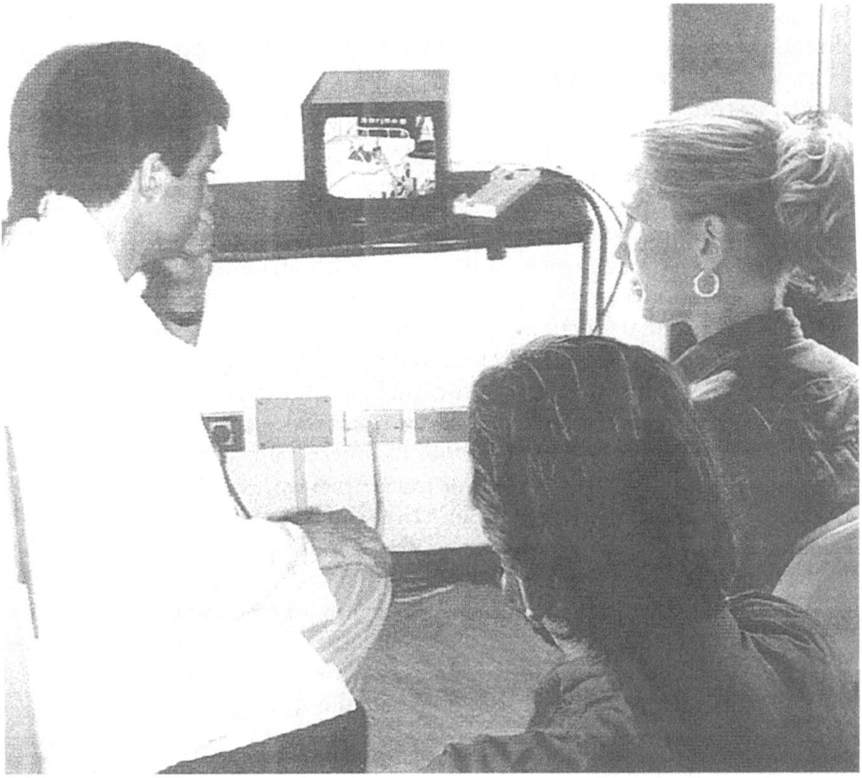

Photograph 3. An internal TV system could be used by physicians during the interview with the relatives of the monitored patient

could easily accommodate one or two visitors. Next to the window, one or two telephones could be used to talk with the patients or with the nursing staff. In some ICUs without corridors or galleries, an internal TV circuit allowed visitors to see their patients and to even talk to them from the visitors' room. On arrival in the room and after calling for authorization from the nursing staff, the TV system is activated and focused on the required patient. The possibility existed, at least in one ICU, that more than one patient could be displayed during one visiting session, depending on the number of different visitors. With short intervals, the camera would automatically focus on another patient and the cycle initiated again and again. The TV system could also be used by physicians during interviews with relatives. Corridors and galleries were used in those ICUs not allowing the physical bedside presence of more than one visitor per patient and also reduced the number of persons inside the ICU to once each day while maintaining a more liberal schedule of "corridor visits."

Particularly in the ICUs with an open visiting system much attention was dedicated to the comfort and facilities available to visitors. A dedicated family room was provided, inside or as an annex to the ICU, often simply but carefully furnished, decorated and clean. This room could, in many ICUs, accommodate with comfort the family of a particular patient during the night. For relatives from afar or needing to be of assistance for longer periods, "hotel" accommodation in the hospital was often possible. The availability of these facilities was less frequent on ICUs with a restrictive visiting system.

Visiting Rules

The visiting system was restrictive in about 50 ICUs, or 65% of all visited units (Table 1). It has to be remembered that, in each country, the EURICUS-I sample pools data from university hospitals and from nonuniversity hospitals of different sizes and regional functions. The visiting system shows a rather clear pattern both regarding countries and European regions. In the open system visits would in principle be discouraged during the night hours or early in the morning. In the other visiting systems the total visiting time was divided into two or three (exceptionally four) equal and fixed periods of time, usually at midday and during the evening. As a rule these periods of time coincided with the general visiting schedule of the respective hospital. Since the visitors' rooms, when existing, were usually rather small, before each visiting period there was an unusual and rather cumbersome concentration of people waiting to enter the ICUs. In case the visiting period was longer than 15 min, each visitor would not be allowed to stay more than 10 min, thereby giving others the chance to visit. However, this could also be regulated in other ways. Consistent across European ICUs was the number of two visitors per patient allowed each time onto the ICU.

Background to the Visiting System

Visits of relatives to hospitalized patients is an ancient practice and all hospitals have regulated this carefully. With few stated exceptions all departments submit to these regulations. The staff of some ICUs like visits by relatives of patients; the staff of the majority of those ICUs surveyed do not. Therefore, many ICUs simply follow the regulations of the house without adapting them to the specific characteristics of care in the unit.

Complaints concerning the presence of visitors in the ICU were particularly vivid on those ICUs using fixed visiting schedules. In these cases, as noted above, all patients received visits simultaneously. Some comments were: "The less visits the better"; "It is difficult for doctors and nurses to work with foreign people in the room"; "Families disturb the work because they ask too many questions"; a head nurse said: "I have to protect my nurses: they are not free to act when the visitors are there"; "We are against more and/or longer visiting periods"; "When the families come in, the work stops and the nurses go out for coffee" (this statement was frequently confirmed during the site visits). On many occasions ICU leaders would spontaneously agree with the advantages of visits but still the disadvantages weighed heavily on their opinions: "The more visits allowed, the less problems with the families and the more problems with the work".

These issues were common and were discussed at length with the ICU leaders. Sometimes the visiting system was simply influenced by architectural circumstances such as lack of space. However, defenders of the restrictive vs the open system argued often with cultural differences regarding the involved populations: "There should be only one information moment each day. The less information we provide the better because we may create more confusion and misunderstandings"; "Families can react strangely when faced with the use of ICU technology"; "This is a rural area, people don't know anything about intensive care"; "In this country everybody has the tendency to interfere with what we are doing. In northern Europe it is different".

The visiting system was often a sensitive problem to approach. People were frequently aware of the insufficiencies of their own system and of the existence of friendlier approaches to visitors. Frustration and some cynicism was therefore not always absent from the exchanged dialogues. During one interview a vivid discussion was raised between the head nurse and a psychologist giving professional assistance to the unit. Finding some support in our questions and, as she said, among the younger nurses of the unit, the psychologist defended her opinion that the visiting system should be drastically liberalized and "humanized". Should the system be changed? ICUs including this last one did collect large amounts of questionnaires among the relatives of patients and the reactions were in general very positive towards the ICU, the personnel, the treatment and the way visitors were received.

The Main Entrance Door of the ICU

The entrance door of the ICU is the place where visitors make the first contact with the unit. In this context, it therefore seemed important to survey, in a standard manner, the first impressions which each ICU conveyed to visitors upon arrival at the unit. The main entrance door was chosen as the first standard

Table 2. Main entrance appearance on site visits

	Restricted/no entrance	Other information	Clean
European area			
Poland	1	5	3
Germany	3		
Denmark	4	1	1
Finland		2	3
Holland	2	4	1
Belgium	4	2	
France	3	2	
UK	7	1	1
Italy	5	1	1
Spain	22	3	3
Portugal	1	1	3
Overall	52	22	16

interface between the ICU and its visitors. Doors were divided into "clean" and "with message". Clean were those doors at which only the identification of the department was indicated. When messages to the visitors were affixed to the door they concerned limitations to entrance or other information.

As can be seen in Table 2, the main entrance door was clean in only 16 ICUs. In more than 80% of the units visited the door was used to communicate messages to visitors. In 52 ICUs the message concerned interdiction to enter and/or information regarding visiting times. The ICU staff did feel that this way of communication was important and improved it whenever necessary. Instructions (sometimes justified: "In the interest of your relative ...") were often difficult to understand, such as "No entrance"; "Push"; "Ring", or even rather misplaced ("Warning! Access to foreign persons is forbidden including representatives of any kind").

Various information was provided at the doors of 22 ICUs concerning the ICU itself, for example, instructions to be followed after entering the ICU; the philosophical rules of IC nursing; educational material including extensive AIDS information, 50 ways to quit smoking; the daily cost of one ICU bed with and without supplement; an appeal to solidarity (blood or organ donation); safety regulations (burglars around; in case of fire keep this door closed).

Strikingly, there was no association between the visiting system of the ICU (open or restrictive) and what was found on the respective door.

The doors were often made of glass. Seven of them were fully transparent and were, in our opinion, the kindest and most appropriate interface between the ICU

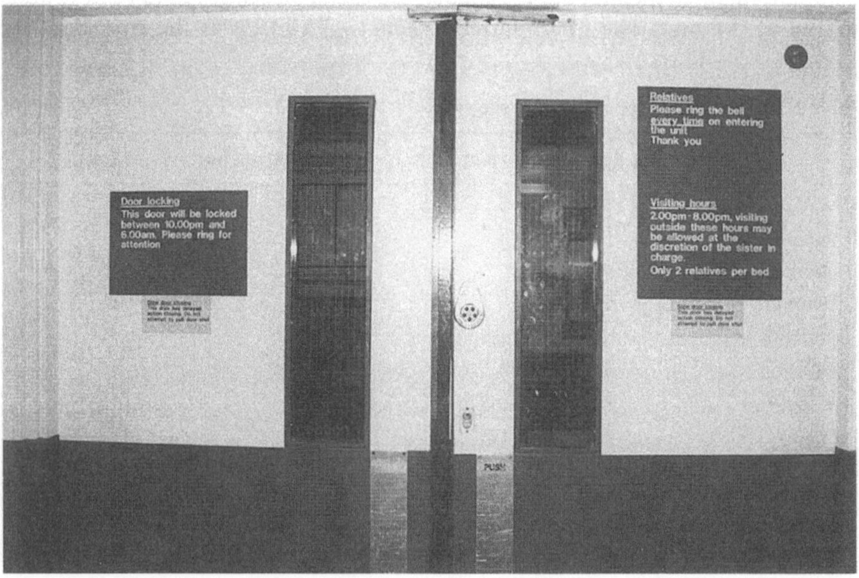

Photograph 4. The ICU main entrance door was often used to convey regulations and various other messages to visitors

and the visitors. While waiting to enter, relatives could observe ongoing professional life on the other side of the door. The existing visiting system is too often the result of the ad hoc solution of isolated problems raised either with the medical or the nursing staff (the providers of care). There is no defining of goals and policies in a system which should have the rights and needs of its users as the major target. In addition because of its specific characteristics of care, the visiting system at the ICU cannot be easily derived from the general visiting rules of the hospital. It was our impression that the open systems were the expression of an attitude towards visitors that was more elaborate than the mere liberalization of visiting times.

Comment

The great importance of visits to patients was generally appreciated and expressed by the ICUs. A deep feeling of dislike concerning the presence of and the contact with visitors was also often observed during the site visits. Notably, this feeling was more frequent and more intensely felt by the nursing staff than by the medical staff. All professional groups indicated dislike regarding precisely those aspects that would entail input of personal effort into contact with visitors. The physicians felt that visitors would misunderstand the clinical information provided and that therefore it might be better to restrain their informative efforts. The nurses felt that visitors would not understand their activities in the ICU and preferred often to reduce their activities in the ICU to the tasks of supervision of visitors and to be absent in the coffee room during the visiting periods.

Table 3. Bed occupancy during site visits

	ICUs (*n*)	Occupancy rate ± SD	ICUs with occupancy rate ≤75%	ICUs with[a] occupancy rate of 100%
European area				
Poland	8	0.6 ± 0.3	2	2
Germany	3	0.4 ± 0.4	1	–
Denmark	6	0.6 ± 0.3	1	1
Finland	5	0.6 ± 0.1	1	–
Netherlands	7	0.7 ± 0.3	4	2
Belgium	4	0.6 ± 0.3	2	–
France	4	0.9 ± 0.1	4	2
UK	8	0.4 ± 0.3	1	–
Italy	7	0.9 ± 0.1	5	3
Spain	24	0.8 ± 0.3	15	11
Portugal	5	0.8 ± 0.2	4	2
Overall	81	0.7 ± 0.3	40	23

[a] The ICUs in this colunu are included in the column >75%.

Since contact with visitors might not be expected to be a natural part of their professional duties, the ICU staff often felt the need to issue general regulations that would assure a certain distance of visitors. The chosen norms were transmitted indirectly to the visitors (such as those affixed to the ICU door).

The Intensive Care Unit as an Organization

Resources Available and Used

"We need more beds, more nurses, more money"

Besides the overall rather low occupancy rate of 70% ± 30% (SD) (Table 3) about 50% of the ICUs were, on the site visit day, functioning with more nurses than judged required based on the number of admitted patients. A shortage of nurses was observed in only 6% of the ICUs (Table 4).

Considering the observed levels of care of the admitted patients, 42% of the ICUs were estimated to have patients of level II, 40% to have level I and only 18% with patients with a very high mean severity of illness, equivalent to level III (Table 5). A shortage of nurses was the single weakness most frequently pointed out during the site visit. In all ICUs the excessive workload was an overriding complaint of the nursing staff, often supported by the medical director. It should be noted that the data correspond to a single observation at each ICU, done at different moments with respect to day and hour.

Table 4. Patient/nurse ratios on site visits

	Nurses > patients	Nurses ≈ patients	Nurses < patients
European area			
Poland	4	3	1
Germany	1	1	1
Denmark	4	2	–
Finland	2	3	–
Netherlands	3	4	–
Belgium	4	1	1
France	2	3	–
United Kingdom	6	1	–
Italy	3	3	1
Spain	10	10	1
Portugal	–	5	–
Overall	39	36	5

Table 5. Classification of level of care

	Levels of ICU care		
	III	II	I
European area			
Poland	1	3	3
Germany	2	1	–
Denmark	2	2	2
Finland	1	3	1
Netherlands	3	1	3
Belgium	–	2	4
France	1	2	2
United Kingdom	1	1	5
Italy	2	4	1
Spain	3	12	6
Portugal	–	4	1
Overall	15	35	33

Protocols

"Protocols are good for juniors"

Except for the Spanish ICUs, where protocols are generally considered an indicator of quality, the existence of protocols did not show a national pattern in the other ICUs. Many ICUs, particularly those operating under anaesthesia leadership, had no or very few protocols (3–10) and, when available, these often concerned the management of postoperative complications. Some ICUs assembled up to more than 100 protocols, some of which were their own protocols others from other departments of the hospital ("nobody can handle them all!"). There was no system to verify the conformance to the protocols in any of the units visited, and in only very few were the protocols submitted to regular revision.

In general, the protocols addressed the treatment of clinical conditions, and the majority were concerned with nursing procedures. Protocols concerning organizational aspects such as admission and/or discharge policies were found in less than 10% of the ICUs. Nobody said that protocols were of no use. The rationale behind the use of protocols, besides that of giving guidance and uniformity to medical treatment and instruction to the performance of nursing procedures, was very often that of training junior staff and/or allowing these to perform intensive care activities in the absence of the senior staff. The most voiced disadvantages of protocols concerned their difficulty and the danger of applying them strictly ("protocols are no cook-book"; "each patient is unique"), the conflict between protocols and individual experience and beliefs ("only juniors follow protocols"), and the risk of limiting clinical judgement and creating dangerous

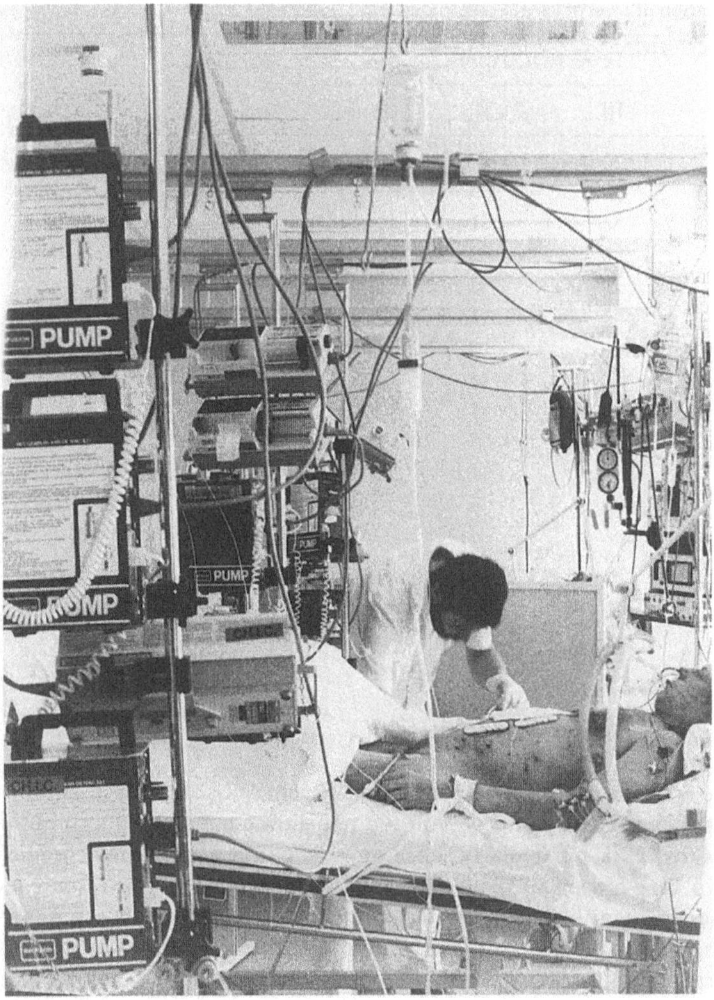

Photograph 5. Some 18% of the ICUs were treating patients at level III

automatisms. In summary, when existing, protocols address exclusively issues of clinical management. They were directly derived from the professional literature and were not prepared to provide feedback for auditing and quality control.

Strengths

During the site visits, the leaders of the ICUs were asked how they felt about the strengths and the weaknesses of their units. The professional team (87 answers) was the first strength mentioned by almost all ICUs. The high quality of teamwork (22) and the enthusiasm and confidence (9), the professionalism (6) and the flexibility (4) of its members were most frequently pointed out as at the origin of

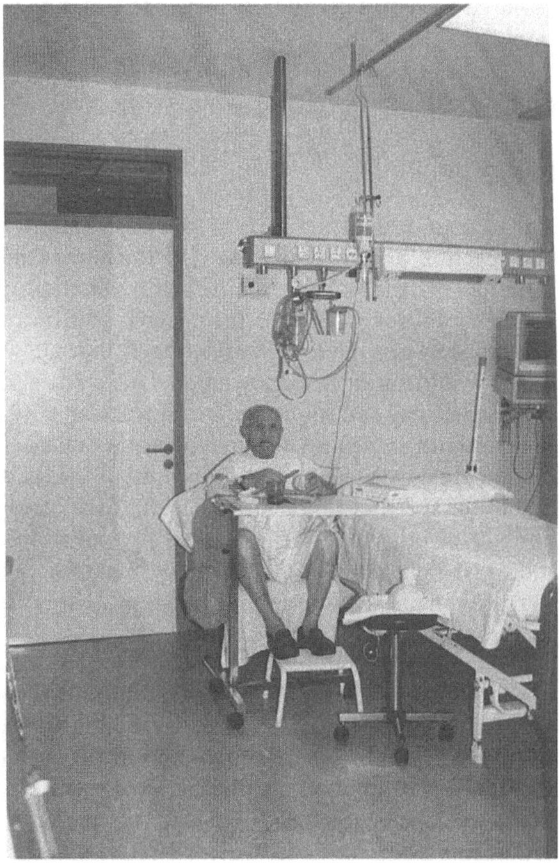

Photograph 6.
Man eating an orange

a successful team. The particular influence of a professional group such as the nursing staff (12) and the medical staff (6) was indicated on occasion. The small size of the team was felt as being beneficial (5) as well low turnover of the staff (3) and good relations with professional groups outside the ICU (8). The importance of recognition of the professional team by the hospital directors was mentioned by nine ICUs. In three units the leaders expressed proudly that their teams were the professional elite of the hospital ("we are the second of none"); though not so clearly spelt, the same message was quite often transmitted during the interviews.

The work developed (41) was the second strength pointed out by the ICUs. The quality of medical care provided (11), particularly in specific situations (8) such as trauma and myocardial infarction, was indicated. A multidisciplinary approach (8) as well as routines and the high technology used (9) were considered relevant assets to the quality of the results delivered. Four ICUs mentioned their efforts regarding good care of the families of the admitted patients.

The organization (20) was the third strength indicated by the leaders of the ICUs. Centralized leadership and/or ("army") discipline was the organization strength most frequently indicated (8). No financial problems (4), teaching and research activities (3), the specialties to which they were bound, etc., were mentioned.

An absence of any strengths was indicated by 11 ICUs. One medical director said "our strength is of not having strong points".

Weaknesses

The organization of the ICU (56) was the weakness most often pointed out. The organization in a general sense (13), the narrow focus of the staff involved with the care (14), the lack of training and research programs (10), the high turnover of nurses and/or physicians (6) the lack of protocols (4) were indicated as relevant weaknesses. Five ICUs mentioned that allowing too much work was the major weakness of the organization. One medical director said: "The chaos here never ends, day and night; we are all working very hard inside the belly of a big boat without somebody to explain us where it goes". The facilities (38) were the second most frequent weakness indicated. The inappropriateness of the building and of the space assigned to the ICU (21), the insufficient equipment (6), and the absence of other facilities (3) were also mentioned. A shortage of money was indicated eight times as the source of weakness. A shortage of staff (33), medical (20); nursing (11) and/or administrative (2), was also frequently pointed out as a major weakness of the ICU.

Concerning human factors (8): bad relations inside the team (2), bad relations with other departments (2), lack of recognition of the work performed in the unit (1), and general dissatisfaction (3) were cited. Very colorful descriptions of chronic conflicts among professionals and or between departments were frequently recounted. The admission or discharge of patients or decisions concerning therapeutic options were often at the origin of periodic explosions of the underlying arguments and emotions. One head nurse, recently appointed because of her record on nursing organization issues, said, after a detailed description of the absurd misunderstandings, she found: "I traveled 400 km upwards and 100 years backwards". Another physician said, after describing his sad experience of management as endless power games: "I stopped telling my family and friends what happens here in the hospital; they just don't understand me. Not only the illnesses in the hospital are different of those out there in the society; people also behave differently inside and outside the hospital".

Some 18 leaders could not recall one weakness of their ICUs.

First Thing to Do

The question was: If you would have the power to change things in your unit, what would be the first thing to do? To get more money! answered eight respondents. Improving the facilities (39) was the priority most often mentioned. Twenty-eight leaders would change the building of the ICU, providing more space and/or more beds; creating step-down units in the intensive care area. The urgent need for more and eventually better equipment was reported on 11 occasions. Other answers were: increase the staff (33): the number of physicians (20);

the number of nurses (12); the administrative staff (1). Some leaders (27) would improve professional aspects including: the general organization of the unit (16); teaching and research activities (8); protocols (3). An improvement of human factors was suggested by some (12), addressing the improvement of relations among professionals inside the unit (7) as well relations of the unit with other departments (5). There were also 15 leaders who were happy with their units as they were.

It seems logical from the afore mentioned that the "first things to do" are related to the weaknesses reported. It was striking that the different nature of the answers regarded the strengths and the weaknesses. "We and our work" was the predominant strength theme whereas the weak points involved mainly "others and things".

Organization Structure

Intensive care units are organizations with predominantly two types of professionals: nurses, who make up 90% of the staff, and physicians, about 10%. Technicians, secretaries and ancillary staff, though considered indispensable to a well functioning ICU, are often not present and, when they are, represent a minority of staff. The nurses and physicians have the same objectives and overlap in many areas of their tasks such as observation, monitoring and caring. Seen from a complementary point of view, these ICU jobs are horizontally specialized. However, because of issues of professional content, the performance of many tasks is dependent on tasks performed by others: the vertical specialization.

This is not only true concerning the work of nurses and physicians together but also regarding some of the work amongst nurses and amongst physicians. The ICUs have usually a simple organizational structure in which the technical structure and the support staff elements are missing (Fig. 1). The strategic apex includes people responsible for general policies in the ICU (e.g. staffing, equip-

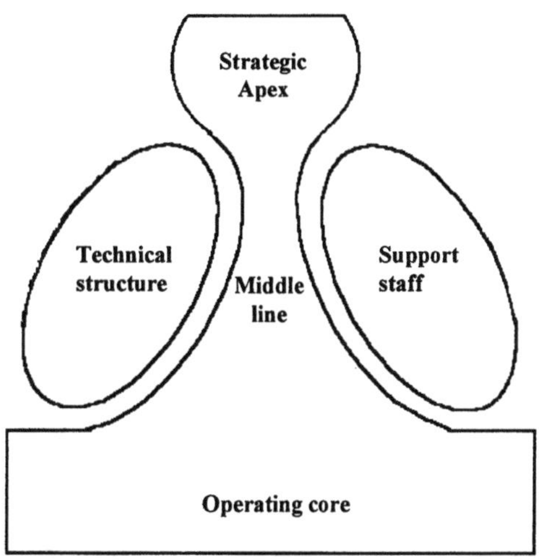

Fig. 1. Basic organisatuion structure of ICUs. [Adapted from: H. Mintzberg (1979). The structure of organisation, Prentice-Hall]

ment, finances, use of facilities). In general the key coordinating mechanisms are: standardization and skills, particularly of the operating core; a focus on horizontal and vertical specialization, much depending on training and indoctrination; little formalization and a bureaucratic behaviour; lack of regulation by the technical system and a complex environment. These are the important benchmarks of a professional bureaucracy. Elements of mutual adjustment, selective decentralization and an organic behaviour may give the character of an adhocracy to the organizational structure of the ICU. "The organizational nature of the ICU is a combination of a professional bureaucracy and an adhocracy. Opposite to other wards, ICU tasks are performed in a team context. Therefore, the overall performance responsibility is delegated to the entire team" (W. van Rossum).

During the site visits ICU leaders were asked to draw the organizational structure of the ICU (the word "organogram" was often used), identifying in particular particularly the positions and the professional interdependencies of physicians and nurses. The request was not always readily understood as many leaders were confronted for the first time with the issue. The drawn systems often represented a complex mixture of the flow of regulated activity with elements of the flow of formal authority. Of 84 ICUs from which the organizational structure was obtained five major models could be constructed.

Model I

The medical director and the head nurse of the ICU are directly dependent on the leadership of a traditional specialty department, e.g. anaesthesia or internal medicine. The strategic apex is outside the unit and the hierarchy line of the nursing staff extends up (usually) to the medical director of this department (Fig. 2).

It may be said that this model represents the traditional approach to the organization and management of departments in the hospital. The impact of the medical profession on hospital care, recognized at the beginning of this century, brought expanded the influence of physicians to all areas of decision-making in the hospital.

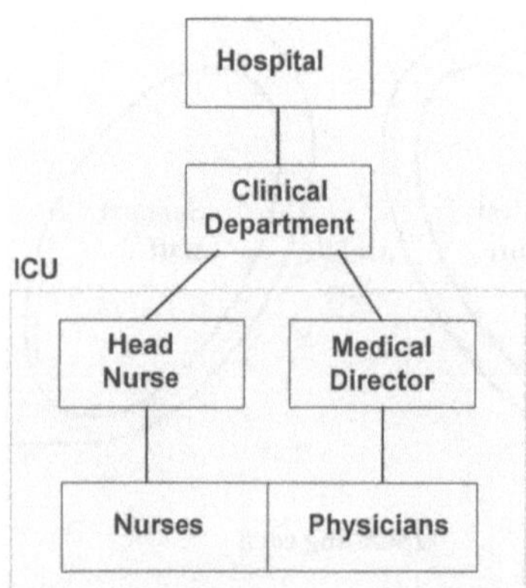

Fig. 2. Organizational structure: Model I

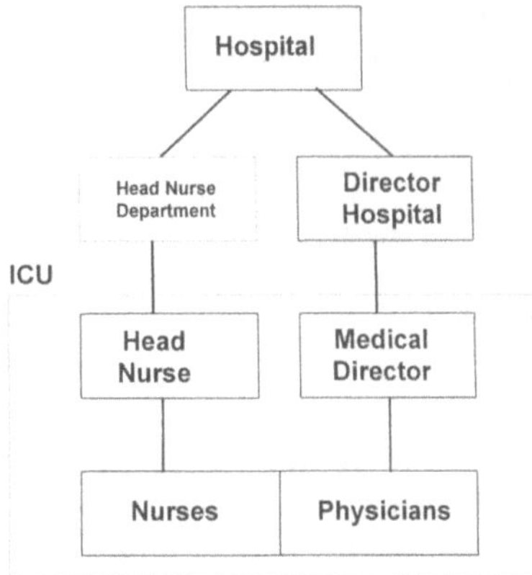

Fig. 3. Organizational structure: Model II

Model II

The strategic apex lies outside the unit. The hierarchy lines of the two professions (nurses and physicians) are separated. If there is no head nurse at the level of the traditional specialty department (Fig. 3, dotted box), then the highest point in the nursing hierarchy may lie outside (above) the department.

This model, clearly derived from the previous one, represents recognition of the impact and importance of the nursing profession on modern hospital care. The direct dependence of the nursing staff on the hospital director seemed necessary in order to reorganize the nursing profession inside the hospital (some would prefer to speak of the emancipation of the nursing profession).

Model III

The strategic apex is inside the unit. The head nurse and the medical director of the ICU share information, leadership and decision-making. Consignment of the various leadership tasks is often based on professional grounds (nurses and physicians). It is however possible, in case one of the leaders is absent (holidays, etc),

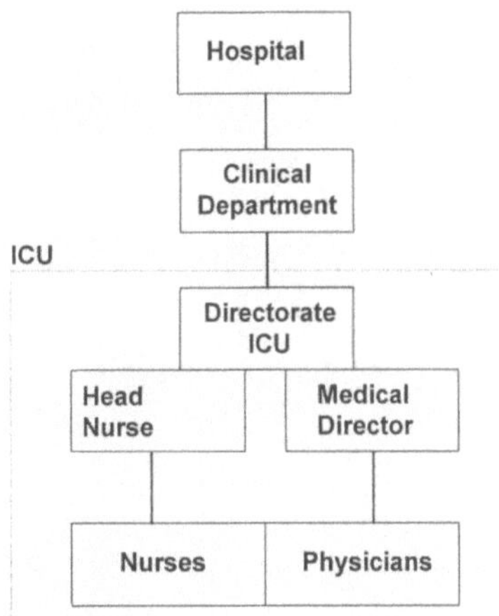

Fig. 4. Organizational structure: Model III

that the other leader is fully responsible for the leadership of the unit. This is particularly the case when the joint leadership is formalized into a directorate (Fig. 4).

Following the logical sequence of the two previous models, this model represents the recognized need to effectively integrate the tasks of nurses and physicians in the ICU.

Model IV

The ICU is governed by a kind of department directorate (medical management and nursing management) placed outside the unit. The middle management level either does not exist or is performed by a pool of professionals on a rotation basis. According to the involved ICUs, the advantage of this configuration is the almost nonexistent intermediate communication steps between the leadership and the operating core. This model, only found in two ICUs, represents probably local views and/or organization and management circumstances (Fig. 5).

Model V

The medical staff work on a private practice basis and is therefore not employed by the hospital. The important decision-making organ is the ICU Committee, consisting of physicians delegated by the medical staff and the head nurse and the medical coordinator of the ICU. The latter is nominated by (is a staff member of) one of the traditional specialties after agreement of the committee (Fig. 6).

This function is often fulfilled on a rotation basis. The ICU nursing staff hierarchy stems directly from the hospital director, that of the ICU medical staff from the committee of the medical staff of the hospital. This model is the consequence of the general organization of the medical staff in some hospitals in the Benelux. The distribution of the various models among the ICUs of 11 European areas is shown in Table 6.

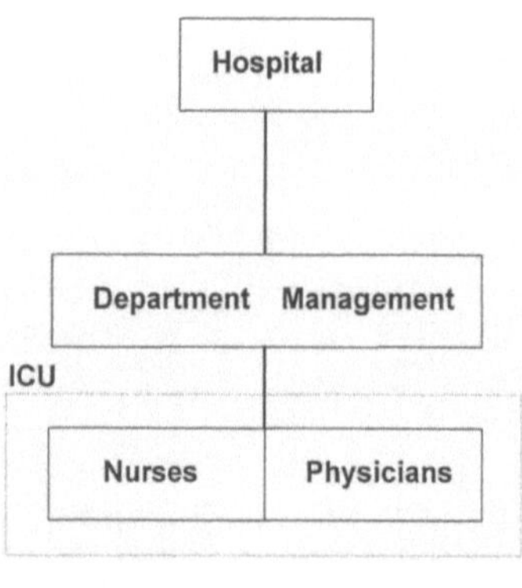

Fig. 5. Organizational structure: Model IV

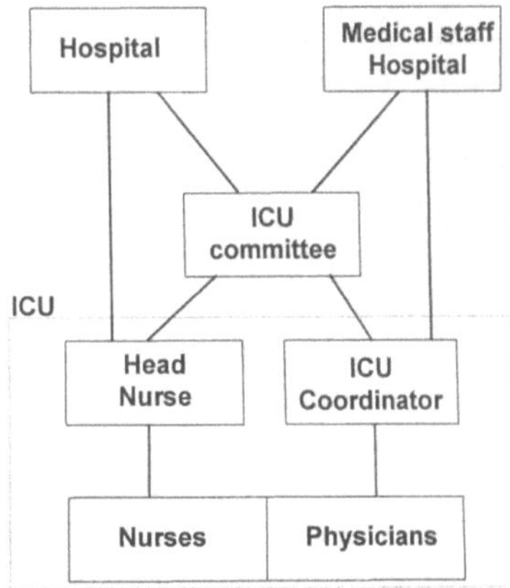

Fig. 6. Organizational structure: Model V

Table 6. Models of ICU organization found on site visits

	Model					
	I	II	III	IV	V	Overall
European area						
Poland	8	–	–	–	–	8
Germany	1	2	–	–	–	3
Denmark	1	–	5	–	–	6
Finland	2	3	–	–	–	5
Holland	–	I	–	1	5	7
Belgium	–	3	–	–	3	6
France	1	1	2	1	–	5
UK	–	2	4	–	–	6
Italy	5	2	–	–	–	7
Spain	4	23	–	–	–	27
Portugal	1	3	1	–	–	5
Overall	22	40	12	2	8	84

Conclusions

It remains to be seen whether the various organizational models can be associated with: (a) the different performance levels of the ICUs when controlling for case mix; (b) output variables of personnel management. If the interpretations formulated above are correct, only 12 ICUs (14%) may be close to an adequate integration of nursing's and physicians' jobs in the ICU. The good news is that 47% have already started the process of reorganizing the nursing staff. The bad news is that 27% of the ICUs in the sample are still attached to a rather archaic organizational model.

Although the professional activities of the staff of the ICUs, both physicians and nurses, are similar across Europe, the attributes of their profession are poorly defined and/or accepted in the hospital. It was also found that there was insufficient communication among the staff of the various ICUs. The ICU staff operated in a professionally limited fashion *vis a vis* the other hospital. A consequence of this was that professional insecurity was identified in a large number of the ICUs.

The level of skill discretion of ICU nurses is insufficiently developed to cope effectively, efficiently and speedily with the multidisciplinary activities involved with the acute care of patients. The nurses' participation in decision-making is poor, despite the fact that they represent 90% of the ICU staff and possess crucial information about the patients. Communication between nurses and doctors is inadequate since nurses are only committed to their specific nursing tasks and activities and lack an overall view of the care of the critically ill.

A limited interaction of the ICUs with the families and visitors of the patients exists in many ICUs across Europe. A "self-protecting" attitude, both of the nursing and the medical staff, rather than workload and high turnover of patients, is at the origin of the intentionally imposed limitations on the visiting system to the ICUs. As a general rule, the ICU announces the imposed limitations in a non-personal manner (doors, leaflets, etc.). This condition is often the cause of inappropriate information conveyed to the families of patients, and sometimes is the source of conflicts between nurses and physicians.

The overall occupancy rate in this study of the ICUs was low and usually dependent on the flow of patients from the operating theatre. Several ICUs were empty and would not receive patients on the day of the site visit. A shortage of nurses to assist the patients on the ICU was rarely found. When existing, the protocols in place were rarely used as instruments for quality control. In the organizational structure of the ICUs, the strategic apex of the units was most frequently located outside the ICU and therefore run by medical professionals not necessarily involved with the professional activities of the units.

In some ICUs, the structured integration of the nurses' and physicians' professional activities deserves the attention of the ICU leadership. On the majority of ICUs, however, this essential process seems to still be far away from reality.

Notes on Intensive Care Medicine Systems in Europe

The country coordinators of EURICUS-I were asked to describe intensive care medicine (ICM) in their countries. No guidelines were provided except that their contribution should include a discussion of those aspects of ICM which would be relevant to the other participants in the study, and that it should not be longer than 1200 words.

Intensive Care Medicine in Poland

M. Sych, J. Pokorski and C. Noworol

The idea of organizing special hospital units for critically ill patients dates back to the late 1950s. The proposal to create ICUs, formulated by Professor Marek Sych, was accepted by the Congress of the Polish Society of Anaesthesiologists in 1960, in Poznán. This can be regarded as the beginning of intensive care medicine in Poland.

It should be noted that pioneer experiments on intensive care techniques and resuscitation were done on animals by Jan Prus, professor of Lwów University, in the years 1899–1900. Direct cardiac massage and artificial ventilation of the lungs of dogs suffering from asphyxia, electric shock or chloroform overdose were performed. Prus demonstrated the efficacy of these procedures in restoring all central nervous system functions.

The first ICUs in Poland were organizationally bound to the anaesthesiology departments and were established in all county hospitals and all other hospitals having at least 1000 beds. They were named "Departments of Anaesthesiology and Intensive Medical Care" and headed by the anaesthesiologists. As the rule the units were organized as general ones (mono-block type) providing a service for all of the hospital wards. The idea of intensive treatment was to combine the knowledge and skills of the referring specialists with those of ICU anaesthesiologists.

The ICUs of university teaching hospitals have more freedom in shaping their functional organization, but usually follow the rules mentioned above. Exceptions are the clinics of the Collegium Medicum at the Jagiellonian University: As they are scattered all over the city, the clinics were forced to develop their own ICUs, which then belonged to the Chair of Anaesthesiology and Intensive Therapy, Collegium Medicum at The Jagiellonian University. Thus, these ICUs are smaller in size and fit the specialty of the ward.

The ICUs in Poland have round the clock medical coverage. In the morning shift the anaesthesiologist is always present. The difference occurs on the late or night shifts. In smaller hospitals <200 beds) the physician of the given specialty is present but may consult the anaesthesiologists regarding more severe cases. In larger hospitals the anaesthesiologists are present on the ICU 24 h a day.

Intensive care medicine does not exist in Poland as a separate specialty. Traditionally it is taught within the specialization of Anaesthesiology and Intensive Therapy. There are very few certified anaesthetic nurses in Poland, i.e. those which have graduated from a 3-year study program. The nursing personnel recruits mostly registered nurses who have completed a 1–3 months training course. The shorter courses include reanimation and intensive therapy while the longer courses include anaesthesiology, catastrophe medicine and treatment of pain.

Supervision of intensive care medicine in Poland is provided by the National Board of Anaesthesiology and Intensive Therapy, headed by Professor Andrzej Nestorowicz from the Lublin Medical Academy, and by the Polish Society of Anaesthesiology and Intensive Therapy, presided over by Professor Andrzej

Kübler from the Wroclaw Medical Academy. The Polish Society of Anaesthesiologists was organized in 1959 and soon joined the World Federation of Societies of Anaesthesiologists. The present name of the society is The Polish Society of Anaesthesiology and Intensive Therapy. Its organ is the quarterly "Anaesthesiology and Intensive Therapy".

Intensive Care Medicine in Germany

W. Kuckelt

For more than 40 years (1953), ICM has been a well established concept in the German medical system, especially in anaesthesiology. However, the first ward for intensive care of postoperative surgical patients was established in the 1930s in Tübingen.

ICM is performed in ICUs as part of different medical disciplines (internal medicine, surgery, neurology) or practiced in interdisciplinary units under the supervision of anaesthesiology.

According to the *Deutsche Krankengesellschaft* [1] in 1992 in all of Germany 2447 hospitals, with a total number of beds of 685976 beds were registered. In the so-called Old Federal States (OFS) of the Federal Republic of Germany 4.0% of all hospital beds were registered as ICU beds and 3.8% in the New Federal States (NFS). At present 21.7% of ICU beds in the OFS are dedicated to anaesthesiology, 31.7% to internal medicine and 30.4% to surgery, with 16.2% dedicated to other disciplines. In the NFS 27.9% of ICU beds are dedicated to anaesthesiology, 22.7% to internal medicine and 26.6% to surgery, with 22.8% dedicated to other disciplines (*Institut für Medizinische Statistik*, Frankfurt am Main, March 1995).

In hospitals with more than 500 beds 91% of the ICUs are headed by anaesthesiologists and in hospitals with 250–500 beds 35% of the ICUs are interdisciplinary [2].

Recently, ICM was introduced by the Germany Society of Anaesthesiology and Intensive Care Medicine as a subspeciality of anaesthesiology. After the initial registration in anaesthesiology, an additional 2 year training course in accredited interdisciplinary ICUs throughout Germany is implemented. Written guidelines are the basis of the training program which passed the Council of the Germany Society of Anaesthesiology and Intensive Care Medicine recently. Similar programs were approved by other medical societies. After finishing the training courses in anaesthesia and ICM and passing the German board examination, one can be registered and licenced as an anaesthesiologist qualified in special ICM in anaesthesiology.

At present about 6500 anaesthesiologists, internal medicine physicians and surgeons act as ICU medical directors, but only approximately 2500 of them can be considered ICM specialists.

Specialized ICU nursing has been available since the mid-1960s. Most ICU nurses are initially trained in anaesthesia and recovery room work. In the mid-1960s the East German government authorized ICU training for nurses as a nationwide integrated part of training in the field of anaesthesiology. Guidelines and standards for training were recommended to program directors.

Today in Germany, as in some other European countries, a division in the ICU establishment exists between physicians and nurses. Although there has been well organized professional development at the nursing level, equivalent medical progress lagged behind. Similar to the situation in The Netherlands, with the exception of university hospitals and major leading hospitals, the medical director of the ICU generally spends only a small amount of time in the ICU during the week. Instead, the medical director often is on duty as an anaesthesiologist or surgeon in the operating room or as an internal medicine doctor in a diagnostic department or out-patient clinic. Traditionally the pay in the ICU is lower than in other wards, therefore the turnover of physicians is higher. ICUs are very expensive, primarily resource consuming departments and therefore not well looked upon by the budgeting organizations, insurance companies, and the officials of other health care-related institutions. Only a few ICUs have an independent status as a Department of Intensive Care Medicine in the corresponding hospital.

The 1995 budget, for example, for the Clinic of Operative and General Intensive Care Medicine at the Central Hospital Links der Weser in Bremen was about 16287000 DM. The workload in 1995, expressed in Therapeutic Intervention Scoring System (TISS) points was 345793 TISS points (1 TISS point = 47.10 DM). During 1995, 3352 patients were admitted; 9442 patient-days were registered. Some 29.5% of the admitted patients (987 of 3352) were identified as long-term patients (mean stay 4.9 days). These patients occupied 51.8% of the patient-days (4890 of 9442) and accounted for 65.1% of the TISS points (224940 of 345793). These patients incurred 65.35% of the total costs (10.6 million DM out of 16.3 million DM).

In this setting, ICU patients consume a large proportion of hospital budgets. As a result, today more than ever, fiscal pressure on the health care system threatens ICM in an extreme manner. As we move into the 21st century, many factors will shape ICM. The aging population, new diagnostic technologies, innovative therapeutic measures, and peoples expectations may increase ICM utilization, while the need to be efficient and contain costs may increase health care rationing.

How can ICM deal with these conflicting demands? There is a nationwide need for development and introduction of standardized instruments which aid in identifying all available treatment alternatives and possible outcomes, weighing the benefits against the risks and costs. In the broadest context, logistical, ethical, economic and legal considerations should also be factored in before deciding who should be treated under what circumstances. For German society, the German government, and the German insurance companies, there has been no clear-cut correlation between the factors mentioned above and the costs of ICM up to now. Since these problems are well known in to ICM doctors, ICU nurses and everyone else involved with ICM, it was not difficult to recruit ICUs into the EURICUS-I study in Germany.

We expect from the results of the study evidence-based arguments and solid ideas to improve the status of ICM as an important clinical discipline. This may also promote a better understanding of ICM problems by politicians and health care policy makers. Ultimately we hope to improve patient care and better combine the needs with the actual possibilities.

Intensive Care Medicine in Denmark

J. Strøm

Intensive care is represented in Denmark (population 5.5 million) in 54 hospitals as multidisciplinary units. There are a total of 481 multidisciplinary ICU beds (figures taken from an inquiry done by Antonsen, Bonde and Thiessen on behalf of the Working Group for Intensive Care of the Danish Society of Anaesthesiologists, published in 1995). If an ICU bed is defined as including both respiratory support and a standardized level of monitoring then the total number of ICU beds is 358 (Table 7). Single discipline units exist at type 3 hospitals within neurosurgery and thoracic surgery wards (40 beds) and as neonatal beds (30 beds).

Table 7 shows that ICU beds at type 3 hospitals are full ICU beds whereas an increasingly higher number of ICU beds are used for postoperative recovery/coronary care in nonuniversity hospitals. The table also shows that we have one hospital bed per 290 inhabitants, but only one ICU bed per 15500 inhabitants.

Hospitals in Denmark are the responsibility of county authorities, and the number of inhabitants per ICU bed varies from 9600 to 25000 between counties. The mean number of patients admitted per bed per year, the mean occupancy rate and mean length of stay in 1994 according to hospital size are given in Table 8.

Multidisciplinary ICUs are managed by anaesthesiologists. Some 90% of type 3 and 44% of type 2 hospitals have a full-time ICU directors; otherwise ICUs are managed on a rotation basis by senior anaesthesiologists. Duty hours in type 3 hospitals are mostly staffed with specialists, whereas more junior doctors are involved in type 2 and type 1 hospitals. The working week is 37 h and doctors normally follow a two-shift schedule. No ICU has a staff of physicians of its own. This means that up to five different anaesthesiologists (attached to intensive care or to anaesthesia) may be responsible for an ICU over a weekend from Friday afternoon until Monday morning.

Table 7. Multidisciplinary ICU beds according to hospital size

	Number	Beds	ICU[a] beds	ICU[b] beds	ICU[b] beds (%)
Type 1	26	4286	170	89	2.08
Type 2	18	6587	188	137	2.08
Type 3	10	8279	130	130	1.57
Overall	54	19152	485	356	1.90

Type 1, local hospitals; type 2, regional hospitals; type 3, university hospitals
[a] Total number of ICU beds.
[b] ICU beds with respiratory assistance and a standardized level of monitoring.

Table 8. Admissions, rates of occupancy and length of stay

	Admissions/bed/year	Occupancy rate (%)	Length of stay (days)
Type 1	153	81	2.2
Type 2	122	74	2.2
Type 3	94	85	3.7

Type 1, local hospitals; type 2, regional hospitals; type 3, university hospitals.

There is no formal education in intensive care in Denmark. Intensive care is included in the anaesthesiology training program, and the length and content of intensive care training may vary from one education centre to another.

The majority of ICU beds in Denmark are technical beds, which means that the patient still is registered in a ward of the primary specialty and that the primary specialty holds the final responsibility. This kind of arrangement demands a high degree of cooperation between the ICU and the primary specialty (Fig. 7). The higher the integration is developed the better the services provided to patients. The main area of dispute normally concerns admission policies and seldom therapeutic issues. ICU beds are for critically ill patients and not for hopelessly ill patients whether critically ill or not.

The number of nurses per ICU bed and the patients/nurse ratios according to hospital type are given in Table 9. The numbers given in the table are based on the budget; however, we have always had a shortage of nurses in Denmark and the actual figures are less than those stated. The number of nurses educated per year has been claimed to be too low for several years. An arrangement in which employees may take leave for up to 1 year to take care of children or for educational purposes while still being paid a very reasonable salary by the government has further added to the problem. The idea was to get the unemployed to work; how-

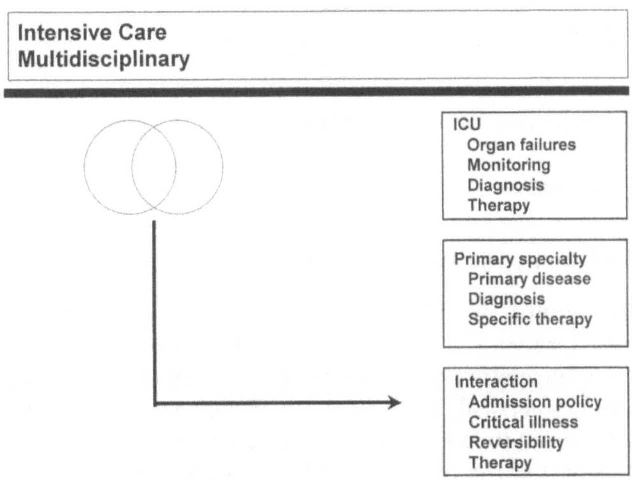

Fig. 7. Interaction between ICU and primary specialty

Table 9. Nursing staff according to hospital size and budgets

	Nurses/ ICU bed	P/N Day	Evening	Night	Education ICU course
Type 1	2.4	0.61	0.34	0.33	47%
Type 2	3.0	0.69	0.36	0.34	69%
Type 3	4.9	1.08	0.80	0.77	45%

Type 1, local hospitals; type 2, regional hospitals; type 3, university hospitals.

ever, there has never been an unemployment problem for nurses in Denmark. Since the arrangement started in 1994, several wards, especially in internal medicine, have been reduced or even closed for short periods, and the majority of type 3 ICUs has been forced to reduce the number of active ICU beds on the order 20%–33%. There is no specific education in intensive care for ICU nurses in Denmark, but the majority of counties offer a 4-week in-service course.

In general, hospital budgets have been reduced by about 2% each year over the last 10 years, and so have ICU budgets. The margin of expenditure for new equipment or to replacement old equipment has likewise been cut back. This development has resulted in a marked increase in productivity, and it has been stated that no bigger private company has increased its productivity to the same degree in this period. However, budgetary constraint has a limit at which productivity no longer increases but instead quality is reduced, and equipment does get worn out.

In this situation we urgently need a method to measure quality of ICU outcome and it is our hope that EURICUS will provide us with a valid tool in this respect. It has been an inspiration for us to take part in the EURICUS project, and consensus has now been obtained among ICUs in Denmark to start a national Danish database in late 1996 (DANICUS, of course) based on the EURICUS framework.

Intensive Care Medicine in Finland

M. Niskanen

The Intensive Care Unit at Kuopio University Hospital

The Finnish part of the EURICUS-I project was conducted from Kuopio University Hospital. The department of intensive care serves as a tertiary referral centre for a population of 870 000 people in Eastern Finland and simultaneously as a primary referral centre for about 250 000 people. Eastern Finland is internationally known for a high frequency of cardiovascular diseases and the population of this part of the country is widely scattered. Our ICU in Kuopio is a multidisciplinary unit with 23 beds and eight full-time physicians (three intensivists, three residents, and two research doctors). Approximately 50% of patients are admitted for postoperative care after open heart surgery. Other major causes of admission are acute respiratory failure of various etiology and postoperative neurosurgical patients. Our ICU is also a nationwide centre for treatment of severe ARDS and major burns. A unique feature of our unit is the computerized patients' data management system, which is used for clinical, administrative and research purposes. Contrary to what might be expected, this system really does make the work of physicians and nurses easier. Scientifically our ICU is known as the Critical Research Program and is led by Professor Takala. The major research topics include various aspects of multiple organ failure, especially septic shock, the splanchnic circulation and vasoactive drugs. This active research work is reflected in the clinical practice, making our ICU a leading centre in the treatment of severe ARDS and major burns. These patients are referred to us from all over the country. Extracorporeal oxygenation techniques are available; transfer of these patients poses extra demands on the ambulance facilities.

The four central hospitals, secondary referral centres, which are participating in EURICUS I are also situated in mid-eastern Finland (Joensuu, Jyväskylä, Mikkeli and Savonlinna). They cooperate closely with the ICU of Kuopio University Hospital. The directors of these ICUs have been educated in Kuopio and there are continuous clinical and scientific collaborations between Kuopio and these ICUs.

Finnish Intensive Care Study

The largest nationwide study characterising Finnish intensive care was carried out in 1986–1987 during a 14 month period. This study comprised a total of 14951 ICU admissions, which was 75% of all intensive care admissions in Finland at that time. A total of 25 medical, surgical and mixed ICUs were involved, 13 being in university hospitals. The mean age of the patients was 56.3 years. The ICU and hospital mortality rates were 9.7% and 18.8%, respectively. The 5-year survival of ICU patients in different diagnostic subgroups and a comparison to the survival of the age- and sex-matched general population is currently in press. This study allowed comparison between the observed and expected mortality rates. It also provided information about the intensity of treatment compared to the severity of illness in different units, thus enabling improved patient selection for intensive care in Finland.

The mean length of stay nationwide was 3.3 days (medium 1.8 days; range 0–154 days). There were considerable variations between ICUs in the lengths of stay: the mean lengths of stay varied between 2.5 and 6.1 days. A total of 8.8% of all patients stayed in the ICU more than 1 week. These patients consumed 46% of all patient-days.

Another interesting approach was to analyze factors predicting prolonged (lasting >7 days) intensive care, and on the basis of the results, it was possible to describe a typical patient who consumes most ICU resources in Finland: Thispatient is is treated intensively (receives a high TISS score) in the beginning of the

ICU stay in an ICU of a central hospital, and the typical reason for the intensive care is respiratory failure, pancreatitis, or multiple/burn trauma.

National ICU Policy

The mean availability of ICU beds is 0.6 beds/10000 inhabitants. These beds of 35 adult ICUs are located in tertiary and secondary referral centres, making up a total of 1.6% of all beds in these hospitals. In general, the directors of the ICUs are anaesthesiologists. In central hospitals, it is customary for one physician to have responsibility for the whole multidisciplinary ICU, consisting of eight beds on the average. Various specialists work as permanent consultants. The anaesthesiologists on duty are responsible for ICU patients at night and on weekends. At the moment, approximately ten ICUs are participating in a national quality control program which produces, for instance, standardized mortality ratios for the ICUs. In the near future, this service is likely to expand. In addition, the Finnish Society of Intensive Care is starting a national project, the aim of which is to standardize the data collection in ICUs for economical, administrative and clinical purposes.

Intensive Care Medicine in The Netherlands

P. Hulstaert

Intensive care medicine is a well recognized phenomenon in the Dutch medical society. Recently ICM has become a subspecialty. After initial registration in anaesthesiology, internal medicine or surgery an additional 1 year training course in accredited ICUs throughout The Netherlands is implemented. After finishing the ICU training course and passing the Dutch board examination as well as the European Society for Intensive Care Medicine examination one can be registered as intensive care physician.

There is only one ICM board and over the past 2 years it has defined standards to recognize already working physicians as intensivists. From a total of 560 registered anaesthesiologists, internal physicians and surgeons who covered ICM in the past, 400 were considered as ICM physicians. ICU nurses have been recognized for many years. In the mid-1980s, the Dutch government authorized ICU training and education for nurses.

Thus in the past few years there has been a tendency to divert the ICU establishment, separating physicians and nurses. There was well established professional development for nursing without a strong and stable medical structure. Apart from medical management of ICU structure in university hospitals and the major leading hospitals throughout the country, the medical director of the ICU spends little time in the ICU. He/she is expected to spend most of the time working in the operating theatre, polyclinics or on the ward. In part this is due to the fact that ICM is not recognized by budgeting organizations, the Dutch government or the insurance companies. Therefore ICM is poorly compensated, especially in those hospitals where physicians work as consultants and are not on the payroll of the hospital. In other words, physicians working in the intensive care department have to earn their money somewhere else.

There is a general expectation that with recognition of the ICM subspeciality the professional development of management may have its start. Although the Dutch standard of ICM is high, there is no, or at least a not well defined, ICU medical management structure. This is due to the fact that, in the view of management, the ICUs, especially those in smaller hospitals, are relatively small. In the majority of hospitals the ICUs are combined with either coronary care units, polyclinic departments, recovery rooms or major hospital departments to form larger management structures.

Through the work of Miranda it is generally accepted that there are three levels of care. The Dutch government however recognizes only one level of care. There are at least 1500 ICU beds throughout the country; only 600 are fully equipped, level III beds, according to Miranda. According to Dutch government standards all ICU facilities are considered as being the same. From this it may be concluded that the case mix among the ICUs will differ tremendously; however, this may give way to false interpretations and wrong conclusions. The major hospitals, with facilities for cardiac surgery, neurosurgery and advanced trauma care, cannot do without high care or step-down units. Because of their inevitably high number of ICU level III beds, they are not allowed to initiate additional level I or II beds. The above results in highly equipped beds, a fully staffed unit and a mismatch in patients case mix due to the presence of relatively healthy patients with only a need for monitoring and an additional nurse. These patients occupy beds for patients in need of level III intensive care. This is considered a relevant and cost-consuming ICM issue.

While one could object to such a mismatch by wondering about the amount of money that is involved, politicians do not recognize this as a problem because no one knows the exact costs of ICM. Miranda and Rutten calculated the daily costs per ICU patients in several different ICUs throughout The Netherlands and found that the daily costs per patient in university hospitals exceeds $ 1800. Any physician fees, special therapy such as haemodialysis or surgical procedures are excluded in this price. As a result of the lack of budgeting tools concerning ICU beds insurance companies have refused to pay for intensive care facilities, paying instead the normal ward bed price, i.e. $600. Thus the average loss per level III bed per patient per day is $1200. In my hospital, with 42 fully equipped ICU beds, there is a daily loss of $ 50 000. The hospital cannot bear that enormous deficit and thus claim an increased overhead for a normal ward bed, thereby disguising the problem. For the Dutch government as well as for the insurance companies there is no clear-cut correlation between wrong case mix and the loss of ICU money. This is a problem well recognized by ICU physicians, ICU nurseing/management staff members and the ICM society. Therefore there was no difficulty in finding cooperative ICUs in other hospitals to initiate the EURICUS-I study in The Netherlands.

The contributing ICUs consider the EURICUS-I study as a basis, not only for gaining insight into current standards of budgeting, management development, input and output with respect to ICM but also for comparing those aspects in each country and between participating countries. Moreover it is a start for further studies of each individual aspect of the intensive care environment with the goal of enhancing the level of management, increasing professionalism and improving the outcome of ICM. Furthermore it is important to provide insight to politicians and health care policy makers into the effective and efficient use of ICM facilities in accordance with the recognition of the level of care. This includes attaining the appropriate case mix per level of care and increasing cooperation between intensive care departments throughout the country and across the border.

The EURICUS-I project and further studies should lead, in the long run, to a full-grown entity of ICM throughout Europe.

Intensive Care Medicine in Belgium

J.-P. Alexander

In Belgium, 1996 was a crucial year for intensive care medicine, as long expected regulations were converted into laws and published one by one. Criteria for accreditation of medical specialists in anaesthesiology, internal medicine, surgery or pediatrics to the corresponding professional title in intensive care was published in October 1995. Accreditation can be obtained after 2 years of full-time training in intensive care, up to 1 year can be done during basic specialty training. A minimum of 3 months to a maximum of 6 months training in emergency medicine and an oral presentation or publication on a intensive care subject is also mandatory. In order to keep the professional title in intensive care, one has to be mainly active in an ICU at least 6 half-days a week. A physician must also prove continuing training, and submit his/her medical activities to the evaluation of experts. Criteria for the accreditation of registered nurses to the attendant professional title in intensive care and emergency care were published in August 1996. Accreditation can be obtained after 450 h theoretical training and 450 h practice in an accredited intensive care and emergency department. Here also, in order to maintain her/his professional title, a nurse has to work in an ICU or emergency department and has to attend a continuing education program at least 2 days/year.

Definitive accreditation criteria for the ICUs, describing architectural, functional and organizational elements, are expected in December 1996.

The first attempts to regulate intensive care medicine started in 1966. Architectural, functional and organizational criteria were published but never brought into practice, mainly for fear of the financial consequences. A second attempt was made in 1986. Accreditation of intensive care beds was linked to the accreditation of "heavy" medical equipment (e.g. CT scan) and medical units (e.g. neurosurgery, cardiac surgery). The new accreditation criteria will almost certainly include the following elements:

- The ICU is a medical department with a clear architectural unity.
- The unit consists of at least six beds, with visual control to all beds, isolation facilities, enough equipment and logistic space.
- The medical staff and doctors on duty have to be specifically trained and in sufficient number in accordance to the activities of the unit.
- The nursing staff also has to be specifically trained, at least 50%–66% of them. The patient/nurse ratio is still a matter of debate.

Up to now, the exact number of units, beds, nurses and doctors involved in intensive care in Belgium is not known.

In 1994, the Flemish Association of Intensive Care Nurses conducted a survey among the Flemish hospitals of Belgium [3], in which 147 ICUs from 114 hospitals could be followed. Of the 147 units, 114 (78%) returned their questionnaires, consequently giving a fairly good picture of the intensive care landscape in the Flanders.

When extrapolating the obtained numbers to all of the Flemish hospitals, we can roughly state that 114 hospitals with all together 29 600 beds amount to 1280 intensive care beds. This is 4.3% of all acute beds for ±6 million inhabitants. Figure 8 shows that the size of the intensive care units varies between 1 and 28 beds, being mostly between 6 and 10 beds. Most units are mixed, i.e. medical and surgical:

- Medical/surgical ICU and coronary care: 48.3%
- Medical/surgical ICU: 19.6%
- Surgical ICU: 11.6%
- Medical ICU: 6.3%
- Medical ICU and coronary care: 5.4%
- Coronary care: 4.5%
- Neonatal ICU: 2.7%
- Pediatric ICU: 0.8%
- Surgical ICU and coronary care: 0.8%

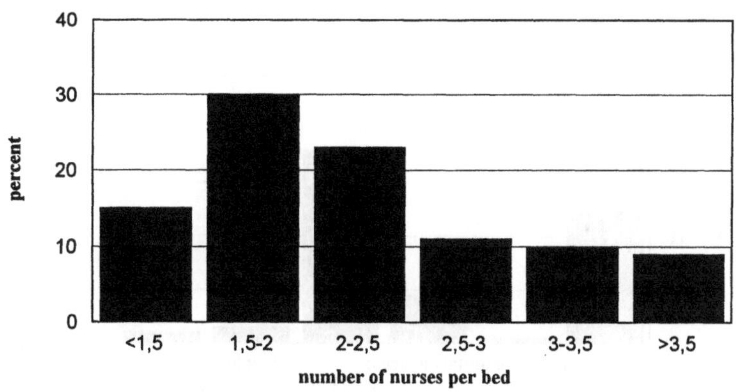

Fig. 8. Number of beds per ICU

The nurse per bed ratio varies widely (Fig. 9).

The director of the ICU is more often trained in one of the subspecialties of internal medicine or in anaesthesiology (Fig. 10).

ICUs being big spenders, it is consequently not surprising that the financial system is under discussion. Until now the payments to an ICU consist of reimbursements by the national health insurance of patient-days and medical procedures, e.g. ventilation, invasive monitoring. This system includes the inherent risk of unnecessarily long stays and medical overreacting. Even then, the income is far below the costs necessary to correctly run an ICU, so every unit is by account bankrupt.

A possible new financial system could consist of "financial packages" calculated on the basis of structural and procedural elements, while taking into account the size of the hospital. Many questions remain to be answered: Will the package be sufficient to meet the needs and allow for some autonomy? Will the system be fully objective? Will there be resources for new (and more expensive) techniques? Intensive care medicine in Belgium is on the move. Hopefully the era of uncertainty, uncontrolled growth and financial ambiguity will come to an end. It is time now to focus on quality and cost-effectiveness.

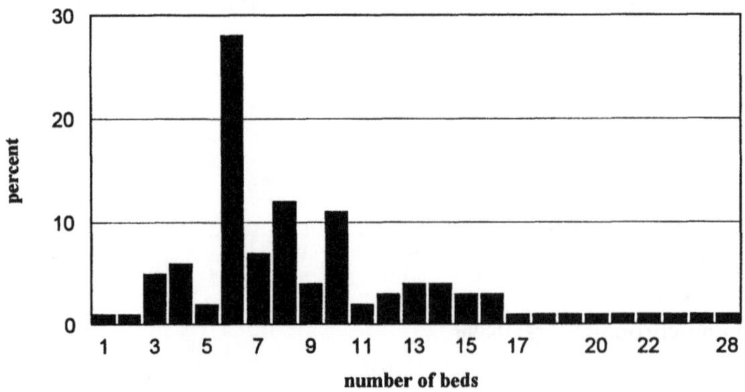

Fig. 9. Nurse per bed ratio

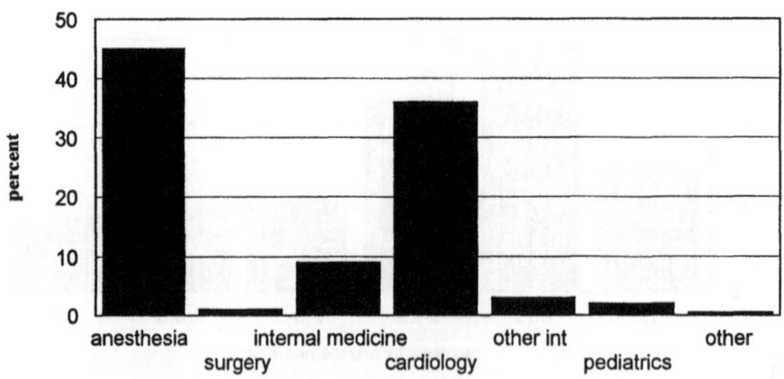

Fig. 10. Basic training of the medical director

Intensive Care Medicine in France (With Special Attention to Medical ICUs)

B. Guidet

The ICU network in France is heterogeneous and based on hospital size, type (teaching or not teaching) and location. Large teaching hospitals usually have two types of ICUs: medical and surgical, while in smaller hospitals, there is usually no specific medical ICU (MICU). This separation between surgical and medical ICU has a historical background. Soon after Denmark in 1954, the first MICUs were created in France. These units were mainly devoted to the treatment of patients with severe infectious diseases, e.g. the Claude Bernard hospital in Paris. Then, in less than 10 years, these units spread out all over France. Nowadays, MICUs coexist with anaesthesiology departments in charge of operating rooms, recovery rooms, and surgical ICUs. There are also specialized units annexed to cardiology, respiratory medicine or nephrology wards. This separation between medical and surgical units is specific to France and explains many apparent redundancies such as:

- Two different national university councils representing two different specialties: medical intensive care/anaesthesiology and surgical intensive care
- Two different scientific societies: Societé de Réanimation de Langue Française (SRLF)/Societé Française d'Anesthésie Réanimation (SFAR)
- Two different journals: Réanimation et Urgences/Annales Française d'Anesthésie et Réanimation.
- Two different trade unions

Table 10. Structure of ICUs in France

	Regional hospital	Local hospital	Both
Medical ICU	32%	6%	16%
Medical + surgical ICU	18%	81%	58%
Surgical ICU	20%	7%	12%
Pediatric ICU	23%	5%	11%
Other ICU	8%	1%	4%
Mean number of ICU beds	13.9	8.5	10.5
Mean number of intermediate care beds	4.4	1.3	2.4
Mean number of patients/year	455	344	3.5
Mean full-time physicians	4.1	3.2	3.6
Mean part-time physicians	1.6	0.9	1.2
On site physician during the night	96%	67%	78%
Haemodialysis equipment	66%	48%	54%

As a medical intensivist, I will now focus upon the structure of MICUs and on the training and scientific activity of physicians working in these units in France. A survey was performed by the Syndicat national des médecins réanimateurs des hôpitaux publics, in 1991–1992, on 184 ICUs. As seen in Table 11, the information is clearly different according to the size of the ICU. Medical intensive care physicians originate from different basic training programs (anaesthesiology, cardiology, respiratory medicine, pediatrics, internal medicine, nephrology, microbiology). These physicians undergo specific complementary training in ICM with at least 2 years of ICU experience (fellowship) and eight courses of 20 h. This theoretical training is organized by MICU university professors and validated by an examination and a written report.

The SRLF was founded in 1971 and includes French-speaking intensive care physicians. SRLF has several activities: A 3 day congress that takes place in Paris every January attracts more than 1100 physicians, 1200 nurses and 300 therapists. This meeting has scientific and educational aims with lectures, a 500 page book and over 300 original scientific papers. Emergency medicine is also substantially represented. The scientific quality is attested to by the fact that 40% of the communications have been published, half of them in international journals. A spring meeting held every year in a different city outside Paris provides an update on a specific subject, for example, in Montreux (Switzerland) in 1994 the subject was cardiopulmonary interactions.

Consensus conferences were introduced in France by SRLF as early as 1987. Fifteen conferences have been already organized plus three in collaboration with the European Society of Intensive Care Medicine. A new collection of ICU books was launched by the SRLF last year, four books have already been published: pulmonary artery catheterization; artificial ventilation; acute circulatory insufficiency, neurology. The editors of these books are internationally recognized French-speaking intensive care physicians. A total of over 12 books are scheduled and translation into Spanish, Germany, and English will be available.

Table 11. Size of ICUs in France

	Number of beds			
	1–7	8–11	12–20	>20
Nurses/bed				
Regional hospital	2.7	1.8	1.8	2
Local hospital	1.7	1.6	1.8	1.2
Mean length of stay (days)				
Regional hospital	6	9	8	10
Local hospital	5	7	9	7
Mechanically ventilated patients (%)				
Regional hospital	42	63	65	70
Local hospital	39	51	51	51

Evaluation of patients was introduced in the early 1980s with the use of SAPS-I. Activity is generally estimated with the Omega score. Most MICUs use severity and work load indexes. A computerized national data base has existed since 1993. In the Paris area, all the MICUs use the same software and the same data collection tools. An annual report allows comparison of the 22 units of this region.

Some years ago, ICM was considered very costly and this prompted us to create specific scores to justify our activities. Nowadays, other medical activities have been developed (oncology, haematology, CABG) which are much more expensive than intensive care. We should not be ashamed of the money we spend for our patients since we can justify our work, unlike other units in the hospital. Evaluation is time-consuming and costly in itself and can have important consequences in terms of budget and accreditation. Therefore the methodology must be correct and the aims clearly identified. In that respect, the EURICUS-I study with its global approach of ICU organization and management is essential.

Diseases have changed. Nowadays we are dealing with more immunocompromised (AIDS, chemotherapy, organ transplant), older patients sometimes with multiple organ dysfunctions and nosocomial infections. The new challenge is to treat more efficiently the right patients at the lowest cost. This amplifies the necessity of an ethical think tank involving not only physicians working in ICUs but also lawyers, economists, philosophers and religious representatives. Such a group should be able to rely on information gathered on a scale such provided by the EURICUS-I population.

Intensive Care Medicine in Luxembourg

M. Hemmer

Doctors

1. There is no scientific society for ICM.
2. There is no ICM subspecialty.
3. All anaesthesiologists (42) who work in Luxembourg are somehow involved in intensive care and emergency medicine and bear the title Anesthésiste-Réanimateur.
4. The Cercle des Anesthésistes-Réanimateurs is the part of the medical syndicate of Luxembourg representing the interests of intensive care medicine and is a dialogue partner for the Ministry of Health.
5. A limited number of internists and cardiologists run small units of intensive surveillance where no mechanical ventilation is available. They have no formal training in ICM.
6. Two internists have formal training in intensive care medicine (French certificate) and run a medical ICU in a central hospital.
7. Five pediatricians run a neonatal ICU in central hospital.– they are part-time pediatricians and part-time neonatologists – and are competent in neonatal intensive care.

8. Three neurosurgeons (without formal training in intensive medicine) run a Réanimation Neurochirurgicale unit in a central hospital.

Intensive Care Units

1. The number of ICU beds is strictly regulated by the Ministry of Health. There are no official standards for either equipment or medical and paramedical personnel.
2. There are 17 ICUs in 11 hospitals: 13 ICUs where mechanical ventilation can be performed; four surveillance units (cardiology, medicine, neurosurgery) without the possibility of mechanical ventilation.
   There are a total of 116 ICU beds; of these 83 are "real ICU" beds, i.e. in ICUs that are completely equipped, including mechanical ventilation devices.
3. Eleven of the ICUs are run by anaesthesiologists; one medical ICU is run by internists; one neonatal ICU is run by pediatricians/neonatologists. There are also two medico-cardiologic units; these are surveillance units without mechanical ventilation and are run by internists/neurosurgeons. A neurosurgical surveillance ICU (no mechanical ventilation) is run by neurosurgeons and a coronary ICU (no mechanical ventilation) is run by cardiologists.

Emergency Medicine

All regional hospitals have a SAMU (medicalized emergency units) run by anaesthesiologists. There are three ICUs with around the clock care: one is located centrally (five hospitals), one is in the north and one in the south.

Conclusions

While there are a good number of ICU beds, there are too many hospitals and too many small units. A centralization would be more efficient in a small country of 380 000 inhabitants. There is good equipment in all ICUs, but insufficient medical and paramedical coverage in smaller units, and no standards concerning personnel and equipment. Excellent SAMU coverage (Table 12).

Intensive Care Medicine in the United Kingdom

D. Ryan

The failure to establish the necessary administration staff and a data collection system or to provide a sophisticated national database means that costs, usage, outcome and demand depend very much on individual initiatives and interest. The result is in an inability to know what the real situation is, outside your own locality. Faced with almost daily crises and the absence of information urgent strategic planning is required. Some things are clear. There is an uneven distribu-

Table 12. ICUs in Luxembourg

ICU	Medical (number of beds)	Surgical	Medicosurgical (number of beds)	Medicocardiologic without MV (number of beds)	Coronary care (number of beds)	Neonatol (number of beds)	Neurosurgical without MV (number of beds)
Hospital C Centre	Internists (6)	Anaesthesio-logists (12)			Cardiologists (7)	Pediatricians (6)	Neurosurgeons (6)
Hospital R Centre		Medical staff	Anaesthesiologists (9)	Internists/ cardiologists (5)			
Hospital R Centre		Medical staff	Anaesthesiologists (8)				
Hospital R Centre		Medical staff	Anaesthesiologists (7)				
Hospital R Centre		Medical staff	Anaesthesiologists (6)				
Hospital R South		Medical staff	Anaesthesiologists (12)	Internists/ cardiologists (7)			
Hospital R South		Medical staff	Anaesthesiologists (6)				
Hospital R South		Medical staff	Anaesthesiologists (5)				
Hospital R South		Medical staff	Anaesthesiologists (4)				
Hospital R North		Medical staff	Anaesthesiologists (14)				
Hospital R North		Medical staff	Anaesthesiologists (3)				

C, central hospital; R, regional hospital (bigger); G, general hospital (smaller); MV, mechanical ventilation.

Table13. Intensive care costs per person

Country	Health care (% GDP)	Health care (£/per capita)	Intensive care (£/per capita)	Intensive care as percent of health care
USA	12.4	1443	144	10
France	8.9	1050	53[a]	5[a]
UK	6.1	582	6	1

GDP, Gross domestic product, market prices 1990 [9]
[a] Estimated

tion of ICU beds throughout the UK, between 1.8 and 3 per 100 000 population. There is a different demand according to clinical specialties be it neuroscience, renal support or burns, which leads to a separate admission criteria and refusal policy for each unit. There is a range of mortality in the different units in the UK within the same case mix group. Starved of resources compared to other health systems (Table 13), most hospitals have had to apply a system of rationing. Finally inter-ICU hospitals transfer is common to meet surges of demand. A recent report [5]on the provision of intensive care in England highlighted other problems. In the units studied only 48 (28%) had a full-time director, 117 (69%) had a nominated consultant but four (2%) had no one at all. Some 72% of ICUs had less than ten funded sessions a week and 32% had fewer than one session consultant/bed.

In sharp contrast is the finding that there was a median of 5.2 nurses/bed per day and over 80% of all senior nursing staff working in an ICU had post-registration qualification pertaining to ICU work. The discrepancy between nursing and medical availability is a worrying anomaly. The conclusion must be that in the majority of cases clinical decision-making and innovation has to be nursing led. This is not how doctors perceive their role but the shortfall in medical coverage appears to be compensated for by high nursing levels. The failure to provide adequate resources to provide medical cover is a historical one but this is clearly an unacceptable situation for everyone. It therefore remains unclear whether the shortfall in resources, be it physical bed space or medical input, leads to units "freezing" beds, or failing to screen inappropriate admissions or place a limitation on total patient throughput. It is likely all three occur. There is a difference between the smaller hospital and the specialist referral centre.

Large centres rarely have a shortfall of demand and are under-bedded. Small hospitals probably cope well within existing resources for short-term management problems. The different pattern of work between these two hospital types needs recognition in any solution, and the preliminary results from EURICUS-I already highlight this.

There are only 15% of hospitals equipped with both high-dependency units (HDUs) and ICU beds provision in England. The HDU offers a "form of patient management, intermediate between conventional ward care and intensive care. HDU involves patients at risk of developing organ or system failure, and includes short term resuscitative measures or physiological support lasting less than 24 hours" [4]. In other words step-up and step-down care between the acute ward and the ICU. Currently only selected medical groups receive this opportunity; e.g. thoracic, liver cases, whereas the demand is more far reaching. The availability of HDUs to all patient types makes sense as it takes the load off the already stretched acute ward, frees up some bed space in the ICU and provides better care for more sick patients and at lower cost. It should lead to better practice. Cases in which a clear decision on whether a patient will deteriorate or not are not infrequent, and the HDU provides a safe place to watch and wait. A proportion of elective major surgical cases could also be processed via the HDU rather than the ICU. There is also a mortality after ICU discharge, somewhere between 6% and 16% in the UK APACHE 2 study. In some cases this is a predictable event but in others the HDU may arguably have an impact on survival in this particular group. To really be successful the ICU nursing and medical team should control care in the HDU, which leads us back to the medical shortfall in sessions.

Hub and Spoke Solutions

The consequences of these findings require a defined plan to meet the current shortfall and permit a way forward for the future. Small units (< 4 beds) with less than 200 admissions/year should be aligned with larger centres. All would gain by such an arrangement. There would be an interchange of ideas, an easier referral pattern, initiatives on training and educational development, mutual support and a uniformity of approach. The transfer of critically ill patients should become the responsibility of regional teams so smaller units would not be in the predicament of having to release their limited medical cover for hours at a time, as well as proving a tried and tested service. It is no longer acceptable for ill patients to arrive without skilled medical and nursing staff in attendance but just be sent in with paramedics regardless of condition.

There is a temptation to be seduced by the power of technology and believe this is the answer. In fact much of the value of technology has not been tested, and over 30% is probably inappropriate. A more critical appraisal of working practice based on proven therapy will lead to more realistic perception of clinical achievement. The public and profession need to be more open and honest about what is reasonable to achieve and what is not. The resources are limited therefore they need to be used to the best effect. No one wants to prolong a hopeless situation but the mechanics of how to withdraw or stop treatment without an abrupt end or appearing callous has not really been provided for in terms of hospital resources, and remains a problem to be addressed. The ICU doctor needs to be a good communicator, a computer expert, a sound clinician, a good people person. The need to have well trained clinicians leading the ICU is a pressing need. The opportunity for later professional development is equally important. Recruitment of doctors into specialist training is an urgent priority.

Conclusion

I began by stating there are not enough beds in the UK, in fact the problem is much more complex. We are no longer a fledgling speciality, nor can we command the interest of government unless we have a concerted plan to improve on the current situation. Each region providing integrated groups, providing coherent care, and speaking the same medical language to each other and to central authority will achieve a powerful focus for change. The other fact of life that is always with us is that knowledge is the key to solve our predicament. It is here that EURICUS-I will stand us in good stead.

Intensive Care Medicine in Italy

G. Iapichino

The formation in 1987 of the ESICM working group on the management of intensive care resulted in the growing interest of Italian intensivists in organizational issues such as identification of patient characteristics, severity of illness, analysis of personnel and equipment and the quality of medical care.

At the end of 1987 the first group of 14 metropolitan north Italian ICUs was ready to start a collaborative epidemiologic study on nursing workload. This study (1988) enrolled 2710 patients and resulted in the first picture of ICM in Italy. Other studies promptly followed. In 1991 the European and North American Multicenter Study enrolled 20 ICUs of a countrywide metropolitan area. At the same time, the proposal to analyze the quality of Italian ICUs from a point of view of structure, procedures and patient's outcome was accepted with enthusiasm. There were 114 ICUs, spread across the country, that participated in this study, which enrolled 5111 patients (GIVITI) during a 2 month period in 1992. This is the largest ICU sample ever assembled in Italy and represents the best description available of ICM in Italy. Some 75% of these patients received at least one intensive therapy option (mechanical ventilation, Swan-Ganz catheter, catecholamines, or haemofiltration), of which mechanical ventilation was the most common; 48% of the patients received two or more therapeutic options during their stay. Although the mean length of stay of patients in the Italian ICUs is not larger than in other European countries, the severity of illness and the corresponding mortality rate are higher [6].

Three consecutive studies (GIRTI I, GIRTI II and GIVITI) gave some insight into the appropriateness of care and the allocation of resources to ICUs. Some 30% of patients were admitted for "intensive observation", and specific intensive care therapeutic options were not used in about 25% of the ICU days. However, and probably related to the samples studied, the clinical indications for admission to the ICU and the pathology involved was rather different in the three surveys. In a study done in 301 multipurpose ICUs, it appeared that 75% of the units had between five and nine beds and that 24% of the units had less than one ventilator per bed. In 37% of the units, the patients/nurse ratio was larger than 2.5 (GIVITI 1993). This means that 95 ICUs had insufficient equipment, and that 146 of the 301 ICUs had insufficient nurses to allow a high level of care.

Step-down units for assisting patients discharged from the ICUs were not reported. One of the conclusions of these studies was that the availability of intermediate units would allow the observation of a higher number of patients requiring intensive care (usually insufficiently surveyed on the general wards), reducing therefore the rate of complications and mortality in the ICUs. This would facilitate earlier discharge from the ICUs and therefore facilitate their efficient use. Administrative official data made available in 1991 reports:

1. Italy has 1130 hospitals providing, overall, 6.7 beds/1000 inhabitants.
2. The mean availability of ICU beds is 0.9 beds/10000 inhabitants, ranging among the different regions from 0.4 to 1.6 beds per 10000 inhabitants.
3. The overall allocation of hospital beds to intensive care is 1.7%; however this number is reduced to 0.7% when excluding intensive care beds allocated to neonatal and coronary care units.
4. The mean occupancy rate of Italian ICUs is 70%.

In an ad hoc survey of 1093 hospitals, Martinelli [7] found that only 37% had intensive care facilities: one third of these were CCUs, one third were multidisciplinary ICUs, and the remainder were specialized ICUs. Very recently, the Italian authorities recommended national implementation of levels of care to the ICUs, taking into account regional needs.

These studies did not approach organization and management issues. However, the rules of the Public Health Administration in Italy are changing, creating a new situation that requires more professional management of ICUs and a deeper cultural comprehension and knowledge of the factors influencing their efficiency and effectiveness. EURICUS-I became therefore mandatory.

The area selected for EURICUS-I is the Milan metropolitan area. This area is one of the best organized of the country (1.2 ICU beds/10000 inhabitants). The hospitals involved in the study are: one tertiary university hospital and five other hospitals along the peripheral ring around the city. All the selected ICUs are multidisciplinary, have interactive transfer of patients and hopefully offer an adequate distribution regarding levels of care.

Intensive Care Medicine in Spain

R. Abizanda i Campos

In 1988 we celebrated in Spain 25 years since the first ICU was opened. Intensive care medicine in Spain is well known. Nevertheless, some special characteristics exist that make our specialty rather distinct and referred to as "the Spanish model for intensive care units". One feature is the medical professionals. In Spain, the first ICUs were under the responsibility of physicians coming from other medical specialities, mainly internal medicine and anaesthesia. In 1973 the National

Health Service created the possibility of independent training in ICM: after qualifying in medicine and passing a national examination, applicants were eligible for specialization in ICM, involving extensive hospital training. The qualified physician then would search for an appointment at any hospital suiting his/her personal interests. This professional option, quite different from the possibilities offered to physicians in other European countries, led to Spain offering specific training in ICM beginning in 1973. At that time, no diploma was obtained after training, and even when diplomas in ICM were issued they were not recognized. Finally, in 1978 ICM was officially recognized, and a specific teaching program for the speciality was approved. The duration of the program was fixed to be 5 years: the first 2 years must be spent in an internal medicine department followed by 3 years in an ICU, acquiring experience and being taught ICM. If some very particular activity related to critical care is not performed in a given hospital (e.g. postcardiac surgery), the trainee must spend certain preestablished periods of time in other centres, where these aspects of training can be fulfilled. The result of these two periods of time (1973–1978, 1978 until today) is that it is possible to find in the ICUs two different kinds of specialists in Spain: those with recognized traditional specializations (anaesthesia, internal medicine, cardiology, etc.) other than ICM; those who have the ICM diploma. Since 1986, the number of new trainees entering the teaching program is about 80–90/year.

Another peculiarity of the Spanish model is that ICUs, or, better said, intensive care departments, are conceived as central attending services, hierarchically independent from any other hospital department. This central concept of ICUs results in the majority of Spanish hospitals having ICUs which are multidisciplinary medical/surgical units with an enclosed coronary care unit. Only in large teaching referral hospitals, do some specialities have their own ICUs (e.g. neurosurgery, cardiology, respiratory medicine).

Spain is the only Western European country where ICM is a primary speciality and yet, as in the majority of other countries, the training program does not differ in principle from other training schemes available: basic training in a major speciality (internal medicine for Spain) and specific training for at least 3 years in critical care. However, it is the feature of exclusive commitment that is a major benchmark of the Spanish model. In Spain, ICUs are run and ruled by specialists in intensive care. They are fully committed to critical care and their medical activities do not include any other attendance responsibilities, only the one devoted to medical activities in the ICUs, no matter the professional level or title. Therefore, this exclusive dedication, 365 days/year, 24 h/day, to critically ill patients represents one of the most important characteristics of our activities.

Most Spanish intensivists (more than 1400 now) are affiliated with the officially recognized Spanish Society of Intensive Care Medicine and Coronary Care (SEMIUC), in which working groups (e.g., infections, cardiology, respiratory failure, patients classification and quality control) are very active. The referred differences between Spain and other European countries make Spanish intensivists very sensitive to those projects that allow comparison of results of our ICUs with those from other countries. This is particularly the case in the context of the new autonomic development of the country, by which administrative and sanitary responsibilities are transferred to local governments, with resultant differences between different parts of the country. Probably, these differences are greater in some parts of the nation, as in Catalonia, that will participate in EURICUS on a national basis, including six to seven hospitals in the study. Catalonian coordination will be held by Dr. A. Artigas, from Sabadell (Barcelona). The rest of Spain (whose national coordinator is Dr. R. Abizanda, from Castelló) will contribute with a larger number of hospitals than any other participating country (more than 20 hospitals have claimed the possibility of contributing to data collection). Problems to be handled are: from the Spanish point of view the regional representativeness of the 20 hospitals from at least six autonomic areas; and from the more general point of view, skewing resulting from the Spanish contribution.

Considering the European Community as a gathering of regions, the integration of the Spanish sample will not pose serious difficulties. The same is true when looking at the pure dependence of nonclinical managerial variables on the clinical variables. There will always be the possibility of, whenever necessary, reducing the Spanish sample to an equivalent and predetermined group of ICUs from a given region, as is the case with all other participating countries.

EURICUS is a very ambitious project that can give some light on not yet solved problems related to the outcome of critical care patients. It will hopefully provide information regarding nonclinical management aspects and as yet unexplored activities in the ICU, and the possibility of influencing them. At a time when the autonomic development of our country is evolving, and when there is no job perspective because of the high number every year of new specialists, information on the organization and management of ICU facilities is essential and could not be more opportune.

Intensive Care Medicine in Portugal

M. J. Brandão

The first ICUs appeared in Portugal in the beginning of the 1960s. As in other European countries their establishment and activity were especially due to the entrepreneurial efforts of a few individuals in the health care field. This was particularly the case in the three principal Portuguese cities near the Atlantic coast where, in this century, economical and cultural developments have been centralized. These socio-political characteristics have definitely influenced the history of Portuguese intensive medicine.

Three different phases in the development of intensive care may be considered during this 36 years history. In the first phase, at the beginning of the 1960s, polyclinic ICUs were created in Oporto, Coimbra and later Lisbon. The original units were the training centres of a great number of Portuguese intensivists; the polyclinic ICUs from the Hospital Universitário de Coimbra (ICU established in 1960) and from the Hospital Geral de Santo António (ICU established in 1962) should be given special mention here. These ICUs acquired very early on (end of the 1960s) their own organization and management and medical and nursing boards. This autonomy gave them cohesion and a team spirit that formed the basis of a technical and scientific development difficult to achieve otherwise. As a consequence, a large and varied clinical experience was accumulated; however, regrettably, insufficient medical and nursing staff forced these professionals to work under much stress. Therefore, and in spite of the relevance of the often innovative experience acquired, the results of this experience frequently remained scientifically unexplored and very little was published.

In several units,the medical board assumed a multidisciplinary character (e.g. in Hospital Geral de Santo António). An exchange of technology and knowledge became a reality, making possible an otherwise difficult to realize training program in intensive medicine. As the quality of the treatment of patients became better and better, the independence of the ICU became greater. Good examples of this can be demonstrated in areas of diagnostic and therapeutic technology such as bronchoscopy, tracheostomy, epidural and intrathecal catheterisms, or regarding pharmacology such as the use of sedatives and analgesics, muscle relaxants, bronchodilators and antiarrythmics. The relations with other hospital departments were improved, and several divergent practices were minimized. This second phase lasted 20 years. A few more polyclinic ICUs have been created. In general, these units are dependent on other hospital departments. Creation of the existing units has been the product of a lot of hard work and despite various restrictions regarding technology and staff.

The third phase, spanning the last 5–10 years, has brought an increase in number of ICUs. Several have been created, not just in the main coastline towns but also inland, following improvements in Portuguese hospitals, a fact related to Portugal becoming a member state of the European Community. Meanwhile a many of the oldest ICUs are being refurnished. At the moment, it is difficult to estimate the number of existing ICUs, not only because some of them have been opened fairly recently but also because some are being closed down both in general and in private hospitals. If we say that the total number of Portuguese ICUs has doubled during the last 10 years this would be a fair estimate of the situation.

An investigation made in 1992 estimated that there were 83 ICUs (14 coronary units included) and 24 polyclinic ICUs (level III). The units which took part in EURICUS-I were selected according to these standards and can be considered representative of the national panorama (Table 14).

The management and organization of these ICUs cannot be considered uniform. There is a director, usually a physician, who reports directly to the medical staff director of the hospital. The nursing staff works full time in the ICU. The medical staff belong to other services (anaesthesiology, internal medicine and others) have only part-time positions in intensive medicine. Only 10% of the ICUs have their own management and their own full-time, dedicated medical and nursing staff. It therefore became of interest to offer specific medical training in ICM, a program which began in February 1990 within the two named services, which have an independent medical board. Nowadays, four hospitals offer specific training, called Ciclo de Estudos Especiais em Medicina Intensiva (Cycle of Special Studies in Intensive Medicine). It consists of a full-time 18 month training program, following specific guidelines, in intensive medicine. All physicians with

Table 14. Participating Portuguese ICUs in EURICUS-I

Hospital	Number of beds in the hospital	Type of ICU	Years of activity	Beds in the ICU (*n*)
Hospital Geral Santo António Universitário Porto	700	ICU	32	10
Hospital São João Universitário Porto	1308	Emergency room	8	9
Hospital Guimarães	480	Polyclinic ICU	2	7
Hospital Viana do Castelo	377	ICU	5	6
Centro Hospitalar Vila Nova de Gaia	560	Polyclinic ICU	6	9

a specialty in the following areas can apply for this subspeciality: anaesthesiology, cardiology, general surgery, nephrology, internal medicine, pediatrics, respiratory medicine and neurosurgery. More recently, the Ordem dos Médicos (equivalent to General Medical Council) has nominated a multidisciplinary committee for unifying the standards of training and the definition of an intensivist. The subspecialty of intensive care medicine was officially established on July 17, 1996.

There is no doubt as to the role of nursing in a well performing ICUs, and all intensivists are aware of this. Nowadays, there are two different generations of nurses in Portugal: nurses with extensive experience whose training has followed the evolution of the field of intensive medicine and younger nurses with a more specialized form of training. As nurses' training is also changing, perhaps there will also soon be a specialty in intensive medicine.

The Sociedade Portuguesa de Cuidados Intensivos (Portuguese Society of Intensive Care Medicine) was established in 1975 and is a mixed society, composed of 820 doctors and 1210 nurses, 2030 members altogether. The Executive Committee is replaced every 3 years, following proposals from each one of the three above mentioned towns (Porto, Coimbra and Lisbon). Beyond its connection to the European Society of Intensive Care Medicine, it is also a branch of The World Federation of Intensive and Critical Care Medicine and it was one of the societies that founded the Federação Pan-American e Ibérica de Medicina Crítica Y Terapia Intensiva. Every 3 years it organizes the Congresso Português de Cuidados Intensivos, attended by 600–900 participants. In the last few years, there have been 150–200 oral and poster presentations which have been published in a special issue of the Portuguese Review. Every 2 years, the Congresso Ibérico de Cuidados Intensivos takes place, an organization belonging to the Societies of Portugal and Spain. The 2nd Congress was held in Oporto in 1993, under the sponsorship of ESICM (1000 participants). The V Congresso Pan-Americano e Ibérico de Medicina Intensiva was organized in Lisbon, Portugal, on June 4–7 in 1995. The Revista Portuguesa de Medicina Intensiva (Portuguese Review of Intensive Care Medicine) has been published twice a year since 1992.

There has been a warm reponse to EURICUS-I by all members of the intensive care profession who have accepted and helped to realize the proposed aims of the project. We firmly believe in the benefits of the practical applications of this work and in the future of ICM in Portugal.

Comments

The overriding conclusion of the description by the country coordinators of ICM in the various countries participating in EURICUS-I is diversity. The described diversity of the organization of ICM at the country level parallels the diversity between ICUs and countries described in all substudies of EURICUS-I as well the diversity of organization and management observed at the ICU level during the site visits.

The descriptions made by the country coordinators in this chapter coincide to a large extent with the observations made 10 years ago by Burchardi and Atkinson [8] when studying education and training in ICM in Europe. It is noteworthy that many of the problems referred to have not changed over the last decade. It seems important to note that several of the problems and differences reported during the site visits and related to the organization and management of the ICUs have also been reported as problems at the country level:

1. Intensive care medicine as a medical activity: ICM is an independent specialty in Spain; ICM is a subspecialty to the traditional specialties (e.g. anaesthesiology, internal medicine, surgery) in some European countries; ICM makes up part of one traditional specialty (anaesthesiology) in other countries. In France ICM is dependent on two national organizations, the French Society of Intensive Care and the French Society of Anaesthesiology and Reanimation.
2. Teaching and training of ICM: Structured teaching and training of ICM exists in very few countries. In the majority of the European countries teaching and training depends on locally organized programs. Differences exist concerning the duration and the content of the programs, and the professionals (nurses and/or physicians) at whom the courses are aimed.
3. Professional organization: Generally speaking nurses are better organized as intensive care professionals than physicians. In about the half of the participating countries, ICU nurses do have a recognized intensive care specialty. This is not the case for physicians. The hospital management always allocates resources to the nursing staff but only rarely to the medical staff of the ICUs. The nursing staff works full-time in the ICU, while the medical staff rarely does. One important consequence of these contrasts is the differences regarding ICM qualification and the continuity of medical care on the ICU level, reported by several country coordinators.

References

1. Deutsch Krankengesellschaft (1994) Zahlen, Daten, Fakten 1994/1995. Deutsche Krankenhaus Verlagsgesellschaft, Düsseldorf, p. 33
2. Peter K, Dietrich HJ (1991) Stand und Perspektiven der Intensivmedizin. Anästh Intensivmed 32:343–347
3. Somers Y, Van Aken P, Bossaert L (1994) Minisymposium: Intensieve Zorgen in Vlaanderen, Vlaamse Vereniging Intensieve Zorgen Verpleegkundigen
4. Stoddart JC, personal communication
5. McPherson K, Metcalfe A (1995) Study of provision of intensive care in England, 1993. HMSO, London
6. Le Gall JR, Lemeshow S, Saulnier F(1993) A new simplified acute physiology score (SAPS II) based on an European/North American multicenter study. JAMA 270:2957–2963
7. Martinelli G(1990) Il terapia intensiva in Italia oggi. I Quaderni del Venotto 43:65–70
8. Burchardi, Atkinson (1990) In: Reis Miranda, Williams, Loirat (eds): Management of intensive care; guidelines for better use of resources. Kluwer Acad, Dordrecht pp 125–162
9. Chew R (1992) Compendium of health statistics 1992. Office of Health Economics, London

7 Substudies

Patients and Facilities

D. Reis Miranda, J. van der Veen, and R. Moreno

Introduction

The EURICUS-I substudy *Patients and Facilities* was aimed at making a survey of clinical activity in the ICUs and the physical environment in which those activities take place. The survey explored the differences in these characteristics between ICUs and aggregated groups of ICUs in Europe. The focus was on variables which may be influential and representative of daily clinical activities in the ICUs from a medical perspective.

The clinical data surveyed included: admission and discharge data, severity of illness at admission to the ICU, daily nursing workload. These variables were collected at the patient level and included all consecutive admissions at the ICUs during the 4 month period of field research of EURICUS-I (October 3, 1994 through January 31, 1995). Two forms were developed for the collection of these data on the ICUs. A detailed protocol covering all aspects concerned with collection and administration of the clinical data was written and translated into the native languages for use in the ICUs. The anonymity of patients was assured (code numbers were used at ICU level). The protocols also considered quality control of the data collected at ICU level (double checks by independent and blind raters), at country level and at data entry level. The data was centrally pooled at the University Hospital in Groningen, the Netherlands, where final (logical and consistency) checks were performed. The data related to the physical environment of the ICUs provided information about the hospitals in which the ICUs functioned (e.g. type, size, clinical activities, other ICUs) and information concerning the ICU itself (e.g. number of beds, staffing). These data were collected by means of a questionnaire administered to the ICU leadership. Site visits to the participating ICUs took place during the field research. These visits, performed by the project leader and other research staff are reported on in Chap. 6 ("Site Visits"). The description of how ICUs were selected at the country level and their representativeness in the sample are discussed in Chap. 1 ("Selection of ICUs"). It is important to underline that Spain participated in the study with more ICUs than any other country. The participation of the Spanish ICUs was prospectively organized in the following way: two European areas (Catalonia with eight ICUs and Valencia with nine ICUs) and ten additional ICUs not integrated into a particular geographic area. The two Spanish geographic areas participated as such in all analyses in this substudy. The other Spanish ICUs received the reports concerning the data analyzed at ICU level and participated in only a few of the analyses performed, as indicated in the respective text and tables.

The Hospitals

The data presented in this substudy concerns the findings in 89 ICUs from 86 hospitals. Of these, 84% were public and 16% were private hospitals; 38% (33) were university hospitals. There was a large variation in the size of the hospitals; as expected, nonuniversity hospitals were smaller. In this sample, the mean size of hospitals in Poland was the smallest in the sample and different from the mean size of those in Italy, Denmark, the UK and Germany (on average the country with the largest hospitals) (Table 1). The hospital size and type were expected to determine several of the organizational characteristics of the hospital, such as the type and volume of the services provided, which in their turn determine many other ICU characteristics.

Services Provided

All hospitals provided general surgery and internal medicine. Statistically significant differences existed regarding some specialized medical activities: neuro-

Table 1. Size of hospitals and numbers of ICU in each geographical locality used in the EURICUS study

	Number of ICUs	Mean size hospital ± SD
European areas		
Poland	8	299 ± 258
Germany	3	1161 ± 548
Denmark	6	774 ± 321
Finland	5	578 ± 316
Netherlands	7	502 ± 208
Belgium	5	372 ± 248
France	4	650 ± 448
United Kingdom	8	762 ± 204
Italy	7	699 ± 274
Spain	19	547 ± 445
Spain-Catalonia	8	416 ± 267
Portugal	5	685 ± 368
Overall	86	582 ± 364

logy, psychiatry, cardiac surgery, obstetrics, neurosurgery, organ transplantation and vascular surgery. Table 2 gives the frequency distribution of these activities showing that their provision is in general associated with the size and type of the hospitals.

Other Critical Care Facilities in the Hospital

Table 3 shows that the existence of other ICU facilities next to the ICU participating in the study is largely dependent on the type and size of the hospital considered. Confirming the observation of other studies, smaller nonuniversity hospitals have usually only one ICU. This is often integrated with the coronary care unit (CCU) of the hospital. This integration is frequent in the hospitals of southern Europe, particularly in Spain, independent of the size and type of the hospital. EURICUS-I did not address specifically the appropriateness of the association of ICUs with CCUs.

Table 2. Hospital size and medical specialties

	Type and size of the hospital (%)			
	<300 Beds ($n=18$)	300–500 Beds ($n=16$)	>500 Beds ($n=21$)	University ($n=33$)
Services provided				
Neurology	50	69	57	46
Psychiatry	22	38	57	52
Cardiac surgery	0	0	33	24
Obstetrics	50	69	100	70
Neurosurgery	11	19	14	36
Organ transplant	0	0	10	33
Vascular surgery	44	25	71	64

Table 3. Hospital critical care facilities

	Type of Hospital				Overall
	<300 Beds	300–500 Beds	>500 Beds	University	
Other ICUs					
No	12	16	12	10	50
Yes	3	2	9	23	37
Recovery rooms					
No	1	4	5	4	14
Yes	14	12	16	28	70
Step-down units					
No	11	13	13	18	55
Yes	2	2	8	11	23

Out of 84 responding hospitals, 14 did not have a recovery room (RR) for immediate postoperative care of patients, and 55 out of 78 hospitals did not have step-down units (e.g. medium care, high care). There were 13 hospitals that reported having between one and six such units, and nine hospitals reported having more than six step-down unit beds. It is noteworthy that, whereas the distribution of RRs correlates significantly with the size and type of the hospitals, a similar association was not found regarding step-down units and their size. It is also important to note that of the existing RRs only 29 hospitals reported having them open 24 h/day.

It was anticipated that diversity in the availability of critical care facilities in the hospital wouldhave an important influence upon the case mix of the units studied.

The Intensive Care Units

Size of ICUs

Table 4 presents the size of the participating ICUs (aggregated into three groups) associated with the hospitals (aggregated according to size and type). As might be expected there is a relationship between size of hospital and size of ICU.

The smallest ICUs were located in the UK, Poland and Italy (Table 5). The mean size of ICUs in the UK was smaller than that of ICUs in Denmark, France, Belgium and Germany. The size of the ICU does influence at least the flow of patients (admission and discharge policies) and the resources required, particularly those concerning the staffing of each unit. An important physical characteristic of the ICU is the existence and number of isolation rooms in the unit, as the number of nurses required will increase proportionately.

Table 6 shows that a large majority of ICUs do not have isolation rooms, that 18% of the ICUs have only one and that 26% have more than one isolation room. The provision of isolation rooms does not seem to follow any particular criteria ($p = 0.8$).

Table 4. Size of the ICU according to type of hospital

	Type of Hospital				Overall
	<300 Beds	300–500 Beds	>500 Beds	University	
Size of ICU					
0–6 beds	8	10	6	8	33
7–9 beds	5	4	7	7	23
>10 beds	2	4	8	20	34
Overall	15	18	21	35	89

Table 5. Size of ICU (number of beds) according to type of hospital of ICU

	Mean size ICU ± SD
European area	
Poland	6.00 ± 1.94
Germany	16.67 ± 10.69
Denmark	8.33 ± 1.51
Finland	10.20 ± 6.76
Netherlands	8.00 ± 4.00
Belgium	12.67 ± 6.98
France	13.00 ± 7.28
United Kingdom	5.75 ± 2.05
Italy	6.86 ± 2.34
Spain-Catalonia	11.00 ± 9.27
Spain-Valencia	11.32 ± 5.55
Portugal	7.80 ± 1.64
Overall	9.55 ± 5.75

Table 6. Isolation wards and hospital size

	Type of Hospital				Overall
	<300 Beds	300–500 Beds	>500 Beds	University	
Isolation beds					
No	7	11	10	20	48
One bed	4	2	6	4	16
>One bed	3	5	5	9	22
Overall	14	18	21	33	86

Type of ICUs

Table 7 shows that the majority of the ICUs in EURICUS-I are "general ICUs", i.e. mixed medical and surgical, and sometimes including the CCU in the same facility. Further analysis of the collected data revealed that denominations such as "medical ICU" and "surgical ICU", are more frequent in university hospitals. This label often represents the organizational structure to which the ICU is connected (medical or surgical department) rather than the type of patients admitted to the respective ICU.

Table 7. Size of the ICU by type of hospital

	Type of Hospital				Total
	<300 Beds	300–500 Beds	>500 Beds	University	
Type of ICUs					
Medical	1	1	1	6	9
Surgical	1		1	4	6
General	13	17	19	25	74
Overall	15	18	21	35	89

The Nursing Staff

The Professionals

All the ICUs had a (deputy) head nurse appointed full-time to the unit. A large difference between ICUs concerned the professional category of the nurses staffing the ICUs. These categories were defined as follows:

1. Certified intensive care nurse: Those nurses who successfully followed additional, recognized education and training in intensive care medicine. Some 57% of the ICUs reported having this category of nurses. Nearly 100% of the staff employed in the ICUs in one country belonged to this category. The presence of these nurses was significantly associated with the variable country.
2. In-service teaching nurse (regular nurse): Those nurses with a general nursing qualification, such as those working at the general ward, and who might receive intensive care training while working. Some 74.2% of the ICUs employed nurses of this category (their presence was not associated with country).
3. Second level of nurse or nursing helper (nursing assistant): Those nurses undergoing education and training to acquire the degree of regular nurse; in some countries the ICUs may use nursing aids; they do not receive any specific nursing education and are only allowed to perform nonspecific nursing tasks. Some 68% of the ICUs reported having this category of nurses. The presence of these nurses was significantly associated with country.
4. Agency nurses: Those nurses had been contracted from outside the hospital to work provisionally at the ICU. Nine ICUs (10%) in four countries regularly hired this category of nurses (distribution significantly associated with the variable country).

The type of nurse was noted by the survey during the site visits, but it was difficult to establish the impact of the various professional categories on the composition of the daily work-shifts of the nursing staff. Except in the very few ICUs hiring exclusively certified intensive care nurses, the overriding situation in the field was that there was a higher percentage of better trained nurses working during the morning shift.

Overall, 33% of the nurses working at the ICUs received intensive care education, varying from 89% in the Netherlands to 0% in Portugal. Prior to being employed by the ICU, 21.6% of the ICUs required that the nursing staff had a certain number of years of experience in general medical/surgical nursing; 29.2% required previous critical care training; 37.5% of the ICUs offered a locally organized orientation course. In 20.2% of the ICUs nurses coming from the general ward regularly joined the staff of the unit. In 36% of the ICUs this situation was rarely the case, and 43.8% of the ICUs never considered this solution in case of a shortage of nursing staff.

Size of Nursing Staff

Table 8 presents the mean number of nurses/bed (N/B) calculated by dividing the total number of nurses in the ICU (full-time equivalents; all professional categories) by the total number of beds in the unit. N/B are stratified by European area, type and size of hospital, and type of ICU. The smaller hospitals did not have all the types of ICUs. The overall N/B was 3.63 with a range of means between 2.38 (Belgium) and 6.46 (UK). Analysis of variance has shown that the differences shown in Table 8 could not be explained by the hospital category nor by the type of ICU and that they could be partially explained by the variable country ($F_{(12,68)} = 5.75$; $p \leq 0.001$).

Available Patient/Nurse Ratios

Patient/nurse ratios (P/N) were computed as indicated elsewhere [1]. P/N ratios, or the mean number of patients that can be treated by one nurse in each nursing

Table 8. Number of nurses per bed by type of ICU and type of hospital

	Type of ICU			Type of hospital				Overall
	Medical	Surgical	General	<300 Beds	300–500 Beds	>500 Beds	University	
European area								
Poland	2.5	4.8	2.9	4.3	2.5	3.9	2.9	3.2
Germany			2.8			2.6	3.4	2.8
Denmark			4.5	3.1		4.3	5.2	4.5
Finland			3.7	3.7		3.8	3.6	3.7
Netherlands		4.5	4.1		3.8	4.6	4.5	4.1
Belgium	2.2	2.1	2.5	2.3		2.1	2.8	2.4
France	2.6	3.5	2.3	2.3			2.9	2.6
United Kingdom			6.5			6.2	6.7	6.5
Italy			3.2		3.0	3.0	3.7	3.2
Spain-Catalonia			3.2	2.8	4.3		3.3	3.2
Spain-Valencia	2.9		3.5	3.0	3.6	4.1	3.3	3.4
Portugal			3.2		2.8	5.0	2.7	3.2
Overall	2.6	3.8	3.7	3.0	3.4	4.0	3.8	3.6

Table 9. Mean patient/nurse ratio by type of ICU and type of hospital

	Type of ICU			Type of hospital				Overall
	Medical	Surgical	General	< 300 Beds	300–500 Beds	> 500 Beds	University	
European area								
Poland	1.80	1.58	1.50	2.52	1.68	1.08	1.24	1.65
Germany			1.51			1.65	1.24	1.51
Denmark			1.05	1.34		0.98	1.00	1.05
Finland			1.14	1.17		1.10	1.16	1.14
Netherlands		0.93	1.06		1.13	0.92	0.93	1.04
Belgium	1.95	1.98	1.74	1.94		1.97	1.55	1.82
France	1.94	1.20	1.82	1.82			1.69	1.74
United Kingdom			0.71			0.70	0.72	0.71
Italy			1.36		1.40	1.43	1.20	1.36
Spain-Catalonia			1.38	1.58	0.99		1.32	1.38
Spain-Valencia	2.05		1.26	1.46	1.20	1.02	1.47	1.35
Portugal			1.39		1.52	0.84	1.54	1.39
Overall	1.90	1.45	1.25	1.69	1.30	1.17	1.29	1.33

shift, are calculated from the number of nursing full-time equivalents and the number of beds in the ICU. The available P/N ratios are measured at unit level and indicate the general staffing capacity of the unit. They do not indicate the nursing requirements at the individual patient level, as it was anticipated that this varied widely in each ICU. The P/N ratio of each ICU is considered the level of care (LOC) of the ICU.

Table 9 presents the P/N ratios stratified by country, type and size of hospital and type of ICU. The overall P/N ratio was 1.33 with a range of means between 1.82 in Belgium and 0.71 in the UK. The P/N ratio differences shown in the table could not be explained by the hospital category nor by the type of ICU; the variance was significantly associated with the variable country (F (12,66) = 3.77; $p \leq 0.001$).

In the P/N calculations two assumptions were made: (1) 85% is the ideal occupancy rate of the ICU; and (2) 25% of the available manpower time will not be used in the unit (holidays, sicknessof the personnel, etc.).

The Medical Staff

Seven questions on the questionnaire filled out by the leadership of each ICU addressed medical coverage of the units. Out of 88 ICUs, 85 had a medical director (MD) and 47 reported the existence of codirector(s). The time spent by the MD in the ICU was not easy to determine, and the official status of the (co)directors was not always clear. The original medical specialty of the MD varied: 42 from anaesthesiology, 21 from critical care medicine (particularly in Spanish

ICUs), 19 from internal medicine, two from surgery, two from cardiology and one from pulmonary medicine. The mean time span of experience of the MD in the ICU was 16 years. With few exceptions, the ICUs were included in the organizational structure of one hospital department, such as anaesthesiology or internal medicine; this would determine the original specialty of the ICU MD.

A total of 76 ICUs reported the presence of a physician in the ICU 24 h/day. This issue was discussed with the leadership of the ICUs during the site visits. Although efforts were made during the design of the project to define the various categories of physicians working in the ICU (e.g. ICU residents, intensive care fellows, trainees of other specialties) the definitions given were not interpreted unequivocally by the participating ICUs. It could be concluded that the intensive care experience of these physicians varied greatly. In the majority of the cases they were residents of a variety of specialties (anaesthesiology, surgery, internal medicine, cardiology, etc.), and quite often they were also covering medical other wards in the hospital.

Other Staff

The survey assessed the effective presence of technicians and secretaries at least during 8 h on 5 working days during the week. Eleven ICUs (in six countries) reported a technician in the unit. Considering the distribution of technicians according to hospital size and type, a technician was present on 14% of the ICUs of nonuniversity hospitals (in 19% of the hospital >500 beds) whereas only 15% of the ICUs of university hospitals reported having a full-time technician. There were 53 ICUs that reported having a secretary. In Italy none of the ICUs had a technician or a secretary. Analysis of variance showed that the presence of technicians and of secretaries in the ICUs was associated with the variable country.

The Equipment

Medical equipment is an important physical characteristic of the ICU. During the preparation of EURICUS-I it was anticipated that there was a large diversity of equipment (type and number) among the ICUs. Besides the variation of equipment used to direct care of patients (e.g. mechanical ventilators, cardiovascular monitors), the variation in equipment available might include computers, patient data management systems, etc. It was also anticipated that the magnitude of variation in this latter type of equipment would make it impossible to compare ICUs. Therefore, for the comparison of equipment among the ICUs a distinction must be made between the existence of basic equipment necessary for care of intensive care patients and equipment required for the performance of particular modes of care (e.g. radiologic examinations, endoscopies) or other activities such as research. Analysis of the equipment was included in the *Finances* substudy.

In the substudy *Patients and Facilities*, the survey regarding equipment available in the ICUs was concerned with equipment considered indispensable to the monitoring and support of three organ and system functions: respiratory, cardiovascular and renal. The availability to the ICU of relevant diagnostic examinations was also explored.

Respiratory Function

1. Mechanical ventilators. All ICUs reported having mechanical ventilators. Overall these could be used with 90% of the beds in the sample.
2. End-tidal CO_2 monitoring. present in 82% of the units and available to 31% of the beds.
3. Pulse oximeter monitoring. present in 92% of the ICUs and available to 64% of the beds.
4. Portable ventilator. present in 82% of the units; 16 ICUs did not have a portable ventilator.

Cardiovascular Function

1. ECG monitoring: present with all beds of all ICUs.
2. Intravascular pressure modules: present in 95% of the ICUs, up to three or four modules per each ICU bed.
3. Pacemakers: external types present in 79% and A-V sequential types in 44% of the ICUs.
4. Defibrillator: present in all ICUs.
5. Portable ECG and pressure monitor: present in 72% of the units; 23 ICUs did not have a portable ECG and pressure monitor.
6. Intra-aortic balloon pump: reported by18 ICUs.

Renal Function

1. Haemodialysis: present in 55% of the ICUs.
2. Peritoneal dialysis: could be performed in 71% of the ICUs.
3. Haemofiltration techniques, e.g. continuous arterial-venous hemofiltration (CAVH) and systemic continuous venous filtration (SCVF): performed in 75% of the ICUs.
4. Two ICUs did not have infusion pumps.

Diagnostic Examinations

1. Chemistry and haematologic tests: always available. A few ICUs reported that several relevant tests were not available 24 h/day.
2. Blood gases: ICUs in Poland reported difficulty in getting blood gases analysis 24 h/day.
3. Chest/abdominal X-rays: ICUs in Poland reported difficulty in getting these examinations performed 24 h/day.
4. Ultrasound and CT scan: The ICUs of eight of the 12 countries reported that ultrasound and CT scan examinations were not available 24 h/day. These were often only available during regular working hours.

Analysis of variance showed that the differences observed concerning: intravascular pressure modules, external pacemaker, haemofiltration techniques, and ultrasound were country-dependent. The presence of an intra-aortic balloon pump was not country-dependent.

The Patients

A total of 16059 patients were admitted to the ICUs during the 120 days of field research of EURICUS-I. The existence of missing values makes the numbers differ between some of the tables.

Hospital and Type of ICU

Table 10 shows the distribution of patients according to type and size of the hospital and type of ICU in each European area. Some 43% of the patients were admitted to university hospitals; 57% patients were admitted to nonuniversity hospitals: 31% in hospital >500 beds, 14% in hospitals between 300 and 500 beds, and 12% in hospitals <300 beds. The large majority of the patients (84%) were admitted on general ICUs, with 9% on medical ICUs and 7% on surgical ICUs.

Table 10. Number of patients from each European area

	Type of ICU			Type of hospital				Overall
	Medical	Surgical	General	<300 Beds	300–500 Beds	>500 Beds	University	
European area[a]								
Poland	364	71	190	56	300	63	206	625
Germany			1459			1177	282	1459
Denmark			1251	246		477	528	1251
Finland			1349	228		346	775	1349
Netherlands		129	1402		595	807	129	1531
Belgium	332	603	1327	319		935	1008	2262
France	480	110	214	214			590	804
United Kingdom			833			343	490	833
Italy			777		124	401	252	777
Spain	483		1527	387	992	272	1399	3050
Spain-Catalonia			2567	464	97		966	1527
Portugal			439		175	84	180	439
Overall	1659	1065	13335	1914	2283	4905	6957	16059

[a] data on Luxembourg are not presented.

Table 11. Mean age (years) of the studied patients

	Type of ICU			Type of hospital				Overall
	Medical	Surgical	General	<300 Beds	300–500 Beds	>500 Beds	University	
European area								
Poland	60	59	52	62	59	52	55	57
Germany			59			62	49	59
Denmark			58	55		60	58	58
Finland		59	58	59		58	57	58
Netherlands		62	61		60	62	59	61
Belgium	64	42	61	65		62	60	62
France	54		59	59			52	54
United Kingdom			59			58	60	59
Italy			58		60	61	52	58
Spain-Catalonia			60	62	63		59	60
Spain-Valencia	62		60	64	61	62	59	60
Portugal			58		62	61	53	58
Overall	60	58	59	61	60	61	57	59

Age

The mean age of the patients is presented in Table 11and is matched with the type and size of hospital and type of ICU. Overall, the mean age of patients at ICU level was 59 years. Surgical ICUs admitted younger patients (mean 58 years) as did university hospitals. Analysis of variance showed that age associated significantly with the variables country, hospital category and the association of both, and with type of ICU whether alone or in association with the variables country or hospital category.

Source of Admission

Table 12 presents the origin of the patients admitted, according to country, hospital type, size and type of ICU. Some 37% of the patients were admitted from the operating theatre, 4% from the recovery room (RR), 30% from the emergency room, 17% from the ward, 2% from other ICUs and 6% from another hospital. This pattern of admission is about the same in all European areas. In Spain, the larger incidence of patients admitted from the emergency room is related to the admission of cardiology emergencies to the ICU. Note the low incidence of patients admitted from the RR (4%). Nearly 50% of the patients were admitted to the ICU directly after surgery. It could be expected that the number of admissions from the RR would be much larger. In another study [2] several admissions were directly from the operating theatre to the ICU in the knowledge, that the RR closed sometime in the afternoon and was not available during the weekends.

Table 12. Location in the hospital before ICU admission (number of patients)

	Admitted from							Overall
	1	2	3	4	5	6	7	
European area								
Poland	76		379	141		24	4	624
Germany	796	31	109	72	26	55	133	1222
Denmark	436	60	303	302	13	59	31	1204
Finland	788	6	271	227	19	13	5	1329
Netherlands	754	190	254	189	25	71	28	1511
Belgium	1084	86	614	295	10	110	29	2228
France	63	10	207	154	34	115	215	798
United Kingdom	330	39	163	205	14	30	30	811
Italy	265	9	154	198	33	97	18	774
Spain	533	19	1559	576	25	226	25	3003
Spain-Catalonia	378	57	549	209	99	158	63	1513
Portugal	164	24	89	66	48	23	17	431
Type of hospital								
<300 Beds	562	13	669	318	15	150	151	1878
300–500 Beds	486	168	1013	357	20	165	34	2243
>500 Beds	2277	129	914	717	94	293	188	4612
University	2383	263	2128	1254	217	385	228	6858
Type of ICU								
Medical	32	7	916	417	37	167	69	1645
Surgical	679	64	86	63	17	63	72	1044
General	4997	502	3722	2166	292	763	460	12902
Overall *n*	5708	573	4724	2646	346	993	601	15591
(%)	(36.6)	(3.7)	(30.3)	(17.0)	(2.2)	(6.4)	(3.8)	(100.0)

Admitted from: 1, operating theatre; 2, recovery room; 3, emergency room; 4, ward; 5, other ICU; 6, other hospital; 7, none of the above.

The admission of patients coming from another ICU is low (2%). This feature is almost nonexistent in the ICUs of small nonuniversity hospitals and rises to 2% in the ICUs of large nonuniversity hospitals and 3% in those of university hospitals. The flow of patients coming from another hospital (overall incidence of 6%) indicates that 5% of the patients admitted to university ICUs are of this category, 6% of admissions of nonuniversity hospitals >500 beds, 7% between 300 and 500 beds, and 8% of admissions of hospitals <300 beds. This suggests the use of the ICU to initially handle the backflow of patients from the wards of larger hospitals where a higher level of care might have been provided. It deserves mention that the operating theatre is the origin of 50% of the patients admitted to the ICUs of large nonuniversity hospitals. This is in contrast with a lower incidence of this group of patients in the other ICUs (37% overall). The high incidence of patients

Table 13. Type of patient by European area, type of hospital and type of ICU

	Admission type			Overall
	Surgical emergency	Surgical scheduled	Medical	
European area				
Poland	41	42	541	624
Germany	216	701	310	1227
Denmark	321	298	588	1207
Finland	263	599	466	1328
Netherlands	296	734	493	1523
Belgium	190	1062	972	2224
France	75	54	661	790
United Kingdom	292	169	356	817
Italy	148	215	413	776
Spain	356	344	2329	3029
Spain-Catalonia	200	312	1013	1525
Portugal	103	114	220	437
Type of hospital				
< 300 beds	327	364	1184	1875
300–500 beds	342	436	1491	2269
> 500 beds	773	1921	1929	4623
University	1115	1988	3783	6886
Type of ICU				
Medical	39	54	1545	1638
Surgical	239	629	181	1049
General	2279	4026	6661	12966
Overall *n*	2557	4709	8387	15653
(%)	(16.3)	(30.1)	(53.6)	(100.0)

coming from the operating theatre may indicate a particular surgery vocation of the large nonuniversity hospitals and is similar to what was observed in the Dutch National ICU Study.

Type of Admission

The association of severity of illness with outcome, led the admissions to be classified into surgical and medical. Surgical admissions were divided into scheduled, i.e. patients whose surgery was scheduled at least 24 h in advance, and unscheduled, i.e. added to the operating room schedule within 24 h of the operation [3]. Table 13 shows the distribution of type of admission according to European area, type and size of hospital and type of ICU. Overall, 54% of the patients were medical and 46% were surgical of which 30% were scheduled and 16% unscheduled. However, it is very important to note that the distribution among the considered stratifications is not homogeneous.

European Areas

The ICUs in Poland, France and Spain (including Catalonia) had a higher incidence of medical patients. The ICUs in Germany, Finland, The Netherlands and Belgium had a higher incidence of surgical scheduled admissions. The ICUs in Denmark, the UK and Portugal had a higher incidence of surgical unscheduled patients.

It must be noted that the definitions of scheduled and unscheduled surgery integrate the influence of three possibly distinct factors: (1) the sudden clinical deterioration of a patient is at the origin of the unexpected decision to operate; (2) insufficient exchange of information among clinicians may lead to the incorrect definition of the type of admission; (3) inappropriate planning of the operative program may reclassify an unscheduled patient who should belong to the scheduled category. In this case, organization and management deficiencies may be at the origin of erroneous computations of severity of illness. These are important limitations of the followed classification system, since unscheduled surgery receives a higher weighting in the severity of illness scoring systems [3].

Hospital Category

Accounting for about 43% of all admissions, the ICUs of university hospitals predominate, to a certain extent, over the overall distribution of the type of admission in the whole sample. Large differences do exist however among the ICUs of nonuniversity hospitals: (a) 60% of the admissions to the ICUs of hospitals >500 beds were surgical, making up 42% of the surgical scheduled category; (b) the majority of the admissions at ICUs of smaller hospitals (respectively 62% and 66%) were independent of the medical category.

Diagnosis

The diagnosis at admission is included in the APACHE severity of illness scoring systems [4, 5]. The rational behind this inclusion is that the outcome of the severity of illness resulting from the physiology derangement considered by the scoring system may also vary depending upon the underlying diagnosis. The severity of illness scoring systems used in EURICUS-I do not consider diagnosis [3, 6]. For each patient enrolled in the study, the primary diagnosis justifying admission to the ICU was registered. The list of diagnoses proposed by Knaus et al [5] was used. This list considers 76 diagnoses grouped into 18 major categories: ten nonoperative and eight postoperative. The rationale behind this decision was that the inclusion of diagnosis may be helpful in a more precise evaluation of outcome in relation to the chosen stratifications of severity of illness. This information, not directly related to the objectives of the project, will be used in later research on the EURICUS-I database. Inclusion of diagnosis may also help to differentiate among ICUs and among hospitals. Relevant aspects of the observed differences are presented below.

Table 14. Diagnostic categories of admission [5] by European area, type of hospital and type of ICU

	Nonoperative diagnostic categories																			
	A		B		C		D		E		F		G		H		I		J	
European area																				
Poland	341	2,2%	39	0.2%	6	0.0%	38	0.2%	3	0.0%	19	0.1%	54	0.3%	2	0.0%	2	0.0%	36	0.2%
Germany	202	1.3%	33	0.2%	33	0.2%	22	0.1%	3	0.0%	7	0.0%	12	0.1%	2	0.0%			3	0.0%
Denmark	91	0.6%	208	1.3%	37	0.2%	64	0.4%	36	0.2%	11	0.1%	126	0.8%	15	0.1%	6	0.0%	24	0.2%
Finland	104	0.7%	76	0.5%	89	0.6%	52	0.3%	20	0.1%	16	0.1%	67	0.4%	16	0.1%	10	0.1%	18	0.1%
Netherlands	112	0.7%	138	0.9%	37	0.2%	45	0.3%	40	0.3%	19	0.1%	84	0.5%	3	0.0%	10	0.1%	22	0.1%
Belgium	553	3.5%	108	0.7%	58	0.4%	78	0.5%	27	0.2%	49	0.3%	59	0.4%	7	0.0%	20	0.1%	30	0.2%
France	78	0.5%	255	1.6%	30	0.2%	97	0.6%	33	0.2%	30	0.2%	86	0.5%	8	0.1%	30	0.2%	21	0.1%
United Kingdom	69	0.4%	131	0.8%	35	0.2%	50	0.3%	23	0.1%	6	0.0%	43	0.3%	5	0.0%	6	0.0%	3	0.0%
Italy	125	0.8%	130	0.8%	18	0.1%	53	0.3%	18	0.1%	39	0.2%	18	0.1%	3	0.0%	5	0.0%	8	0.1%
Spain	1493	9.5%	318	2.0%	57	0.4%	161	1.0%	62	0.4%	104	0.7%	81	0.5%	9	0.1%	8	0.1%	43	0.3%
Spain-Catalonia	605	3.9%	143	0.9%	31	0.2%	101	0.6%	20	0.1%	56	0.4%	26	0.2%	2	0.0%	10	0.1%	17	0.1%
Portugal	25	0.2%	119	0.8%	7	0.0%	18	0.1%	8	0.1%	24	0.2%	7	0.0%	1	0.0%	3	0.0%	11	0.1%
Type of hospital																				
<300 Beds	588	3.8%	190	1.2%	65	0.4%	128	0.8%	25	0.2%	40	0.3%	94	0.6%	2	0.0%	20	0.1%	31	0.2%
300–500 Beds	894	5.7%	207	1.3%	35	0.2%	108	0.7%	44	0.3%	71	0.5%	107	0.7%	7	0.0%	10	0.1%	23	0.1%
>500 Beds	825	5.3%	412	2.6%	133	0.8%	180	1.1%	64	0.4%	74	0.5%	171	1.1%	24	0.2%	17	0.1%	66	0.4%
University	1492	9.5%	895	5.7%	208	1.3%	370	2.4%	161	1.0%	202	1.3%	292	1.9%	40	0.3%	63	0.4%	116	0.7%
Type of ICU																				
Medical	844	5.4%	299	1.9%	35	0.2%	119	0.8%	49	0.3%	5	0.0%	126	0.8%	10	0.1%	27	0.2%	49	0.3%
Surgical	14	0.1%	30	0.2%	14	0.1%	36	0.2%	12	0.1%	59	0.4%	6	0.0%	1	0.0%	1	0.0%	11	0.1%
General	2941	18.8%	1375	8.8%	392	2.5%	631	4.0%	233	1.5%	323	2.1%	532	3.4%	62	0.4%	82	0.5%	176	1.1%
Overall	3799	24.2%	1704	10.9%	441	2.8%	786	5.0%	294	1.9%	387	2.5%	664	4.2%	73	0.5%	110	0.7%	236	1.5%

A, Cardiovascular/vascular; B, respiratory; C, gastrointestinal (GI) ; D, neurologic; E, sepsis; F, trauma; G, metabolic; H, hematologic; I, renal diseases; J, other medical diseases.

Table .14. Continued

	Postoperative diagnostic categories																			
	K		L		M		N		O		P		Q		R		S		Total	
European area																				
Poland	10	0.1%	1	0.0%	54	0.3%	7	0.0%	7	0.0%	1	0.0%	3	0.0%	2	0.0%	–		625	100%
Germany	484	3.1%	47	0.3%	98	0.6%	129	0.8%	43	0.3%	58	0.4%	20	0.1%	38	0.2%	–		1234	100%
Denmark	122	0.8%	57	0.4%	238	1.5%	10	0.1%	38	0.2%	29	0.2%	12	0.1%	91	0.6%	–		1215	100%
Finland	430	2.7%	33	0.2%	170	1.1%	165	1.1%	28	0.2%	6	0.0%	1	0.0%	13	0.1%	16	0.1%	1330	100%
Netherlands	533	3.4%	71	0.5%	262	1.7%	26	0.2%	39	0.2%	41	0.3%	12	0.1%	32	0.2%	–		1526	100%
Belgium	775	4.9%	111	0.7%	125	0.8%	98	0.6%	30	0.2%	22	0.1%	25	0.2%	51	0.3%	–		2226	100%
France	19	0.1%	15	0.1%	30	0.2%	6	0.0%	30	0.2%	9	0.1%	5	0.0%	7	0.0%	–		789	100%
United Kingdom	117	0.7%	48	0.3%	193	1.2%	12	0.1%	38	0.2%	15	0.1%	8	0.1%	18	0.1%	1	0.0%	821	100%
Italy	109	0.7%	35	0.2%	105	0.7%	37	0.2%	25	0.2%	30	0.2%	4	0.0%	13	0.1%	2	0.0%	777	100%
Spain	145	0.9%	80	0.5%	252	1.6%	69	0.4%	89	0.6%	23	0.1%	11	0.1%	13	0.1%	2	0.0%	3020	100%
Spain-Catalonia	207	1.3%	27	0.2%	146	o.9%	61	0.4%	51	0.3%	7	0.0%	3	0.0%	5	0.0%	1	0.0%	1519	100%
Portugal	9	0.1%	20	0.1%	125	0.8%	13	0.1%	35	0.2%	10	0.1%	2	0.0%	–		–		437	100%
Type of Hospital																				
<300beds	90	0.6%	65	0.4%	307	2.0%	32	0.2%	60	0.4%	33	0.2%	11	0.1%	91	0.6%	12	0.1%	1842	100%
300–500 beds	119	0.8%	76	0.5%	355	2.3%	44	0.3%	78	0.5%	50	0.3%	16	0.1%	21	0.1%	2	0.0%	2268	100%
>500 beds	1599	10.2%	177	1.1%	490	3.1%	96	0.6%	102	0.7%	85	0.5%	32	0.2%	75	0.5%	5	0.0%	4425	100%
University	1162	7.4%	237	1.5%	664	4.2%	509	3.2%	235	1.5%	85	0.5%	53	0.3%	103	0.7%	3	0.0%	6631	100%
Type of ICU																				
Medical	46	0.3%	9	0.1%	12	0.1%	9	0.1%	2	0.0%	4	0.0%	3	0.0%			–		1347	100%
Surgical	460	2.9%	55	0.4%	122	0.8%	98	0.6%	68	0.4%	21	0.1%	16	0.1%	14	0.1%	–		1038	100%
General	2464	15.7%	491	3.1%	1682	10.7%	574	3.7%	405	2.6%	228	1.5%	93	0.6%	276	1.8%	22	0.1%	12781	100%
Overall	2970	19.0%	555	3.5%	1816	11.6%	681	4.3%	475	3.0%	253	1.6%	112	0.7%	290	1.9%	22	0.1%	15166	100%

K, cardiovascular/vascular; L, respiratory; M, gastrointestinal (GI); N, neurologic; O, trauma; P, renal; Q, gynecologic; R, orthopedic; S, other surgical diseases.

Table 14 shows the distribution of the 18 major diagnostic categories according to country, type and size of hospital and type of ICU. The majority of the diagnostic categories account for rather modest percentages of all admissions. Four categories, however, predominate in EURICUS-I: nonoperative cardiovascular and respiratory diagnoses (together 35% of the admissions) and the postoperative cardiovascular and gastrointestinal diagnoses (together 31% of the admissions). Cardiovascular diagnoses made up a total of 43% of all admissions during the study.

Table 15 analyzes the distribution of the four high-incidence categories in more detail, considering only those with an incidence above 10% of the admissions for each given stratification. Postoperative diagnoses are for example predominant in the participating ICUs from Finland and The Netherlands, whereas nonoperative diagnosis predominate in the participating ICUs from France and

Table 15. Distribution of most frequent diagnostic categories of admission (above 10%) [5] by European area, type of hospital and type of ICU

	Diagnostic category			
	Nonoperative (%)		Postoperative (%)	
	Cardiovascular	Respiratory	Cardiovascular	Gastrointestinal
European area				
Poland	55			
Germany	16		39	
Denmark		17	10	20
Finland			32	13
Netherlands			35	17
Belgium	25		35	
France	10	32		
United Kingdom		16	14	24
Italy	16	17	14	14
Spain-Catalonia	40		14	10
Spain-Valencia	49	11		
Portugal		27		29
Type of hospital				
<300 Beds	31	10		16
300–500 Beds	39			16
>500 Beds	18		35	11
University	22	13	17	10
Type of ICU				
Medical	51	18		
Surgical			44	12
General	23	11	19	13
Overall	24	11	19	12

Spain. It can also be seen in the table that the incidence of postoperative diagnosis is higher for the nonuniversity hospitals >500 beds, and that nonoperative cardiovascular diagnosis predominates in the smaller nonuniversity hospitals.

It is appreciated that these differences may influence the results of the study, and therefore they will be considered during the analysis to be performed on the database whenever indicated.

Severity of Illness

The Simplified Acute Physiology Score (SAPS-II) [3] and the Mortality Prediction Model (MPM) [6] were used in the study as severity of illness scoring systems. Allowing for stratification of patients according to severity of illness, the scores are able to predict the mortality of the admitted patients in the ICU concerned. This information is important for comparing the observed with the expected mortality, usually expressed as a mortality ratio. The mortality ratios of various ICUs can be compared in this way and used as a measure of their effectiveness, as the compared ratios are controlled for severity of illness. The standardized mortality ratio (SMR) is equal to 1 when the observed mortality matches the expected mortality, and some ICUs will perform better (SMR < 1), and others will perform worse (SMR > 1) than expected. It was decided during the design of EURICUS-I that SMRs would be used as the measure of effectiveness. In other words, the SMRs of the ICUs were to be used as the dependent variable throughout the whole study whenever effectiveness was to be considered. This issue is further discussed in the section "The Multiple Regression Analyses:

Table 16. Mean SAPS-II scores

	Type of ICU			Type of hospital				Overall
	Medical	Surgical	General	<300 Beds	300–500 Beds	>500 Beds	University	
European area								
Poland	35.7	36.4	39.3	37.4	38.9	40.3	33.9	37.1
Germany			28.5			30.2	24.1	28.5
Denmark			29.6	20.9		32.0	32.5	29.6
Finland			30.2	31.4		32.1	27.9	30.2
Netherlands		31.8	29.4		25.8	34.3	31.8	29.7
Belgium	31.5	26.4	30.2	25.0		28.7	32.6	29.8
France	34.7	30.0	38.9	38.9			33.8	35.2
United Kingdom			38.5			38.5	38.6	38.5
Italy			37.3		37.5	35.7	39.9	37.3
Spain-Catalonia			35.4	33.1	32.0		37 0	35.4
Spain-Valencia	36.4		37.5	38.5	36.7	36.5	37.7	37.4
Portugal			37.5		34.4	47.0	35.8	37.5
Overall	34.8	29.4	33.6	31.4	33.1	33.4	34.3	33.5

Testing the Hypotheses". Two reasons for choosing to use two scoring systems with identical capabilities of identifying effectiveness were: (1) SAPS-II is scored 24 h after admission whereas MPM is scored at admission. The use of MPM is therefore complementary to that of SAPS-II for those patients staying < 1 day in the ICU. (2) It was considered opportune to compare the predictive performance of the two scoring systems on a large and multicentre database independent of the database in which the two scores were developed. However, as four ICUs in the study did not collect the MPM scoring system on their patients, only SAPS-II was used to compute the SMRs to be used in the study in order to maximize the number of enrolled ICUs. The MPM data will be used for the research purposes indicated in (2) above, which are not included in the context of EURICUS-I.

Table 16 displays the mean SAPS-II scores in the ICUs of the European regions according to hospital size and type and ICU type. The original SAPS-II did not fit the sample well and the scoring system was customized for the EURICUS-I population (see Chap. 8 "Analysis of ICU Performance"). The mean SAPS-II scores oscillated between 28.5 in the ICUs from Denmark and 38.5 in the ICUs from the UK. The mean SAPS-II score (33.5) increased with the size of the nonuniversity hospitals, and was higher in university hospitals. Medical ICUs had a higher mean SAPS-II score than surgical ICUs.

Mortality

Mortality was used in EURICUS-I as the measurable clinical output of the ICUs. Table 17 presents the overall mean mortality in the ICU and Table 18 the mor-

Table 17. ICU mortality rate (%)

	Type of ICU			Type of hospital				Overall
	Medical	Surgical	General	< 300 Beds	300–500 Beds	> 500 Beds	University	
European area								
Poland	14	30	25	14	21	25	15	19
Germany			6			6	5	6
Denmark			13	6		13	17	13
Finland			8	9		10	7	8
Netherlands		22	9		9	8	22	10
Belgium	11	4	8	5		6	9	7
France	14	29	14	14			17	16
United Kingdom			20			21	20	20
Italy			18		14	19	19	18
Spain-Catalonia			15	10	13		18	15
Spain-Valencia	18		15	12	15	12	18	16
Portugal			14		9	26	14	14
Overall	15	11	12	10	14	11	14	13

Table 18. Hospital mortality rate (%)

	Type of ICU			Type of hospital				Overall
	Medical	Surgical	General	<300 Beds	300–500 Beds	>500 Beds	University	
European area								
Poland	19	32	25	20	26	27	17	23
Germany			9			10	8	9
Denmark			20	8		21	26	20
Finland			14	19		16	12	14
Netherlands		29	15		16	14	29	16
Belgium	17	6	13	8		9	14	12
France	19	32	21	21			22	22
United Kingdom			31			31	31	31
Italy			26		21	26	27	26
Spain-Catalonia			21	16	19		23	21
Spain-Valencia	23		20	15	20	18	23	21
Portugal			21		19	32	17	21
Overall	20	14	18	15	20	16	20	18

tality in the hospital, according to European area, type and size of hospital and type of ICU. The differences between corresponding figures in both tables provide information regarding the mortality observed in the hospital after discharge from the ICU. The overall mortality in the ICU was 13% and that in the hospital 18%. The ICU mortality in university hospitals and in nonuniversity hospitals with 300–500 beds is equal, and about 5% higher than that observed in the other two categories of nonuniversity hospitals. The overall mortality varies between 9% in the German ICUs and 31% in the British ICUs (Table 18).

The overall mortality in the hospital wards after discharge from the ICU is 6%, ranging between 3% in Germany and 10% in the UK. A record of the clinical status was made at the time of discharge from the hospital. The relevant patients were not researched by EURICUS-I after discharge from the ICU, e.g. severity of illness of the patients at discharge, nursing work provided on the wards. The differences among the post-ICU discharge mortality seem however very large to be explained only by differences in severity of illness of the patients at admission at the ICUs. Let us take the example of the ICUs of Denmark, with the lowest mean severity of illness at admission and where the post-ICU discharge mortality was 7%, one of the highest in the whole group. Large differences can also be seen in the other selected stratifications in the table. The reasons for this higher mortality might be, for example, organizational aspects resulting in premature discharge of patients, such as shortage of staff and/or beds; lack of step-down units; poor clinical performance on the wards, such as inappropriate staff coverage.

Table 19 presents the observed mortality and the predicted mortality according to the original SAPS and the customized SAPS. After applying the exclu-

Table 19. Observed mortality rate and mortality rate predicted by original SAPS-II and by a customized version of SAPS-II according to European area, type of hospital and type of ICU

	Observed mortality (%)	SAPS-II predicted mortality (%)	Customized SAPS-II predicted mortality (%)
European area			
Poland	23	27	24
Germany	12	16	15
Denmark	21	19	17
Finland	17	18	17
Netherlands	17	18	17
Belgium	13	16	16
France	21	24	22
United Kingdom	29	29	26
Italy	24	26	23
Spain-Catalonia	22	24	21
Spain-Valencia	23	26	23
Portugal	21	26	23
Type of hospital			
<300 Beds	14	19	18
300–500 Beds	19	22	20
>500 Beds	20	22	20
University	22	23	21
Type of ICU			
Medical	21	23	21
Surgical	19	17	16
General	20	22	20
Overall	20	22	20

Values are presented as percentage.

sion criteria described in the literature: patients < 18 years of age, readmissions, acute coronary disease, burns, postoperative cases after coronary artery bypass surgery, and patients staying in the ICU for a period of less than 8 h, SAPS-II was computed for 10642 patients in EURICUS-I. For each group considered, the overall mean mortality was compared with the predicted mortality using the prediction equation of SAPS-II and a customized version of the system. The important difference between the two tables is that the 5000 patients excluded for the calculation of SAPS-II in Table 19 are included in Table 18. The overall (total) mean mortality in Table 18 is 2% lower than that registered in Table 19 after customization of SAPS-II. The overall range of differences is small and only higher than 2% on the ICUs from Denmark (4%) and the UK (3%), in which the predicted mortality was lower than the observed mortality, and in the ICUs from Germany (3%) and Belgium (3%), in which the inverse observation was made.

These data may suggest that the participating ICUs of the latter two countries contributed a relatively large number of less severely ill patients to the study than did the ICUs from the former two countries. The other important information presented in Table 19 is the differences between observed and predicted mortality in each aggregated group.

Table 20. Differences between observed and predicted (customized SAPS-II) mortality according to type of patient

	Unscheduled surgery		Scheduled surgery		Medical	
	Observed mortality (%)	Predicted mortality (%)	Observed mortality (%)	Predicted mortality (%)	Observed mortality (%)	Predicted mortality (%)
European area						
Poland	42	39	11	14	23	23
Germany	26	29	5	10	13	18
Denmark	20	17	8	6	28	23
Finland	16	19	6	8	24	21
Netherlands	23	20	6	8	25	24
Belgium	17	21	4	9	19	19
France	20	20	9	13	21	22
United Kingdom	30	29	12	11	35	31
Italy	30	26	6	11	31	29
Spain-Catalonia	28	28	17	13	22	21
Spain-Valencia	31	29	15	15	22	23
Portugal	22	28	5	11	28	27
Admitted from						
Operating theatre	24	25	6	10	23	21
Recovery room	27	21	8	8	18	18
Emergency room	17	19	14	16	18	21
Ward	35	27	13	12	33	25
Other ICU	27	25	24	12	40	26
Other hospital	29	30	26	12	25	23
Type of hospital						
<300 Beds	13	20	4	9	18	20
300–500 Beds	26	24	7	10	21	22
>500 Beds	27	26	7	10	25	24
University	26	26	9	10	26	23
Type of ICU						
Medical	23	22	11	12	22	21
Surgical	25	21	5	10	36	19
General	25	25	8	10	24	23
Overall	25	25	7	10	24	23

Table 21. Observed and predicted (customized SAPS-II) mortality by type of hospital

	< 300 Beds		300–500 Beds		> 500 Beds		University	
	Observed mortality (%)	Predicted mortality (%)	Observed mortality (%)	Predicted mortality (%)	Observed mortality (%)	Predicted mortality (%)	Observed mortality (%)	Predicted mortality (%)
Europan area								
Poland	21	23	28	27	27	30	18	19
Germany					14	17	8	11
Denmark	7	9			22	19	28	20
Finland	18	17			16	18	16	15
Netherlands			14	13	20	21	26	18
Belgium	8	11			15	14	15	18
France	19	26					22	20
United Kingdom					30	26	27	26
Italy			20	24	25	22	23	26
Spain-Catalonia	15	19	15	18			27	23
Spain-Valencia	16	24	20	22	22	21	27	24
Portugal			18	19	33	35	18	21
Type of admission								
Unscheduled surgical	13	20	26	24	27	26	26	25
Scheduled surgical	4	9	7	10	7	10	9	10
Medical	18	20	21	22	25	24	26	23
Admitted from								
Operating theatre	7	14	15	17	15	16	15	16
Recovery room	0	12	7	8	16	14	18	14
Emergency room	12	18	17	20	21	23	19	22
Ward	28	22	28	24	30	25	35	25
Other ICU	27	20	36	19	36	29	36	27
Other hospital	20	22	25	26	24	21	29	26
Overall	14	18	19	20	20	20	22	24

It is generally accepted that the use of observed vs predicted mortality ratios (SMRs) provides a reliable benchmark for comparing the performance (clinical effectiveness) of ICUs or groups of ICUs. When applying this methodology to the ICUs in Table 19 the resulting SMRs oscillate between 0.20 (best performance) and 1.99 (worse performance).

Table 20 presents the differences between observed and predicted mortality (customized SAPS-II) stratifying the patients according to type of admission. Table 21 presents the differences between observed and predicted mortality when stratifying the patients according to hospital category.

Type of Admission

The risk-adjusted mortality concerning surgical scheduled patients (SMR = 0.73) is better than the risk-adjusted mortality for surgical unscheduled (SMR = 1.00) and medical patients (SMR = 1.03).

Origin of Patients

The risk-adjusted mortality varies according to the place from where the patients came to the ICUs, with the SMRs oscillating from 0.84 (ori-gin was the emergency room or operating theatre) to 1.45 (origin was other ICU).

Hospital Category

The SMRs increased with the size of the nonuniversity hospitals from 0.78 to 1.01 and were higher for university hospitals (1.06). These figures might suggest that better clinical performance is achieved with surgical scheduled patients and with those originating from the emergency room and that the smallest nonuniversity hospitals are the best performers of all hospitals. That the ICUs from Denmark and from the UK are among the worse performers in the sample may indeed be associated with the reduced or even absent recruitment of ICUs of small nonuniversity hospitals in their country samples.

Workload

The Therapeutic Intervention Scoring System (TISS) [7, 8] is currently used to measure nursing workload in the ICU. During the preparation phase of EURICUS-I it was decided that a simplified version of TISS-28 items [8] should be used. The Nine Equivalents of Nursing Manpower Use Score (NEMS) was developed and validated in the TISS-28 database of the Foundation for Research on Intensive Care in Europe (FRICE) [9]. NEMS was used in EURICUS-I as the measure of daily nursing workload at patient level. The mean values of NEMS and TISS-28 are not different, and the mean scores of both therapeutic indexes are about 4 points higher than the mean score of the original TISS.

Table 22 shows the mean first-day NEMS and the mean overall NEMS of the ICUs of each European area, also according to type and size of the hospitals. Overall, the mean NEMS first-day is slightly higher (26.8) than the average NEMS of the units (26.5). In the ICUs of some countries the difference between these two means is inversed, and the mean first-day NEMS is lower than the average

Table 22. First day NEMS and mean overall NEMS

	Day 1 NEMS	Average NEMS of ICUs
European area		
Poland	24.9	22.1
Germany	28.0	28.6
Denmark	23.5	26.2
Finland	27.2	28.4
Netherlands	28.0	28.0
Belgium	27.9	27.0
France	26.0	23.8
United Kingdom	29.3	29.2
Italy	28.4	27.1
Spain-Catalonia	27.0	27.3
Spain-Valencia	25.5	25.2
Portugal	28.0	27.7
Type of hospital		
<300 Beds	23.2	24.0
300–500 Beds	24.3	24.5
>500 beds	28.7	28.1
University	27.3	26.8
Overall	26.8	26.5

NEMS, Nine Equivalents Manpower Use Score.

ICU NEMS. This is probably related to a high turnover of less severely ill patients in some units.

Figure 1 shows the relationship between the first-day NEMS score and the length of stay (LOS). In this figure the patients who died were excluded. A large percentage of mortality occurred during the first 48 h and the graphic expression of the relation of NEMS with LOS is difficult. The mean first-day NEMS was higher for surgical patients than for medical patients. It appears that the first-day NEMS score is a predictor of LOS. Figure 2 shows the decay of mean NEMS over LOS for all types of ICUs, showing that NEMS decreases over time.

Table 23 lists the percentual distribution at patient level of the nine activities registered in NEMS, according to country, ICU type and hospital category. Overall, as expected, the incidence of basic monitoring and intravenous medication was about 100% in all groups. The incidence of the other items varied between 3% (dialysis) and 61% (supplementary ventilatory support). The variance of the incidence of the various items could be explained by the variables country, ICU type and hospital category or by the interactions between these explanatory variables.

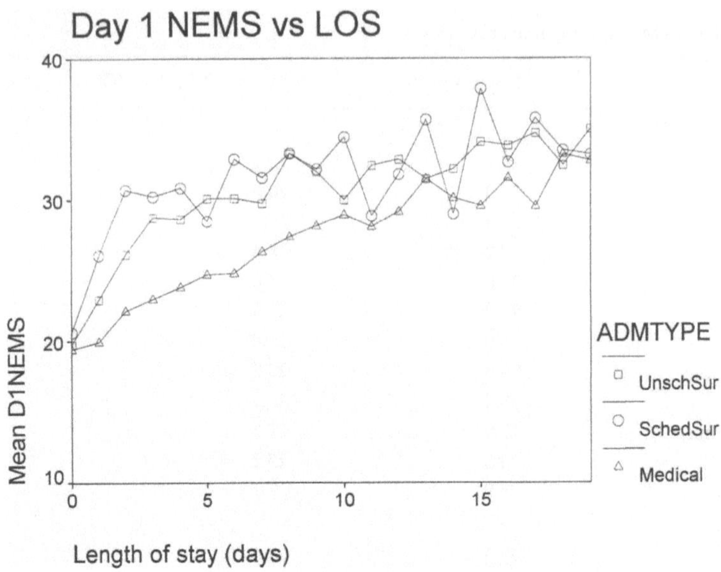

Fig. 1. First day Nine Equivalents Manpower Use Score (NEMS) and length of stay (LOS): survivors

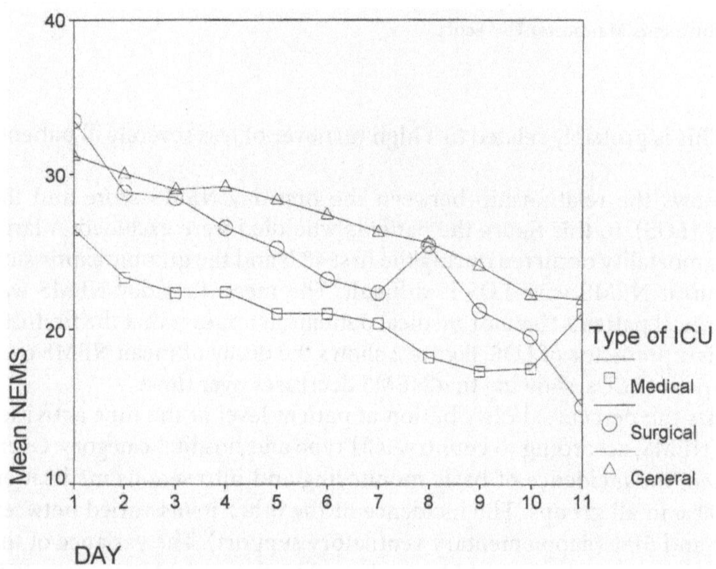

Fig. 2. Mean Nine Equivalents Manpower Use Score (NEMS) and types of ICU

Table 23. NEMS, European area, type of ICU and hospital

	Activities (%)								
	Basic moni-toring	Intravenous medication	Mechanical ventilation	Supplementary ventilatory support	Single vaso-active medication	Multiple vaso-active medication	Dialysis techniques	Interventions inside the ICU	Interventions outside the ICU
European area									
Poland	100	95	31	47	40	19	2	40	17
Germany	100	97	52	58	49	25	4	34	15
Denmark	99	90	35	63	24	16	2	22	13
Finland	100	95	61	42	36	16	4	24	15
Netherlands	99	86	55	52	21	45	5	20	16
Belgium	100	98	47	63	46	25	3	25	15
France	100	94	50	56	30	15	8	39	26
United Kingdom	100	94	59	54	35	24	6	42	31
Italy	100	96	62	66	41	23	4	39	33
Spain-Catalonia	100	95	48	70	49	26	4	26	22
Spain-Valencia	98	96	35	68	49	22	2	32	22
Portugal	100	100	66	78	47	21	5	37	15
Type of ICU									
Medical	100	96	23	54	28	14	4	32	14
Surgical	100	98	76	61	48	22	2	23	25
General	99	94	48	62	40	25	4	30	20
Type of hospital									
<300 Beds	100	92	32	61	33	15	2	24	16
300–500 Beds	100	93	31	70	40	17	3	27	16
>500 Beds	100	95	56	58	42	33	4	28	18
University	99	96	52	60	40	22	4	33	23
Overall	99	95	48	61	40	24	3	30	20

Use of the Facilities

Length of Stay

The patients enrolled in EURICUS-I spent 82894 days in the ICUs, a mean of 5.2±10.1; median of 2 days; interquartile range between 0.9 and 4.9 days. LOS oscillated between 0 (<1 day) to 291 days.

Table 24 presents the distribution of LOS (ranking of median) according to European region, size and type of hospital, type of ICU and origin of patients. As might be expected, patients admitted from other ICUs stayed longer (median 8.4 days) than patients coming from the operating theatre the RR (median 1 day). The median LOS of scheduled surgical patients was also smaller than that of the other types of admission. There was a regional pattern observed in the median of LOS when aggregating the patients by European area. Except for the ICUs of Poland, the median LOS of the ICUs to the south of (inclusive) France was larger than the median LOS of those ICUs in northern Europe. This pattern of LOS does not exactly parallel the SAPS-II differences displayed in Table 16.

Table 25 shows the percentual distribution of patients (survivors and nonsurvivors) in relation to LOS. Some 30% of the survivors had a LOS <1 day and a total of 64% of these patients stayed in the ICUs for a period <3 days. Nonsurvivors stayed longer in the ICU than patients who were alive at discharge from the hospital. The pattern of LOS in the nonsurvivors group of patients was similar to that of the group of survivors, 48% of the patients who died stayed in the ICUs for a period of time <3 days.

Length of Stay and Age

Stratifying the patients by age, the median LOS increased significantly with age: 2 days in the group of patients between 18 and 24 years, and 2.2 days in the group of patients between 65 and 74 years. The LOS decreased in patients older than 84 years of age.

Length of Stay and Type of Admission

The median LOS was significantly shorter in the group of surgical scheduled admissions (1 day) than in the group of surgical unscheduled patients (2.4 days) and medical patients (3 days). The difference in LOS between the latter two groups of patients was also statistically significant.

Length of Stay and Origin of Patients

The patients admitted from the operating theatre and from the recovery room had a shorter LOS (median 1.2 days) than patients originating from the emergency room (2.8 days), the ward (3.1 days) and other ICUs/other hospitals (4.8 days). The differences between these groups were statistically significant (with and without correcting for SAPS-II score). These differences can be seen in Fig. 3, which presents the decrease in the percentage of patients in each of the considered categories in relation to LOS in the ICUs.

Table 24. Length of stay (LOS) according to European area, type of hospital, type of ICU, type of patient and location in the hospital before ICU admission

Length of stay	N	Median	Percentile 25	Percentile 75	Mean	≤D
All patients	16056	2.04	.94	4.88	5.16	10.10
European region						
Portugal	438	5.59	1.90	13.83	10.75	16.63
Poland	625	3.50	1.67	7.81	6.31	8.38
France	804	3.72	1.69	7.92	7.65	15.87
Spain	3050	3.50	1.88	6.08	6.06	8.73
Spain-Catalonia	1527	3.27	1.81	6.92	7.51	12.15
Italy	777	3.00	1.08	7.24	7.23	13.12
Belgium	2262	1.88	0.95	3.00	3.30	7.27
United Kingdom	833	1.72	0.85	3.98	4.29	9.08
Germany	1458	1.21	0.84	3.00	4.09	9.04
Denmark	1251	1.01	0.75	2.92	3.07	5.96
Finland	1348	1.00	0.84	2.39	3.42	7.98
Netherlands	531	1.00	0.79	3.02	3.97	10.29
Type of hospital						
300–500 Beds	2282	2.73	1.04	5.19	5.06	8.25
University	6957	2.29	0.95	5.69	5.96	11.28
<300 Beds	1913	2.13	0.96	4.65	4.71	10.43
>500 Beds	4904	1.88	0.91	3.87	4.29	8.81
Type of ICU						
Medical	1659	3.17	1.67	6.00	5.51	8.58
Surgical	1065	1.99	1.06	4.33	5.25	9.48
General	13332	1.99	0.92	4.75	5.11	10.32
Type of patient						
Medical	8386	2.98	1.33	3.02	6.04	10.88
Unscheduled surg.	2557	2.36	0.90	6.73	6.61	11.86
Scheduled surg.	4709	1.04	0.88	2.30	3.01	7.02
Admitted from						
Other ICU	345	8.38	3.17	20.73	14.39	15.85
Other hospital	993	4.06	1.92	9.85	8.79	14.61
Ward	2646	3.12	1.35	7.17	6.83	11.15
Emergency room	4724	2.75	1.20	4.93	4.75	7.64
Operating theatre	5708	1.27	0.88	2.90	3.72	8.68
Recovery room	573	1.04	0.82	2.96	3.90	9.09

Table 25. Length of stay (LOS) and hospital outcome

	Number of patients	Mortality rate (%)
Length of stay (days)		
1	4846	15.4
2	3036	12.6
3	1968	14.0
4	1355	13.7
5	888	16.2
6	617	19.0
7	475	20.4
8	351	27.1
9	277	22.4
10	211	32.2
11	164	32.9
12	176	29.5
13	112	36.6
14	115	35.7
15	84	36.9
16	1207	40.3

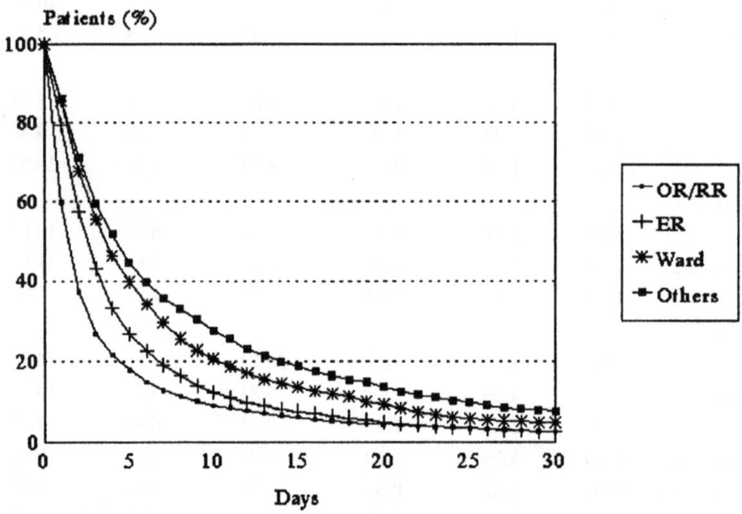

Fig. 3. Length of stay (LOS) and origin of patients ($n = 16056$)

Length of Stay and Diagnosis

The major diagnostic categories in the study were significantly associated with LOS after correcting for severity of illness. For all the diagnostic categories, LOS was shorter in the surgical groups of patients (scheduled/unscheduled) than in the medical group of patients. This pattern was however not observed regarding gastrointestinal and trauma diagnostic categories.

Length of Stay and Severity of Illness

Length of stay was correlated positively with severity of illness measured 24 h after admission (SAPS-II score). For example, patients with LOS <1 day had a mean SAPS score of 26.7; patients with LOS >30 days had a mean SAPS score of 43.5. However, this relationship fit only into a logistic curve as it did not follow a linear pattern. Using logistic binomial regression with random effects it was shown that the association of LOS and severity of illness did vary between the individual ICUs when controlling for severity of illness. In other words, LOS varied among the ICUs for patients with the same severity of illness.

Length of Stay and Workload

Patients with longer LOS had higher NEMSs. This association was observed both for: (a) the NEMS for the first 24 h (mean of 24.7 NEMS points for patients with LOS <1 day and 31.8 NEMS points for LOS >30 days); and (b) the mean NEMS score during the entire stay in the ICU (24.5 NEMS points for LOS <1day and 28.2 NEMS points for LOS >30 days). When introducing SAPS-II scores into the same equation, the explanatory power of the variance of NEMS was only slightly improved.

Using logistic binomial regression with random effects the variation in LOS was studied at patient level in relation to NEMS first-day score. As for the severity of illness, it could be shown that this relationship presented different patterns depending upon the ICU. In other words, the variation of LOS, when controlled for NEMS, was much larger among ICUs than within each ICU.

Prediction of Length of Stay

By regression analysis, age and SAPS-II score explains 10% of the variance of LOS at patient level. Aggregating LOS at ICU level, age and SAPS-II score explains 45% of the variance of LOS. However looking at the percentages in Table 25 the question asked is whether a patient will stay shorter or longer than 3 days in the ICU. Logistic regression analysis has shown that the combination of age and SAPS-II (independent variables) enables a correct prediction in 70% of the patients [$\text{logit}(\text{LOS} < 3 \text{ days}) = -1.5397 + (0.0624 \cdot \text{SAPS-II}) - (0.0156 \cdot \text{age})$]. Adding the 18 diagnostic categories used in the study, the prediction power of the equation at patient level increased to 72%. (Note: The prediction of LOS <3 days was calculated for the group of patients who survived until hospital discharge.)

Table 26. Mean annual volume by type of ICU and type of hospital

	Type of ICU			Type of hospital				Overall
	Medical	Surgical	General	<300 Beds	300–500 Beds	>500 Beds	University	
European area								
Poland	275	107	191	84	302	190	207	209
Germany			1467			1775	851	1467
Denmark			629	742		719	531	629
Finland			814	344		522	2338	814
Netherlands		389	705		449	1217	389	660
Belgium	1001	1819	1001	481		1410	1520	1137
France	724	332	323	323			593	485
United Kingdom			314			259	370	314
Italy			335		374	302	380	335
Spain-Catalonia			576	467	293		728	576
Spain-Valencia	728		455	389	427	820	528	484
Portugal			265		264	253	271	265
Overall	556	535	544	385	383	705	600	544

Patient Turnover

Volume of Annual Admissions

Table 26 shows the volume of annual admissions in the participating ICUs of the various European areas, according to hospital size and type and ICU type. Overall mean volume is presented in the Overall column. The annual figures were extrapolated from the volume of admissions registered during the 120 days of the field research. With a mean value of 544, there is a large variation in the volume of admissions of patients ranging from about 209 (Poland) up to a mean of about 1500 patients annually admitted to the participating ICUs from Germany. Volume has been negatively associated with the overall severity of illness and mortality at ICU level [10].

Number of Admissions per Bed per Year

The appropriateness of volume as a measure of turnover of patients remains to be determined. The admissions per bed per year (ABYs) seem however a rather convenient measure as they index volume by the number of beds in the ICU, thereby making turnover comparable. Table 27 presents the ABYs in the same format as in the previous table. With an overall mean ABY of 57, the range of the mean ABYs varied from about 34 in the ICUs in Poland to 87 in those in Belgium. At individual ICU level, the variation of ABYs was much larger, ranging from 11 (Polish ICU) up to 117 (Dutch ICU). A high turnover of patients (ABY >75) is associated with the number of surgical scheduled admissions and with the RR function of some ICUs.

Table 27. Mean number of admissions/bed/year (ABY) by type of ICU and type of hospital

	Type of ICU			Type of hospital				Overall
	Medical	Surgical	General	<300 Beds	300–500 Beds	>500 Beds	University	
European area								
Poland	44	20	30	21	45	21	36	34
Germany			77			73	86	77
Denmark			76	94		83	66	76
Finland			71	62		63	107	71
Netherlands		39	86		82	95	39	80
Belgium	78	108	84	81		93	87	87
France	44	33	46	46			40	43
United Kingdom			60			55	64	60
Italy			51		75	47	48	51
Spain-Catalonia			60	59	74		57	60
Spain-Valencia	50		45	52	48	32	44	46
Portugal			35		41	37	29	35
Overall	49	43	59	56	57	62	53	57

Occupancy Rate

Table 28 presents the mean occupancy rate (OR) registered in the ICUs in each European area during the field research period of the study, and according to hospital type and size and ICU type. The OR was computed by relating the total possible number of nursing days in the ICU (number of beds x 120 days) and the total number of patient-days registered during the period of study. Patient-days were calculated based on the dates and times of admission and discharge. When fractions of a day resulted from the difference between these two registration moments, the following criteria were applied: (a) for patients with a LOS <3 days only the dates of admission and discharge were used; (b) periods of time ≥ 12 h were rounded up to 1 day; (c) periods of time ≤ 12 h were rounded (up or down) to one fourth of 1 day.

ICUs with a high turnover do often admit more than one patient to the same bed on the same day. The use of this criterion, developed in other studies, should avoid the computation of ORs above 100%; however an OR above 100% was computed for three ICUs in the study (101%, 108% and 110%) and were rounded down to 100%. The overall OR was 71%, ranging between 56% and 85%. At ICU level (not shown in the table), 11 ICUs had an OR $<50\%$ of which one was lower than 25%. The ABYs on these ICUs were <35 except in one (ABY $=67$).

Table 28. Occupancy rate by type of ICU and type of hospital (%)

	Type of ICU			Type of hospital				Overall
	Medical	Surgical	General	<300 Beds	300–500 Beds	>500 Beds	University	
European area								
Poland	66.4	37.8	60.4	37.3	69.8	57.2	60.4	58.1
Germany			84.7			91.6	71.0	84.7
Denmark			61.3	60.1		63.7	60.2	61.3
Finland			70.4	73.8		67.4	69.7	70.4
Netherlands		90.4	79.0		78.1	80.9	90.4	80.6
Belgium	63.3	76.9	68.2	67.7		70.1	68.7	68.8
France	63.3	80.1	79.9	79.9			68.9	73.3
United Kingdom			58.5			54.3	62.8	58.5
Italy			79.7		78.2	76.7	86.3	79.7
Spain-Catalonia			82.7	76.1	66.5		91.6	82.7
Spain-Valencia	73.8		63.6	64.3	61.3	44.3	70.3	64.7
Portugal			84.7		74.9	109.8	82.1	84.7
Overall	67.0	63.1	71.0	66.6	69.2	70.6	71.7	70.1

Work Utilization Rate

Work utilization rate (WUR) establishes the ratio between the nursing work expended in the unit, as measured by the therapeutic index NEMS, and the nursing work available in the unit during the same period of time. The nursing work expended was computed by the total sum of NEMS points produced [2]. The NEMS score corresponds to a period of 24 h; a criterion similar to that used for OR was used for the computation of NEMS. Missing values (600 out of 80000) were handled in the following way: (a) the mean daily NEMS value of the unit was attributed to the missing first-day NEMS; (b) the missing last-day NEMS was attributed the NEMS value of the previous day; (c) a missing NEMS during the stay of the patient was assigned the mean value of the two known NEMSs, before and after that particular date. The available nursing work in the unit was derived from the total number of nursing full-time equivalents (FTEs) and admitting that: (a) one nurse (FTE) works 200 days per year, after discounting for holidays, illness, etc; (b) 1 day of nursing work corresponds to 46 NEMS points [8]; (c) 1 day nursing work corresponds to three nursing shifts.

Table 29 presents the mean WUR computed for the ICUs in each European area during the field research period of the study and according to hospital type and size and ICU type. With an overall mean of 72%, the WUR ranged between 40% and 112%. At ICU level (not shown in the table) WUR ranged between 30% and 172%. Abnormal values were rechecked at ICU level and two were discarded (12% and 480%). Eleven ICUs had a WUR >100% (of which six were above 120%); 19 ICUs had WUR below 50%.

Table 29. Work utilization ratio by type of ICU and type of hospital

	Type of ICU			Type of hospital				Overall
	Medical	Surgical	General	< 300 Beds	300–500 Beds	> 500 Beds	Uni-versity	
Euopean area								
Poland	0.62	0.47	0.62	0.60	0.73	0.35	0.52	0.59
Germany			1.12			1.51	0.74	1.12
Denmark			0.49	0.52		0.55	0.45	0.49
Finland			0.65	0.67		0.60	0.70	0.65
Netherlands		0.85	0.74		0.77	0.68	0.85	0.76
Belgium	0.88	1.34	0.94	0.88		1.11	0.99	1.00
France	0.72	0.80	1.12	1.12			0.74	0.89
United Kingdom			0.40			0.39	0.40	0.40
Italy			0.86		0.80	0.86	0.88	0.86
Spain-Catalonia			0.91	0.82	0.65		1.04	0.91
Spain-Valencia	1.12		0.59	0.66	0.54	0.37	0.77	0.64
Portugal			0.91		0.90	0.78	1.00	0.91
Overall	0.78	0.80	0.71	0.77	0.68	0.70	0.74	0.72

A WUR above 100% might have been caused by: (a) a miscalculation associated with a high turnover of patients and not fully corrected for by the criteria indicated above; (b) the use of nursing manpower from outside the ICU (additional FTEs) to cope with workload demands. The utilization of the ICU is often evaluated by the value of the OR. It is however important to include the WUR as a measure of the utilization of the ICU. Five examples of the database are displayed in Table 30.

Table 30. Examples of work utilization ratio and utilization of ICUs

ICU example[a]	A	B	C	D	E
Number of beds	16	12	8	6	5
Work utilization ratio	80	81	69	74	96
Occupancy rate	74	56	87	56	72
Length of stay	2.7	6.4	4.5	6.5	2.9
Admissions per bed per year	117	39	72	29	94
Mean NEMS	37	25	23	31	21
Mortality	11	11	25	32	12
Medical + surgical unscheduled (%)	35	57	66	57	61

NEMS, Nine Equivalents Manpower Use Score.
[a] For explanation, see text.

Examples

ICU A is a large unit admitting predominantly surgical scheduled patients. Having one of the largest turnovers registered in the study, the OR and the WUR of the ICU are rather low. ICU A is an example of a high turnover and underutilized unit.

ICU B is a large general unit. Having a low turnover, the WUR of the ICU is proportionally high when associated with the low OR. This suggests that the low turnover and OR of this unit may be related to a shortage of nursing staff. A rather similar picture appears with the example of ICU D, although this unit is much smaller than ICU B. ICU C is a small unit admitting predominantly medical patients. With a median turnover, the ICU has a high OR and a reduced WUR. In other words, as the beds are physically well utilized, the nursing manpower available to this unit is underutilized. The leadership of this ICU might wish to consider whether increasing the utilization of manpower could have any impact upon the high mortality in the unit. ICU E is an example of a very small unit with a high turnover of patients and a full utilization of the nursing manpower available. Maybe because of reasons pointed out in ICUs B and D, the OR in this unit is rather low. ICUs D and E illustrate the frequent difficulty of coordinating the use of resources (beds and nurses) in small sized units. Admitting that these particular units are appropriately sized, the hospital management might wish to consider the integration of them together with other critical care areas in the hospital (e.g. RR, emergency room) into a larger organization, the Critical Care Department of the hospital.

Conclusions

The substudy *Patients and Facilities* gathered a large database of ICUs in Europe. The analysis of the collected data presented in this report was aimed at making a survey of the ICUs with the focus on differences between ICUs and European areas. Other analytic strategies are therefore possible. The design of the study will not allow inferences to be made regarding differences between European countries; however, several analyses performed indicated that significant differences may exist. One important consequence of the selection of ICUs made at country level regards the inclusion criteria concerning hospital categories. Besides the documented differences between ICUs of university and nonuniversity hospitals, the results of the survey made suggest that ICUs of the large nonuniversity hospitals (>500 beds) have distinct characteristics, consistent with lower severity of illness and a high turnover of patients.

The differences concerning the professional grade and number of both nursing and physician staffs is very large among ICUs. These differences are associated with the European areas in the study rather than with the characteristics of the patients admitted to the ICUs. This suggests that the currently used guidelines for staffing the ICUs should be revisited.

The medical or surgical type of admission and the origin of the patients (operating theatre, ward, other ICU, etc.) are relevant markers of severity of illness of the admitted patients and a predictor of outcome of the patients in EURICUS-I.

The clinical management of patients differs between the ICUs in essential aspects, after controlling for severity of illness. One relevant aspect concerns LOS: the pattern of LOS vs severity of illness was rather constant at ICU level, but exhibited a large variance between the ICUs. Another aspect concerns the use of nursing manpower vs severity of illness, in which the same pattern was found as for LOS. Next to LOS and OR, controlled for variables of case mix (e.g. severity of illness), the indexed utilization of nursing manpower (WUR) has proved to be a good indicator of the use of resources on the ICU.

Organization

W. van Rossum

Introduction

In order to reach its medical objectives, an ICU should be adequately managed and organized. The goal of this section is to investigate the extent to which managerial and organizational factors contribute to the medical performance of European ICUs. The relationship between managerial and organizational factors and medical performance has in the past been extensively studied. These studies focused upon particular wards, i.e. emergency rooms [11]; hospital wards in general (although emphasizing the treatment of surgical patients [12]; and ICUs [13, 14]. Although the researchers pointed out the importance of adequate organizational and managerial arrangements, nevertheless, their findings with respect to the relationship between managerial and organizational factors and medical performance were not conclusive.

One could not, definitively, indicate that particular managerial and organizational practices are related to better medical performance. By contrast, however, the Dutch psychologist Wagenaar, in a study on risk management, found that the occurrence of mistakes in an ICU was significantly related to organizational factors (Wagenaar, personal communication).

There are several explanations for the inconclusiveness of the findings of these studies. First, although the nature of particular medical and nursing tasks, as well as aspects of (financial) scarcity, presume management and organization of medical tasks, measuring the adequacy of both occurs at different levels. Medical performance is accomplished at the interindividual level of the interaction between medical and nursing personnel and patients. Managerial and organizational factors, however, are measured in terms of and at the collective level of units or subunits within a hospital. The overlap between the two levels is not self-evident. Second, in some cases, i.e. the ICU, the relationship between medical performance and managerial/organizational factors may be expected to be more directly related, as the medical and nursing tasks are more to be considered as team-related efforts. But in this case too, some problems to be solved are specifically at the individual level (such as the sudden deterioration of the health state of a patient) and others are at the level of the work group, such as the uncertainty as a consequence of unpredictable work flows. These problems, as we will see later, can only be solved by different organizational means. Third, the comparability of subunits and units within hospitals is not self-evident. This is especially a case in point regarding the ICU.

An ICU is commonly circumscribed in terms of the (multidisciplinary) treatment of critically ill patients using advanced medical technology. This does not, however, delimit the boundaries of the ICU in organizational terms. Compare, for example, the situation in which the treatment of intensive care patients, though located in an ICU, is predominantly the responsibility of specialists outside the ICU, with the situation of an ICU with its own separate team of physicians responsible for the treatment of intensive care patients. Only in the latter case, can one, in organizational terms, speak of the existence of an ICU. Moreover, there exists a large difference between the nature of ICUs in large, e.g. university, hospitals and the nature of ICUs in small, peripheral hospitals. Although the objective of the ICUs in both cases is similar, the fact that ICUs in the latter type of hospitals can refer patients to the former type of hospitals will most definitely influence the nature of the organization. A large percentage of patients with high severity of illness scores will require another type of organization than a small percentage of such patients.

In this section we therefore start the analysis of the influence of managerial and organizational factors with an indication of the variability of ICUs. This will be done by attempting to formulate profiles of ICUs based upon variables relevant for the nature of its management and organization. The second aspect to be taken care of is the difference between factors influencing performance at the individual and the collective level. We will come back to this distinction between the individual and collective level in the section on the explanation of medical performance.

In the next descriptive section we will deal with an overview of the organizational characteristics of the ICUs in the EURICUS-I data. In the following section we will test some hypotheses with respect to the effects of organizational factors upon the performance of ICUs. First, we will investigate the characteristics of the two performance measures at the level of ICUs. As we found that various types of ICUs – with respect to their score on the B20 and B80 – could be discerned, our objective in this section is to consider to what extent there are organizational differences between: (a) ICUs scoring high on both measures vs those scoring low on B20 and B80; (b) ICUs scoring low on one of the two measures, but higher on the other; and (c) ICUs scoring high on one, and lower on the other. In the final section we will investigate the degree to which managerial and organizational factors determine the medical performance of ICUs, measured by, respectively, B20 and B80.

The Organizational Variability of ICUs

The starting point for this overview is the assumption that ICUs can, from the point of view of organizational analysis, be considered as uncertainty reducing units. Uncertainty refers, in this case, to various aspects of the input of critically ill patients. This substudy on managerial and organizational determinants assumes that uncertainty has to be reduced not only by medical, but also by managerial and organizational means. It is the combination of medical and managerial and organizational means, rather than the medical means alone, which will explain the extent to which ICUs can adequately treat critically ill patients.

In order to study the managerial and organizational characteristics of ICUs, we first have to establish the characteristics of the ICUs in the sample. Although the definition of ICUs as indicated above facilitates a comparison, different types of ICUs were sampled. Before engaging in an analysis of the effects of the managerial and organizational factors on the medical performance of the ICUs, we therefore analyze the variability of the ICUs.

Types of ICUs

The sample comprises ICUs in different types of hospitals. In the presentation of the results of the substudy on organization and management, we have made a distinction between four different categories of ICUs. ICUs within: (a) small (<300 beds), nonuniversity hospitals ($N=14$); (b) medium (300–500 beds), nonuniversity hospitals ($N=15$); (c) large (>500 beds), nonuniversity hospitals ($N=19$); (d) university hospitals ($N=29$).

This variable, types of ICUs, is directly related to the size of ICUs, in terms of the number of beds in each ICU. In Table 4 of the *Patients and Facilities* substudy the distribution of the size of ICUs is indicated for the various types of ICUs. The table shows that ICUs within university hospitals are relatively larger.

ICUs in Terms of Organizational Uncertainty

From a managerial/organizational point of view, uncertainty can be operationalized in terms of several attributes of the patient population of ICUs. (We do not include medical attributes, as we eventually want to study the relationship between managerial/organizational factors and medical performance.) We choose the following variables to measure the organizational uncertainty to be dealt with in the ICUs:

- *Number of patients to be treated related to their LOS*: This variable is operationalized by multiplying the number of admissions (averaging over the years 1991–1993) with the LOS (also the average over 1991–1993) and dividing this by the number of beds of the ICU. Table 31 shows that there is a significant relationship between the complexity of the input of ICUs and the type of ICUs. As can be expected, ICUs in university hospitals are characterized by a more complex input than the other types of hospitals (especially the smaller and medium sized hospitals), whereas the large, nonuniversity hospitals have an overrepresentation of cases on both ends of the continuum.

- *Occupancy rate*: Table 32 shows that there are no large differences between the types of hospitals in terms of the average OR. Only in the case of the university hospitals can a relatively higher OR be discerned.
- *Length of stay*: The types of hospitals do not differ very much in terms of the average LOS of patients in ICUs. There is a tendency of a shorter LOS in the nonuniversity hospitals, and a medium LOS in the university hospitals (Table 33).

Table 31. ICU input: length of stay × number of admissions per bed[a]

	Type of hospital				Overall
	<300 Beds	300–500 Beds	>500 Beds	University	
Input					
50–295	6	3	8	5	22
256–295	2	8	2	10	22
296–456	4	2	7	9	22
Overall	12	13	17	24	66

[a] For details, see text.

Table 32. Average occupancy rate

	Type of hospital				Overall
	<300 Beds	300–500 Beds	>500 Beds	University	
Occupancy rate (%)					
19.4– 63.5	6	4	7	6	23
63.6– 79.2	3	6	5	13	27
79.3–109.8	5	5	7	10	27
Overall	14	15	19	29	77

Table 33. Average length of stay (LOS)

	Type of hospital				Overall
	<300 Beds	300–500 Beds	>500 Beds	University	
Length of stay (days)					
2.26– 4.03	5	5	8	8	26
4.04 6.35	7	6	5	9	27
6.36–16.16	2	4	6	12	24
Overall	14	15	19	29	77

- *Degree of scheduling of patients*: In order to obtain information about the degree to which the work flow of the ICU can be planned, we asked the medical director to what extent - in general - the incoming patients could be scheduled. The variable was operationalized as the percentage of patients that were scheduled (Table 34). This result is consonant with the patterns found for the frequency of admissions without previous knowledge (not presented here). Although there is no significant relationship between the percentage of patients scheduled and the types of hospitals, Table 34 elucidates that relatively more ICU patients in university hospitals were unscheduled than were ICU patients in other types of hospitals.
- *Degree of sudden deterioration of the health state of patients*: At the individual level, organizational uncertainty is a function of the number of patients that experience a sudden deterioration of their health state. We asked the medical director to indicate to what extent this happened in his/her ICU (Table 35). Furthermore, we asked for an indication of how often organs system failure occurred (Table 36). Task predictability, in terms of the frequency of sudden deterioration of the health state, and the frequency of organs system failure, does not significantly differ between the ICUs in the different types of hospitals. The only exception is the university hospitals in which a slightly higher frequency is reported.

Table 34. Percentage of admissions scheduled in advance

	Type of hospital				Overall
	<300 Beds	300–500 Beds	>500 Beds	University	
Scheduled admissions (%)					
1– 11	3	3	5	14	25
12– 39	7	6	9	7	29
40–100	3	5	4	6	18
Overall	13	14	18	27	72

Table 35. Deterioration of clinical condition

	Type of hospital				Overall
	<300 Beds	300–500 Beds	>500 Beds	University	
Weekly incidence of cases					
0– 4 times	6	3	6	9	24
5–10 times	8	8	11	13	40
>10 times		4	2	7	13
Overall	14	15	19	29	77

Table 36. Occurrence of organ system failures

	Type of hospital				Overall
	<300 Beds	300–500 Beds	>500 Beds	University	
Weekly occurrence of OSF					
Always		1			1
Often	3	1	2	2	8
Regularly	6	7	10	15	38
Rarely	5	6	7	12	30
Overall	14	15	19	29	77

In conclusion, one can say that only slight differences, with respect to the characteristics of their input of patients, could be found between the ICUs in different types of hospitals. It is safe to say that only ICUs in university hospitals show higher levels of uncertainty, both at the individual and at the collective level.

The Characterization of ICUs in Terms of Technologies Involved

One of the main characteristics of an ICU is the use of various advanced medical technologies to monitor and treat patients. Besides the organizational technologies which will be dealt with below, these medical technologies are the predominant means by which ICU can reduce uncertainty. In the questionnaire, a list of current technologies was included and ICUs were asked to indicate which medical technologies were available in the ICU. One can comprehend that most of the listed technologies would be available in all ICUs in the sample. In order to get an impression of the differences between ICUs with respect to available technologies, we formulated a scale, Available Advanced Technologies, representing the number of those technologies available within an ICU. These were, in general,

Table 37. Advanced medical technology

	Type of hospital				Overall
	<300 Beds	300–500 Beds	>500 Beds	University	
Number of advanced technologies					
0	2	1			3
1	4	3	3	2	12
2	1	2	5	4	12
3	5	2	6	10	23
4	1	2	1	5	9
5				5	5
Overall	13	10	15	26	64

only available in a minority of ICUs (i.e. <75% of the ICUs). This scale enabled a ranking of the ICUs in terms of most advanced technologies available (Table 37). The following technologies were included: A-V sequential; intra-aortic balloon pump; haemodialysis; peritoneal dialysis; CAVH or SCVF. The scale will also be used in the final explanatory analysis.

In general, most ICUs are remarkably similar with respect to the availability of most IC technologies. Nevertheless, Table 53 shows that there is, in terms of the availability of the less frequently used technologies, a clear distinction between the ICUs of university and nonuniversity hospitals. As we are, in this management and organization substudy, especially interested in the differences among ICUs, we will proceed with this scale. We have to emphasize that these differences only concern a smaller number of advanced technologies.

Theoretical Framework

The ICU is a special subunit of the hospital in which various types of medical expertise and advanced medical technologies are used to treat critically ill patients. What kinds of managerial practices and organizational structure should such a subunit have in order to lead to qualified medical performance? In contrast to many other work groups, in which the application of technologies results in more predictability of tasks and work flows, in the case of ICUs, the availability of advanced technologies will instead result in more uncertainty. The more advanced technologies that are available within the ICU, the more the ICU is able to treat more severely ill patients, and hence a growth in uncertainty which has to be reduced by specific managerial practices and organizational structure. This uncertainty arises at two levels: (1) at the level of the individual tasks to be performed by physicians and nurses and (2) at the level of the work group itself, i.e. in terms of the nature of the work flow. Managerial practices and organizational structure should be such that both sources of uncertainty can adequately be addressed. In a study of the organizational structure of American hospitals, Comstock and Scott [12] have indicated that the main objective of organizations is to reduce the uncertainty in their environment by attempting to increase technological predictability. The latter term refers to the extent to which an organization is able to adequately deal with the uncertainty of the input, i.e. to make it understandable to members of the organization. In the case of ICUs this means that the ICU needs to develop and implement such adequate managerial practices and an organizational structure that it can reach its objective to treat critically ill patients. As Comstock and Scott argue, technological predictability implies, at the individual level, the existence of an adequate degree of task predictability; and, at the collective level, an adequate degree of work flow predictability. In other words, more task and work flow predictability imply more organizational effectiveness and hence a better performance of the organization. In their view, the degree of task predictability is related to the degree of standardization within the organization (or work group) via two other variables, the degree of task differentiation and the level of the qualifications of the staff. The work flow predictability influences standardization via yet another variable, the degree of centralization of decision-making. Finally, Comstock and Scott presumed a relationship between the size of the organization or work group and the degree of centralization (a larger organization or work group will have less centralized decision-making); more differentiated staff roles and a lower level of qualifications of the members of the organization or work group.

Whereas Comstock and Scott applied their theory in an empirical analysis of the relationships between organizational structures of different wards in (American) hospitals, there are reasons to expect that the situation of ICUs is in this respect a special one. In general an increasing degree of implementation of technologies with the execution of tasks will result in an increasing degree of task and work flow predictability. However, in the case of the ICU, an increasing level of implementation of technologies will in itself result in a decrease of task and work flow predictability. The more advanced the medical technologies that are implemented in an ICU, the more severe the patients that can be treated. As a consequence, task and work flow predictability will decrease. This has specific consequences for the relationship between task and work flow predictability and the organizational and managerial variables. First and foremost, the level of standardization of tasks within an ICU will, in general, be less high than in other work groups. Moreover, at the level of the individual tasks, the level of qualifications of ICUs should be relatively high, in order to reduce the effects of the low level of task predictability. The same applies to the degree of task differentiation: the nature of the tasks implies a low level of task differentiation (or – as stated in other organizational studies of ICUs – the ICU should have a team-like structure). High qualifications and low task differentiation simultaneously imply a low level of standardization (Fig. 4).

A similar argument can be formulated regarding the nature of work flow predictability within an ICU. One may expect that the effect of the implementation of more advanced medical technologies will be a lower level of work flow predictability. Rather than centralizing decision-making (which would be the effect of a high degree of work flow predictability), the low degree of work flow predictabi-

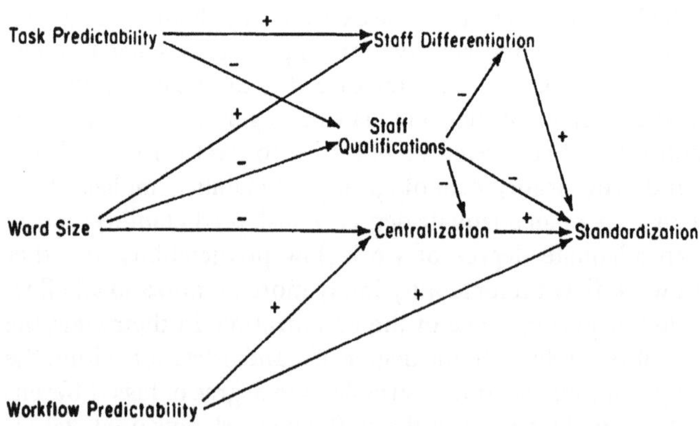

Fig. 4. Predicted relations between technology and structure in wards. (Adapted from [12])

lity of an ICU implies a lower degree of centralization of decision-making (or – as stated in other organizational studies of ICUs – a form of democratic decision-making). Finally, the effects of the variable size are difficult to establish in the case of an organizational analysis of ICUs. Not only is the range of the various sizes of ICUs not too great; but there is also a direct relationship between increasing size and increasing number of technologies employed in an ICU. As a consequence, the effect of the latter variable is difficult to separate from the size effect.

The central analysis of the *Organization* substudy started from the presumption that ICUs will differ in terms of the nature of the input; available technologies, and hence should have different types of organizational structures. In line with Comstock and Scott's theory, as described above, we will therefore formulate for each managerial and organizational variable a specific hypothesis regarding its contribution to differences in ICU performance. But first we will give a brief sketch of these variables.

The Variables

Task and Work Flow Predictability

As indicated above, we used, at the individual and collective level, several measures of the input of ICUs. These measures were used as, respectively, indicators of task and work flow predictability. We expect relationships between the measures of task and work flow predictability and the scale representing the number of advanced technologies.

- *Hypothesis 1*: Task and work flow predictability are negatively related to the number of advanced medical technologies available in the ICU.

In Table 38 the correlations are given between the Available Advanced Technologies scale and the operationalizations of task and work flow predictability. Work flow predictability is operationalized via the two variables indicated above, i.e. input and the percentage of scheduled patients (% scheduled). Task predictability is operationalized by an index calculated by adding the scores on the two questions indicating, respectively, the frequency of sudden deterioration of the health state of patients and organ systems failure (TASKPRED).

The table shows only a small (not significant) relationship in the predicted direction of the advanced technology scale with task predictability. There are no relationships with the two operationalizations of work flow predictability. However, when we calculate the same correlations for only the ICUs within university hospitals, the findings are completely reversed. Now we find a negative relationship with work flow predictability, operationalized as the product of admissions and LOS, divided by the number of beds (INPUT). This indicates that ICUs with many of the advanced technologies have relatively more patients staying for a shorter time in the ICU. The advanced technology scale is now positively related to the percentage of scheduled patients. This refers to the fact that in ICUs within university hospitals with more of the advanced technologies, more patients will

Table 38. Correlations of advanced technology scale (TECH) with INPUT; %SCHEDULED; TASKPRED

All hospitals[a]	%SCHED	INPUT	TASKPRED	TECH
%SCHED	1.00	−0.05	−0.03	0.08
INPUT	−0.05	1.00	0.15	0.09
TASKPRED	−0.03	0.15	1.00	0.20
TECH	0.08	0.09	0.20	1.00
Correlations **only for ICUs within university hospitals**[b]				
%SCHED	1.00	−0.28	−0.05	0.36
INPUT	−0.28	1.00	0.21	0.20
TASKPRED	−0.05	0.21	1.00	−0.11
TECH	0.36	0.20	−0.11	1.00

[a] N of cases: 52; 2-tailed significance: * 0.01, ** 0.001
[b] N of cases: 20; 2-tailed significance; * 0.01, ** 0.001

be coming from the operating room. In the case of ICUs within university hospitals, the relationship to task predictability disappears. Apparently, more advanced technologies in this case do not result in a higher frequency of sudden deterioration of health states of patients and/or organ systems failure. Given these results, we will include in the final explanatory analysis the variable ICU within university or nonuniversity hospital (UNIV) and the advanced technology scale (TECH).

Task Differentiation

The ICU directors were asked to indicate to what extent tasks of various types of staff members (physicians, residents, head nurse, nurses) were done by other staff members. The more this is the case, the less task differentiation exists in the ICU. At the one extreme (complete differentiation) each staff member with a specific function has his/her own set of tasks; at the other, all tasks within the ICU are shared among all staff members. Although this operationalization does not exactly represent the extent to which a team-like structure exists, one may presume that the more an ICU has a team-like structure, the more tasks among various types of staff members are shared. We calculated a scale of task differentiation by adding the scores for the various types of personnel involved. A high score on this scale refers to a larger degree of task differentiation.

The ICUs within small nonuniversity hospitals predominantly have a medium level of task differentiation, whereas for the other types of ICUs large differences exist with respect to task differentiation (Table 39). As low values on this scale refer to more sharing of tasks, we may expect better performance of those ICUs with a relatively low differentiation score. Therefore, we expect a negative relationship between this variable and the medical performance of the ICUs:

Table 39. Task differentiation

	Type of hospital				Overall
	<300 Beds	300–500 Beds	>500 Beds	University	
Differentiation[a]					
19.9–27.1	2	4	8	9	25
27.9–29.1	11	3	5	8	27
29.9–33.1	1	6	6	11	24
Overall	14	13	19	28	74

[a] For explaration, see text.

- *Hypothesis 2*:The degree of task differentiation (DIFFTOT) is negatively related to the medical performance of the ICU.

Qualifications

The level of qualifications of the ICU should be established by aggregating the individual measurement of the qualifications of each staff member. The problem of a European comparative study, however, is that the nature of qualifications differs among the various nations. This is especially the case with the education of physicians. Whereas in some countries intensive care is a separate specialty, in others it is not. Consequently, we cannot take the number of physicians in the ICU with a formal training in intensive care, as, for example, an indicator of the degree of professionalism of the ICU (medical) staff. We therefore restricted the operationalization of the level of qualification of the ICU to a specific measurement of the percentage of nurses within the ICU having critical care training. Although this restricts the analysis to only one type of staff member, it still gives an adequate indication of the differences between ICUs in terms of qualifications. In Table 40 the distribution of this variable (QUALIF) is indicated for the various types of ICUs. The three categories stand for: (1) <5%; (2) 5%–50%, and (3) >50% nurses with critical care training.

Table 40. Percentage of nurses with special intensive care education

	Type of hospital				Overall
	<300 Beds	300–500 Beds	>500 Beds	University	
Level of ICU education					
1	4	7	6	9	26
2	4	1	9	10	24
3	6	7	4	10	27
Overall	14	15	19	29	77

1, <5%; 2, 5%–50%; 3, >50%.

It is surprising to note that there are no large differences between the various types of ICUs regarding the distribution of the percentage of nurses with critical care training. In the final explanatory analysis we expect that the variable QUALIF is positively related to the medical performance of ICUs (more adequately trained nurses will result in a higher performance):

- *Hypothesis 3*: The level of qualifications of an ICU, in terms of the percentage of nurses with specific critical care training, is positively related to the medical performance of the ICU.

Centralization

Several questions were asked regarding the way decisions were handled within the ICU. We asked, with respect to two specific policies (antibiotics and decubitus prevention) and with respect to admission and release of patients, who was involved in the decision-making. Tables 41 and 42 refer to, respectively, the nature of decision-making within the ICU regarding two policies: antibiotic prophylaxis and decubitus prevention. In Table 41, centralization refers to the extent to which the director, alone or with other physicians, makes decisions regarding this policy (the table refers to the policy at the patient level). In Table 42, centralization refers to the extent to which nurses and physicians are involved in decision-making concerning decubitus prevention (more centralization meaning less nurse involvement). Tables 43 and 44 refer to decision-making regarding, respectively, the admission of patients to the ICU or the release of patients from the ICU.

Table 41. Centralization of antibiotic prophylaxis

	Type of hospital				Overall
	< 300 Beds	300–500 Beds	> 500 Beds	University	
Director and physician	11	10	8	20	49
Director	2	5	11	9	27
Overall	13	15	19	29	76

Table 42. Centralization of decubitus prevention

	Type of hospital				Overall
	< 300 Beds	300–500 Beds	> 500 Beds	University	
Nurses involved	11	7	15	20	53
Director and physician	2	5	1	5	13
Director		3	3	4	10
Overall	13	15	19	29	76

Table 43. Centralization of the decision to admit a new patient

	Type of hospital				Overall
	<300 Beds	300–500 Beds	>500 Beds	University	
Nurses involved	1	5	2	8	16
Director and physician	4	1	5	4	14
Director	9	9	12	17	47
Overall	14	15	19	29	77

Table 44. Centralization of decision to remove a patient

	Type of hospital				Overall
	<300 Beds	300–500 Beds	>500 Beds	University	
Nurses involved	2	3	3	9	17
Director and physician	5	1	3	2	11
Director	7	11	13	17	48
Overall	14	15	19	28	76

Only in the case of decision-making concerning antibiotics prophylaxis do we find a clear and significant relationship between the extent of centralization of decision-making and the types of ICUs. In ICUs within small, nonuniversity hospitals, it is more often the director and the other physicians who make the decision. In ICUs within large nonuniversity hospitals, decision-making is relatively more centralized in this respect. Table 42 shows that in most cases, with respect to decision-making regarding decubitus prevention, nurses will be involved. There are no significant differences between the various types of ICUs. Tables 43 and 44 show that in all types of ICUs both centralized decision-making (only the director makes the decision) and decentralized decision-making (nurses and other physicians are involved) occur. There are in this respect no significant differences between the various types of ICUs.

Based upon these variables and those measuring centralization of decision-making on antibiotics prophylaxis and decubitus prevention on the unit level, we calculated an index (CENTRAL) that measures the level of centralized decision-making within the ICU. A high score on this variable implies more centralized decision-making. In Table 45, the scores are summarized in three categories.

The variable centralization of decision-making is not significantly related to the types of ICUs, although, as could be expected there is slightly more centralized decision-making in the large, nonuniversity hospitals. We expect that this variable is negatively related to the performance of ICUs. We indicated above that the specific uncertainty of ICUs implies more team-like work and hence less centralized decision-making. This results in the following hypothesis:

Table 45. Centralization of decision-making

	Type of hospital				Overall
	< 300 Beds	300–500 Beds	> 500 Beds	University	
Centralization[a]					
5.9– 9.1	6	5	5	10	26
9.9–10.1	4	5	7	14	30
10.9–15.1	3	5	7	4	19
Overall	13	15	19	28	75

[a] For details, see text.

- *Hypothesis 4*: The more ICUs are characterized by centralized decision-making, the lower the performance of ICUs.

Standardization

Standardization has been measured in essentially two different ways. First we tried to establish to what extent ICUs had written descriptions and written criteria for the various functions. Tables 46–50 indicate to what extent these written descriptions and criteria are available in the various hospitals. Only in the case of the written criteria of physicians can one discern a significant relationship with

Table 46. Description of the function of ICU director

	Type of hospital				Overall
	< 300 Beds	300–500 Beds	> 500 Beds	University	
Present					
No	7	6	12	17	42
Yes	7	8	7	12	34
Overall	14	14	19	29	76

Table 47. Description of the function of the head nurse

	Type of hospital				Overall
	< 300 Beds	300–500 Beds	> 500 Beds	University	
Present					
No	3	4	10	14	31
Yes	11	11	9	15	46
Overall	14	15	19	29	77

Table 48. Description of the function of the nurse

	Type of hospital				Overall
	<300 Beds	300–500 Beds	>500 Beds	University	
Present					
No	3	4	7	13	27
Yes	11	11	12	16	50
Overall	14	15	19	29	77

Table 49. Written criteria for evaluation of nurses

	Type of hospital				Overall
	<300 Beds	300–500 Beds	>500 Beds	University	
Present					
No	7	6	5	6	24
Yes	4	5	8	16	33
Overall	11	11	13	22	57

Table 50. Written criteria for evaluation of physicians

	Type of hospital				Overall
	<300 Beds	300–500 Beds	>500 Beds	University	
Present					
No	6	5	9	6	26
Yes	1		2	13	16
Overall	7	5	11	19	42

the type of hospital: In the case of ICUs within university hospitals, there is a significantly higher frequency of such criteria.

Previous organizational research has, however, made clear that the presence of a formal structure, or, as it is operationalized here, the availability of written descriptions and criteria does not imply that these descriptions/criteria are also used. More importantly for the standardization of activities within an ICU is the extent to which medical protocols are available and used. We asked the medical director to indicate to what extent such protocols were used within his/her ICU. The distribution of this variable (STAN) is indicated in Table 51. Also in this case the scores of the variable are summarized in three categories.

The table shows that in all types of ICUs protocols are rather frequently used. Further analysis indicated that there is no correlation between the score

Table 51. Formal use of clinical protocols

	Type of hospital				Overall
	<300 Beds	300–500 Beds	>500 Beds	University	
Use					
Frequently	10	10	11	17	48
Sometimes	3	3	4	8	18
Seldom	1	2	4	4	11
Overall	14	15	19	29	77

on this variable and the availability of written descriptions/criteria of functions. Therefore, we only included the variable STAN (the use of protocols) in the final explanatory analysis. We expect that ICUs that use more protocols will have a better medical performance (in our case indicated by a negative relationship).

- *Hypothesis 5*: Standardization will result in a better medical performance.

Before we turn to the explanatory analysis, we have to deal with the dependent variable in our analysis, i.e. medical performance. Considering the fact that we use two indicators for medical performance (B20, the score for patients with a low level of severity of illness, and B80, the score for patients with a high level of severity of illness), we first have to analyze the distribution of these variables over the ICUs.

The Dependent Variable: Medical Performance of ICUs

In the EURICUS-I study two different measurements of medical performance are used (B20 and B80; see Chap. 8 "Analysis of ICU Performance" for the background of these measures). The measurements are made on the individual patient data and aggregated to the level of ICUs. Our first analysis of these medical output measures concerns establishing whether there are systematic relationships with the various types of ICUs. To what extent are their significant variations between the various types of ICUs regarding the measurement of medical performance in terms of B20 and B80? In order to answer this question, we did a one-way variance analysis (ANOVA) with B20 and B80 and the types of ICUs. Table 52 summarizes the findings of this analysis.

As this table shows, there is no significant variance of both B20 and B80, comparing the various categories (size and type) of the ICUs. The second analysis concerns the differences between the scores of ICUs on the two performance measures. One of the reasons to use two measures of medical performance (instead of one, the SMR) was the unequal distribution of the SMR. Consequently, scores on B20 and B80 will not always be in the same range. Although there is a (significant) correlation between B20 and B80, still there are ICUs with incon-

Table 52. One-way variance analyses of B20 and B80 with respect to the types of ICU

Variable B20 (by variable type) and performance B20 (type/size hospital)					
Source	*D.F.*	*Sum of squares*	*Mean squares*	*F ratio*	*F probability*
Between groups	3	3.4679	1.1560	1.2674	0.2920
Within groups	72	65.6672	0.9120		
Total	75	69.1350			
Variable B80 (by variable type) and performance B80 (type/size hospital)					
Between groups	3	0.8660	0.2887	0.7058	0.5517
Within groups	72	29.4472	0.4090		
Total	75	30.3132			

sistent scores on both measures. One can then, with respect to the scores on B20 and B80, distinguish between four groups of ICUs. First, one can distinguish between ICUs with a consistently high or low score on both measures. Second, there are also ICUs with either a low score on one of the measures and a higher one on the other, or a high score on the one, and a lower one on the other.

We performed three different analyses to investigate if there are organizational variables comparing: (a) consistently high scoring with low scoring; (b) inconsistently low scoring (either B20 or B80 low and on the other a higher score), and (c) inconsistently high scoring (either B20 or B80 high and on the other a lower score). It proved difficult to find managerial and organizational determinants either for distinguishing consistently high vs low scoring ICUs or for comparing the inconsistently low or high scoring ICUs. Only a slight relationship can be discerned between the variable country and the inconsistent performance of the ICUs on the two measures (indicating that inconsistency occurs more frequently in some countries). Furthermore, the only organizational factor that distinguishes (albeit slightly) between the consistently low and high scoring ICUs is the variable measuring the number of patients/nurse. One of the reasons for this lack of adequate findings is the small numbers of ICUs than can be compared. As a result of this analysis we decided to perform two separate explanatory (multiple regression) analyses to test hypotheses 2–5; one with B20 as the dependent variable and the other with B80 as the dependent variable.

The Multiple Regression Analyses: Testing the Hypotheses

In the paragraphs above, we hypothesized relationships of the following variables with the dependent variable medical performance: task differentiation (DIFFTOT; hypothesis 2); qualifications (QUALIF; hypothesis 3); centralization of decision-making (CENTRAL; hypothesis 4), and standardization (STAN; hypothesis 5). For reasons outlined above, we also included in the analysis the following other variables: SIZE (of the ICU), TECH (the advanced technology scale) and UNIV (indicating if the ICU is located in a nonuniversity or university hos-

Table 53. Equation number 1: dependent variable B20; ,performance B20 [a]

Variable	B	SE B	β	T	Significance T
CENTRAL	−0.14	0.066	−0.25	−0.211	0.039
UNIV	0.19	0.27	0.10	0.73	0.471
QUALIF	−3.1	0.0034	−0.01	−0.09	0.927
STAN	−0.34	0.14	−0.30	−2.51	0.015
DIFFTOT	−0.070	0.040	−0.21	−1.75	0.086
TECH	−0.23	0.10	−0.30	−2.21	0.031
SIZE	0.051	0.026	0.28	1.93	0.059
(Constant)	0.64	1.62		0.39	0.70

[a] For explanation, see Text.

Table 54. Equation number 1: dependent variable. B80; performance B80

Variable	B	SE B	β	T	Significance T
CENTRAL	−0.070	0.045	−0.20	−1.54	0.130
UNIV	0.089	0.18	0.07	0.49	0.628
QUALIF-2	−1.71	0.0023	−0.01	−0.08	0.941
STAN	−0.048	0.094	−0.07	−0.52	0.609
DIFFTOT	−0.076	0 .027	−0.36	−2.78	0.008
TECH	−0.0099	0.070	−0.02	−0.14	0.888
SIZE	0.0035	0.018	0.03	0.19	0.848
(Constant)	1.95	1.11		1.76	0.085

pital). The dependent variable in the analysis is either B20 or B80. The findings of the analyses are indicated in Tables 53 and 54.

The first equation (Table 53) explains 31% of the variance of B20; the second equation (Table 54) only explains 19% of the variance of B80. Apparently, the managerial and organizational variables better explain the performance of ICUs with respect to less severely ill patients than the performance of ICUs with respect to more severely ill patients.

Using B20 as the dependent variable, it is clear that the hypotheses regarding task differentiation, centralization and standardization are confirmed. The more an ICU works with a team-like structure - indicated by less task differentiation and less centralization - the better the performance with respect to less severely ill patients. Furthermore there are separate effects upon performance with respect to the variables SIZE and TECH. In other words, as measured with the variable B20, the performance of larger ICUs with more advanced technologies is better. However, if we turn to the other measure of performance, i.e. B80, it is clear that only one determining organizational variable can be discerned (i.e. less task differentiation). Considering that there is also (although not significant) an effect of the variable centralization, one may conclude that also with respect to performance regarding more severely ill patients, a team-like structure is a major determinant of the performance of ICUs. But apparently (considering the lower explained variance), the effect of managerial and organizational variables diminishes when medical performance of ICUs regarding more severely ill patients is taken into account. One may presume that, in this context, medical attributes of the ICU become more important.

Conclusions

In conclusion, the findings of the substudy *Organization* once more underline the necessity to emphasize the specific nature of the ICU as a work group. The analysis showed that, in contrast to other work groups, the implementation of technologies within the ICU did not result in more centralization, more task differentiation and more standardization, but instead resulted in the development of team-like working. In the final analysis we could prove that this resulted in better medical performance of the ICUs.

Personnel*

W. Schaufeli and P. Le Blanc

Introduction

Aims of the Substudy

The EURICUS-I *Personnel* substudy was designed to study the working situation and well-being of ICU nurses, who proportionally are the largest group of employees in an ICU. The aim of this substudy is twofold: First, a detailed job analysis is performed. The jobs of nurses in the participating ICUs will be described in terms of nursing staff characteristics, job characteristics (especially nurses' workload), and nurses' level of job-related stress (burnout). Potential risk factors for ICU nurses' well-being at work as well as specific high-risk groups will be identified. Second, a model on the relationship between ICU nurses' workload (inputs), their levels of job-related stress or burnout (throughputs) and the medical performance of their ICU (outputs) will be tested both on the individual (subjective) level and on the aggregated ICU (objective) level. This research model will be expounded on below.

* The authors would like to express their appreciation to Tom Cox (Centre for Organizational Health and Development, University of Nottingham) for his insightful comments on an earlier draft of this chapter.

Research Model

The basic research model used in the *Personnel* substudy is depicted in Fig. 5. The main hypothesis underlying this model is that when workload is too high this will induce feelings of chronic job stress (burnout) among ICU nurses, which in turn are expected to lead to impairments in nurses' performance levels. Accordingly, nurses' performance is supposed to be influenced by their level of job demands, both directly and indirectly through the development of burnout symptoms. The latter effect is supposed to be stronger than the former. Nurse burnout was selected as the focal mediating variable since it is not only characterized by feelings of exhaustion, but also by a lack of commitment to the patients and by feelings of insufficiency and incompetence. All three aspects are expected to impair performance. Besides, burnout is a long-term stress reaction that is particularly observed in human services such as health care, in which employees do "people work" of some kind [44]. Last but not least, already more than a decade ago, burnout was viewed as one of the top research priorities for ICUs [37]; however, only few studies have been conducted since.

This basic research model has been refined in two ways. The first refinement deals with the relationship between workload and burnout. It is assumed that certain positive conditions, so-called coping resources [25], can help nurses to cope with a high workload, thereby preventing the occurrence of long-term stress reactions such as burnout. These coping resources can be characteristics of the working situation as well as personal characteristics of a nurse. An example of a situational coping resource is the level of autonomy [31] in ICU nurses' jobs. If nurses have sufficient autonomy to cope with demanding job situations (e.g. to solve problems), these situations are less likely to lead to stress reactions. An example of a personal coping resource is a high level of self-efficacy, or perceived personal competence [15]. Nurses who feel competent in their jobs will be less upset by high demands, because they can rely on their capabilities to handle them. So, high demands are only expected to lead to stress reactions such as burnout if situational or personal coping resources are lacking.

The second refinement concerns the relationship between burnout and performance. This relationship is expected to be influenced by a nurse's level of involvement in the job, i.e. the importance that she/he attaches to the job [26, 39]. Specifically, nurses with a high level of job involvement are expected to be more motivated to exert themselves under stressful circumstances than nurses with a low level of job involvement. Therefore, we assume that high levels of job involvement will prevent performance from deteriorating under stressful circumstances.

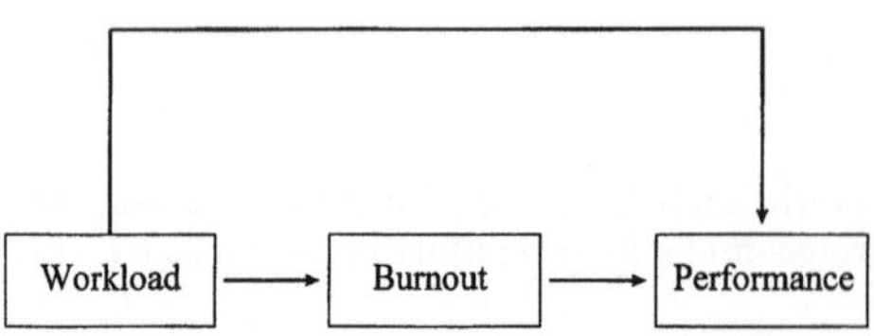

Fig. 5. Basic research model

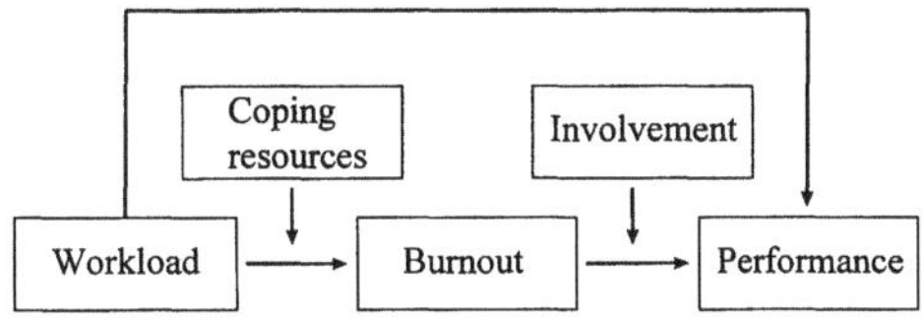

Fig. 6. Extended research model

The above-mentioned refinements lead to the extended research model that is depicted in Fig. 6. In Appendix A, a definition of all variables that are included in the extended research model is given.

Structure of the Chapter

In the remaining part of this section, the following topics are addressed: "Method" deals with the method of data collection. First, the instruments that were used to assess the variables in our (extended) research model are presented and their psychometric properties are discussed. Second, the study sample is described in greater detail ("Respondents"). In the "Results" sections ("Job Analysis" and "Work and Well-Being Questionnaire"), results of the descriptive analyses will be presented and discussed. The results of the job analysis and the identification of risk factors for ICU nurses' well-being at work are discussed. Then, the specific subgroups are compared with respect to their scores on the key study variables in order to identify high-risk groups. In the next section ("Results: The Basic and Extended Research Models"), the basic and extended research models are tested. More particularly, results of multilevel analyses are presented, in which the total amount of variance in each variable is partitioned into variance accounted for on the individual, the ICU and the area level ("Multilevel Analysis"). Next, the basic research model (Fig. 5) is tested using subjective (individual) and aggregated objective (ICU) data ("The Basic Research Model"). Finally, the extended research model (Fig. 6) is tested at the ICU level ("The Extended Research Model").

The chapter ends with a concluding section that draws together the most important findings of the *Personnel* substudy.

Method

In October and November 1994, two questionnaires were distributed among the nursing staff of the 89 ICUs participating in the EURICUS-I project: the so-called WEBIC questionnaire for job analysis, and the Work and Well-Being questionnaire.

Job Analysis: The WEBIC Questionnaire

A systematic approach, based on sociotechnical systems theory (for an overview, see [46]), was used to perform a detailed job analysis of ICU nurses' jobs. For this purpose, the so-called WEBA method (*welzijn bij de arbeid* – well-being at work [50]) was adapted for analyzing ICU nurses' jobs. The resulting instrument, the WEBIC questionnaire, is particularly tailored to the work of ICU nurses, i.e. the activities they perform. WEBIC is an acronym that stands for well-being of ICU nurses. Sociotechnical systems theory postulates that a job must integrate four categories of tasks in order to be carried out adequately and not impair the workers' well-being. These four types of tasks are:

1. Operational tasks: e.g. nursing care of patients, activating patients
2. Organizing tasks: e.g. contact with physicians, patient meetings
3. Preparatory tasks: e.g. transport of patients, replenishing medical supplies
4. Supportive tasks: e.g. writing reports, calibrating equipment

Ideally, the task mix in ICU nurses' jobs should be balanced, i.e. a nurse should perform each of these four types of tasks in order to enhance her/his well-being and performance.

As depicted in Fig. 7, operational tasks make up the core of the ICU nurses' job, with all other categories of tasks contributing to this core activity.

In the first part of the WEBIC questionnaire, a listing of about 40 tasks, or activities, is presented. This listing is based on an earlier study among Dutch ICU nurses [8]. For each of these tasks nurses have to indicate: (a) how demanding and (b) how satisfying the performance of this particular task is. Scores range from 1 (undemanding/dissatisfying) to 5 (demanding/satisfying). Accordingly, this first part provides information about ICU nurses' qualitative workload in terms of perceived demands and perceived satisfaction. In the second part of the questionnaire, ICU nurses' task mix is assessed by asking them to estimate the percentage of time they spend in performing each of the four main categories of tasks.

When carrying out the different tasks, ICU nurses may encounter several problems, e.g. unclear instructions from superiors, inadequate planning of personnel, insufficient quality of materials, becoming emotionally "touched" by the death of patients. However, these problems are only expected to lead to an impairment of well-being (e.g. by inducing psychological strain) or performance (e.g. by

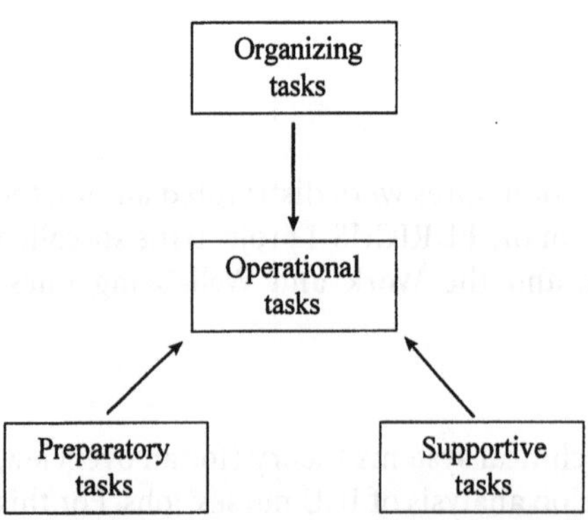

Fig. 7. Task-mix in ICU nurses' jobs

interfering with task completion) when the level of autonomy in ICU nurses' jobs is insufficient to tackle these problems. So, problems at work do not cause stress reactions per se, but only to the extent that nurses are unable to solve them because of a lack of autonomy [31]. Accordingly, as long as nurses have enough autonomy to deal with problems at work, negative effects on well-being and performance are likely to be prevented. Therefore, in the third and last part of the WEBIC questionnaire a detailed list of about 30 potential problems in ICU nurses' jobs is given, pertaining to: (1) patients, (2) norms and instructions, (3) equipment, (4) nurses' mental and physical condition, (5) supply of information, (6) feedback, (7) planning and (8) the physical working environment. This list is also based on the above-mentioned study by Reis-Miranda et al. [8]. For each of these potential problem areas, nurses are asked to indicate: (a) how often it occurs (an indicator of problem frequency) and (b) how it is usually solved (an indicator of autonomy). Scores on the frequency items range from 0 (never) to 4 (often); scores on the autonomy items range from unsolvable to solved independently.

Workload, Burnout and Performance: The Work and Well-Being Questionnaire

The questionnaire on work and well-being of ICU nurses is composed of several scales, corresponding to the variables in the research model. Each of these scales has been used and validated in earlier studies. First, a more detailed description of the content of each of the scales is given, followed by a discussion of their psychometric properties.

Workload

Perceived Quantitative Job Demands. This scale is derived from a Dutch version [20] of Karasek's [30] Job Content Instrument. The job demands scale is made up of four items that refer to quantitative demanding aspects of the job (e.g. time pressure, working hard). Because of a low factor-loading, one of the items of the job demands scale was removed. Items are scored on a four-point Likert scale, ranging from 1 (never) to 4 (always).

Imbalance Patients and Imbalance Team. In earlier studies on burnout (e.g. Van Dierendonck et al. [49]; Schaufeli et al. [45]), it was found that a so-called negative exchange relationship with either patients or colleagues, in which a care provider continuously feels that she/he invests much more than she/he gets back, is positively related to the development of burnout. Therefore, nurses are asked to evaluate the investments (I) and outcomes (O) in the relationship with: (a) their patients and (b) their team on a 7-point Likert scale, ranging from 1 (very little) to 7 (very much). Based on this information, two ratio scores are computed ($I_{patients}/O_{patients}$) and ($I_{team}/O_{team}$), respectively. The higher a ratio score, the more negative or imbalanced the respective relationship with either the patients or the colleagues in the ICU is perceived.

Stress Reactions

Burnout. Burnout is assessed with three subscales of the Maslach Burnout Inventory (MBI [38]): (1) emotional exhaustion (eight items), referring to the draining of emotional resources; (2) depersonalization (five items), i.e. a callous and cynical attitude towards the recipients of one's care; and (3) personal accomplishment (seven items), or feelings of work-related competence. High levels of emotional exhaustion and depersonalization and a diminished sense of personal accomplishment are indicative of burnout. Two original items of the MBI have been eliminated because of their poor factorial validity (see [17]). Scores on the items range from 1 (never) to 7 (every day).

Job Dissatisfaction. Nurses' overall dissatisfaction with their job is measured with a one item rating that is scored on a 5-point faces measure [34]. This measure is strongly correlated (r=7..75) with a multi-item questionnaire that assesses nurses' general job satisfaction [18].

Performance

Perceived Unit Performance. Perceived unit performance is measured by a six item scale, developed in the USA by Shortell et al. [48]. This scale has also been used in an earlier study on the effectiveness and efficiency of Dutch ICUs [32] and assesses nurses' judgement on the performance of their ICU. Items are scored on a 5-point Likert scale, ranging from 1 (strongly disagree) to 5 (strongly agree).

Situational Coping Resources

Autonomy. This scale is also derived from the above-mentioned Dutch version [20] of Karasek's [30] Job Content Instrument. It includes five items concerning skill discretion (i.e. the breadth of skills used by workers in performing their job) and four items concerning decision authority (i.e. freedom of action in accomplishing the formal work task). In earlier studies, factor analyses have repeatedly demonstrated that all nine items load on one factor and can therefore be combined into one scale [21, 22, 29]. However, because of low factor-loadings, two of the items of this scale had to be removed. Items are scored on a 4-point Likert scale, ranging from 1 (never) to 4 (always).

Leadership. Nurses' judgement on their head nurse's leadership behaviour is measured with two different scales: (1) Social emotional leadership [40] is the degree to which the head nurse is friendly and pays attention to his or her subordinates. (2) Task oriented leadership [40] is the degree to which tasks are specified and monitored in detail by the head nurse. All items are scored on a 5-point Likert scale, ranging from 1 (never) to 5 (always).

Personal Coping Resources

Generalized Self-Efficacy. Nurses' perceived personal competence [15], or "judgement of their capabilities to organize and execute courses of action required to attain designated types of performance", is measured by a 10-item scale developed by Jerusalem and Schwarzer [27]. Items are scored on a 4-point Likert scale, ranging from 1 (not at all true) to 4 (exactly true).

Conscientiousness. Nurses' level of conscientiousness is measured with four, 9-point self-ratings [28] reflecting: (1) responsibility, (2) accuracy, (3) efficiency, and (4) skilfullness. Conscientiousness is one of the "big five" personality characteristics that are assumed to constitute an individual's personality [23].

Involvement

Job Involvement. The degree to which the job is at the centre of nurses' lives is measured with a five item scale developed by Ladewich and White [35]. Items are scored on a 5-point Likert scale, ranging from 1 (strongly disagree) to 5 (strongly agree).

Organizational Commitment. The strength of nurses' identification with and involvement in the ICU is measured with a five item scale developed by Shortell et al. [48]. Items are scored on a 5-point Likert scale, ranging from 1 (strongly disagree) to 5 (strongly agree).

Psychometric Properties of the Work and Well-Being Scales

Internal Consistency

Table 55 presents some characteristics of the scales from the Work and Well-Being questionnaire. In general, a Cronbach's α of about 0.70 or higher is consi-

Table 55. Internal consistency (α), range, mean and standard deviation (SD) of the Work and Well-Being Scales ($n = 2090$)

		Number of items	α	Range	Mean ± SD
Scale					
A1	Quantitative job demands (workload)	4	0.60	1.00–4.00	2.69 ± 0.52
A2	Imbalance patients	1	n.a.	0.29–7.00	1.52 ± 0.89
A2	Imbalance team	1	n.a.	0.25–7.00	1.25 ± 0.60
B1	Emotional exhaustion	8	0.86	1.00–6.63	2.89 ± 1.09
B1	Depersonalization	5	0.61	1.00–6.50	2.18 ± 0.95
B1	Reduced personal accomplishment	7	0.73	1.00–6.29	2.56 ± 0.92
B2	Job satisfaction	1	n.a.	1.00–5.00	3.81 ± 0.71
C1	Perceived unit performance	6	0.70	1.33–5.00	3.72 ± 0.54
D1.1	Autonomy	7	0.70	1.00–4.00	2.85 ± 0.42
D1.2	Social emotional leadership	4	0.87	1.00–5.00	3.58 ± 0.86
D2.1	Task-oriented leadership	3	0.63	1.00–5.00	3.13 ± 0.81
D2.1	Generalized self-efficacy	10	0.85	1.50–4.40	3.09 ± 0.42
D2.2	Conscientiousness	4	0.70	1.00–9.00	7.69 ± 0.84
E1	Job involvement	5	0.73	1.00–5.00	2.75 ± 0.65
E2	Organizational commitment	5	0.73	1.20–5.00	3.65 ± 0.61

n.a., not available.

dered to be acceptable [41]. Inspection of Table 55 makes clear that there are three scales which do not meet this criterion, i.e. perceived quantitative job demands, task-oriented leadership and depersonalization. The relatively low α of the first two scales may be due to the small number of items (3). With respect to depersonalization, a low α has also repeatedly been found in other studies [42]. Despite the relatively poor internal consistency of these scales, they are nevertheless included in the analyses since α values between 0.60 and 0.70 are considered borderline [41].

Validity

Inspection of the relationships between the variables in the research model yields some information on the validity of the scales. In Appendix B, the correlation matrix of all variables is given. For survey reasons, the intercorrelations between the variables are discussed in three steps, corresponding to the steps in the research model. However, it should be noted that, due to the large sample size, even small correlation coefficients reach statistical significance.

Workload and Stress Reactions. The first step deals with the relationship between workload and stress reactions, which is assumed to be moderated by situational and individual coping resources. The correlations between the variables concerned are reported in Table 56.

As expected, the relationship between quantitative job demands, and emotional exhaustion, depersonalization and dissatisfaction is positive. Higher job demands are related to higher levels of emotional exhaustion and depersonalization and to more dissatisfaction. However, the relationship of job demands to reduced personal accomplishment turns out to be significantly negative instead of positive, i.e. higher demands are associated with stronger feelings of accomplishment. The perception of imbalance in the exchange relationship with patients is positively related to all three burnout symptoms, whereas the perception of imbalance in the exchange relationship with colleagues (the team) is only positively related to emotional exhaustion. Both measures of imbalance are significantly, positively related to dissatisfaction. So, the more nurses feel that their investments in their relationships with patients or colleagues outweigh the outcomes, the more emotionally exhausted and dissatisfied they will be. The more negative the exchange relationship with patients is evaluated, the higher nurses' level of depersonalization and the lower their feelings of accomplishment. With the exception of the nonsignificant relationships between: (a) autonomy and emotional exhaustion, and (b) task-oriented leadership, and emotional exhaustion and depersonalization, respectively, all coping resources are negatively related to burnout symptoms and dissatisfaction. In general, a lack of either situational or personal coping resources increases the risk of stress reactions such as burnout and dissatisfaction. Both personal coping resources (self-efficacy and conscientiousness) are quite strongly, positively intercorrelated ($r=0.41$), whereas the intercorrelations between each of the three situational coping resources (autonomy, task-oriented leadership and social emotional leadership) are much lower ($r<0.15$).

Table 56. Correlations between workload, stress,reactions and coping resources ($n = 2090$)

	DEM	IOp	Iot	SEL	TOL	Aut	Sef	Con	EE	DP	RPA	Dsat
DEM	1.00	0.17**	0.12**	−0.14**	0.11**	0.18**	−0.03	0.04	0.40**	0.10**	−0.09**	0.19**
IOp		1.00	0.24**	−0.07**	−0.06**	−0.01	0.03	0.03	0.16**	0.10**	0.05*	0.12**
IOt			1.00	−0.10**	−0.01	−0.01	0.02	0.04	0.14**	0.03	0.03	0.14**
SEL				1.00	0.12**	0.10**	0.12**	0.07**	−0.20**	−0.13**	−0.14**	−0.31**
TOL					1.00	−0.05*	−0.03	0.04	0.02	−0.04	−0.08**	−0.08**
Aut						1.00	0.17**	0.14**	−0.01	−0.08**	−0.28**	−0.22**
Sef							1.00	0.41**	−0.13**	−0.07**	−0.28**	−0.18**
Con								1.00	−0.11**	−0.18**	−0.28**	−0.15**
EE									1.00	0.43**	0.13**	0.47**
DP										1.00	0.24**	0.29**
RPA											1.00	0.34**
Dsat												1.00

DEM, quantitative job demands; IOp, imbalance patients; IOt, imbalance team; SEL: social-emotional leadership; TOL, task-oriented leadership; Aut, autonomy; Sef, self-efficacy; Con, conscientiousness; EE, emotional exhaustion; DP, depersonalization; RPA, reduced personal accomplishment; Dsat, dissatisfaction.

* $p = 0.05$; ** $p = 0.01$.

Finally, the relationships between the three burnout symptoms and dissatisfaction are all positive and significant, i.e. higher burnout levels are related to dissatisfaction. In conclusion: the pattern of correlations presented in Table 56 confirms the validity of the measures of job demands, stress reactions, and coping resources used in this study. Only one out of 66 correlations is significant and in the unexpected direction (i.e. job demands and reduced personal accomplishment).

Stress Reactions and Perceived Unit Performance. The second step deals with the relationship between stress reactions and perceived unit performance, which is assumed to be moderated by job involvement and organizational commitment. The correlations between the variables concerned are reported in Table 57.
As expected, the relationship between the three burnout components and job dissatisfaction, and perceived unit performance is significantly negative. Job involvement and organizational commitment are both positively related to perceived unit performance, but this relationship is much stronger for organizational commitment ($r=0.47$) than for job involvement ($r=0.19$). Both measures of psychological identification with the job are moderately, positively correlated ($r=0.33$). Finally, both job involvement and organizational commitment are negatively related to burnout (with the exception of the nonsignificant relationship between involvement and emotional exhaustion) and dissatisfaction (the latter relationship is especially strong for organizational commitment). In conclusion: the pattern of correlations presented in Table 57 confirms the validity of the measures of stress reactions, involvement, commitment, and perceived performance used in this study. None of the significant correlations is in an unexpected direction.

Workload and Perceived Unit Performance. Finally, the relationships between the three workload measures (perceived quantitative job demands, imbalance patients and imbalance team) and perceived unit performance are all – as expected – negative and significant (-0.05^{*}, -0.14^{**} and -0.15^{**}, respectively).

Table 57. Correlations between burnout, dissatisfaction, involvement, commitment and perceived unit performance ($n=2090$)

	EE	DP	RPA	Dsat	Inv	Com	Pup
EE	1.00	0.43**	0.13**	0.47**	−0.03	−0.31**	−0.18**
DP		1.00	0.24**	0.29**	−0.09*	−0.18**	−0.17**
RPA			1.00	0.34**	−0.27**	−0.24**	−0.21**
Dsat				1.00	0.26**	0.44**	0.34**
Inv					1.00	0.33**	0.19**
Com						1.00	0.47**
Pup							1.00

EE, emotional exhaustion; DP, depersonalization; RPA, reduced personal accomplishment; Dsat, dissatisfaction; Inv, job involvement; Com, organizational commitment; Pup, perceived unit performance.
* $p=0.05$; ** $p=0.01$.

Morale and Stress Reactions. In order to evaluate the interrelationships between the scales that measure "human resources outcomes" (i.e. burnout, dissatisfaction, involvement, commitment, perceived performance) more systematically, a principal components analysis that includes the mean scale scores has been conducted. The results of this analysis, after varimax rotation, are shown in Table 58.

As can be seen from this table, the analysis yields a clear two-component structure. The first component is made up of personal accomplishment, perceived unit performance, job involvement and organizational commitment and can therefore be interpreted as morale. The second component comprises emotional exhaustion and depersonalization and can be labeled as stress reactions. Dissatisfaction loads equally high on both factors.

Objective Measures

In addition to the subjective data that were collected by means of the questionnaires, two objective measures were used in testing our research model. However, these objective measures were only available for 80 ICUs. First, per ICU, nurses' objective workload was assessed by the NEMS [9], a validated simplified version of the TISS [7]. NEMS scores specific nursing activities performed during the past 24 h, referring to each patient. For a period of 4 months, NEMS was scored each day for each patient that stayed in the ICU, which yielded an objective indicator of nurses' workload. Second, objective unit performance was assessed using clinical management data of 9300 patients. The ICUs were ranked according to the logits of mortality computed at two levels of severity of illness measured by SAPS-II: B20 and B80 of the distribution of SAPS-II scores in EURICUS-I. Detailed information on this issue is provided in Chap. 8 ("Analysis of ICU Performance").

Table 59 presents the correlations between objective measures of workload and unit performance and the corresponding subjective measures of workload and (perceived) unit performance from the Work and Well-Being Questionnaire. Accordingly, Table 59 yields information about the validity of the objective and subjective data. Note that the subjective variables in this table have been aggregated at the unit level; that is, mean scores across units are used to compute the cor-

Table 58. Principal components analysis of scale means after varimax rotation ($n = 2090$)

	Factor 1: morale	Factor 2: Stress reactions
Variable		
Emotional exhaustion	−0.10	0.85
Depersonalization	−0.08	0.75
Reduced personal accomplishment	−0.56	0.16
Dissatisfaction	−0.54	0.56
Perceived unit performance	0.63	−0.17
Organizational commitment	0.72	0.14
Job involvement	0.72	−0.26
Variance (%)	38.2	16.5

Table 59. Correlations between subjective and objective measures of workload and unit performance ($n=2090$)

	NEMS	Dem	IOp	IOt	Pup	B20	B80
NEMS	1.00	0.17	0.04	0.03	−0.05	−0.23*	−0.12
Dem		1.00	0.45**	0.35**	−0.11	0.03	0.01
Iop			1.00	0.37**	−0.28*	−0.08	−0.07
Iot				1.00	0.01	−0.05	0.10
Pup					1.00	0.09	0.16
B20						1.00	0.38**
B80							1.00

Dem, quantitative job demands; IOp, imbalance patients; IOt, imbalance team; Pup, perceived unit performance; B20, SAPS-II (percentile 20); B80, SAPS-II (percentile 80).
* $p=0.05$; ** $p=0.01$

relation coefficients. Inspection of Table 59 also makes clear that, though correlations between corresponding subjective and objective measures are all in the expected direction, only very few of these correlations reach significance. A possible explanation for this overall lack of significance is the small number of units (i.e. 80 ICUs), which reduces the statistical power of the significance test.

Though the correlations between the subjective and objective measures of workload are in the expected – positive – direction, none of these correlations is significant. The highest correlation with the objective workload measure (NEMS) is found for perceived quantitative job demands, which can probably be explained by the fact that both measures assess the quantity of work (number of activities) nurses perform. The small correlations between NEMS and the two imbalance measures can be explained as follows: Whereas the two imbalance measures (i.e. imbalance patients and imbalance team) include nurses' perception of investments and outcomes in the relationship with patients and colleagues, respectively, NEMS only refers to a specific subcategory of investments in the relationship with patients (i.e. medical care of patients). Positive, though nonsignificant, intercorrelations are also found for the subjective and objective measures of unit performance. This result can probably be explained by the fact that clinical management of patients is only one of several aspects on which nurses base their judgement of their units' performance. In general, it can be concluded that the validity of the subjective measures of workload and unit performance is confirmed by the direction of the relationships with objective measures; however, the magnitude of these relationships is somewhat smaller than expected. These small correlations can probably be explained by conceptual differences in operationalization of the subjective vs the objective measures.

Respondents

The WEBIC questionnaire was filled out by 1954 nurses (response rate: 67%), whereas the Work and Well-Being Questionnaire was filled out by 2090 nurses (response rate: 72%). In Table 60, the distribution of the larger group of 2090 res-

Table 60. Distribution of the respondents over the different areas

	Number of respondents	Percentage (%)
European area		
Poland	127	6.1
Germany	125	6.0
Denmark	163	7.8
Finland	163	7.8
Netherlands	226	10.8
Belgium	180	8.6
France	144	6.9
Luxembourg	24	1.1
United Kingdom	242	11.6
Italy	148	7 1
Spain-Catalonia	250	12.0
Spain-Valencia	179	8.6
Portugal	119	5.7
Overall	2090	100.0

pondents over the different countries is reported. The sample of 2090 nurses is made up of 1618 women (77.4%) and 399 men (19.1%); for 73 nurses (3.5%) information on their gender is missing. Ages range from 20 to 64 years, with a mean age of 32.5 years (SD = 7.1). On average, these nurses have 6.5 years (SD = 5.6) of ICU experience and on average they have been working on the present ICU for 5.6 years (SD = 5.2). Some 80% of these nurses have a full-time position.

Results: Job Analysis (WEBIC Questionnaire)

In the first part of the WEBIC questionnaire, a distinction is made between four categories of tasks, or activities (see also "Job Analysis: The WEBIC Questionnaire"), namely:

1. Operational tasks: nursing and medical care of patients
2. Organizing tasks: job-related cooperation and meetings with others
3. Preparatory tasks: tasks which should be performed before the operational work can start
4. Supportive tasks: activities that should make sure that the operational tasks can be performed undisturbed

Demands and Satisfaction

First, for each of these categories the mean demands score and the mean satisfaction score were computed. These figures are presented in Table 61. Here, it can be concluded that operational tasks are perceived as the most demanding, but also

Table 61. Mean demands score and mean satisfaction score for each of the categories of tasks ($n=1954$)

	Demanding: 1–5 (Mean ± SD)	Satisfying: 1–5 (Mean ± SD)	Correlation Demanding × satisfying
Category of tasks			
Operational tasks	3.51 ± 0.78	3.74 ± 0.69	0.41**
Organizing tasks (tot)	2.38 ± 0.76	2.95 ± 0.73	0.42**
Internal functional contacts	2.61 ± 0.88	3.47 ± 0.75	0.05*
External functional contacts	1.99 ± 0.98	2.41 ± 0.97	0.60**
Meetings	2.55 ± 1.10	2.98 ± 1.12	0.63**
Preparatory tasks	2.81 ± 0.87	2.87 ± 0.78	0.51**
Supportive tasks (tot),	2.68 ± 0.83	2.77 ± 0.79	0.71**
Supportive tasks operational work	2.80 ± 0.92	2.83 ± 0.88	0.64**
Supportive tasks organization	2.53 ± 1.01	2.71 ± 1.00	0.79**

as most satisfying. The nurses' most central (operational) tasks which pose the greatest demands seem to drive nurse satisfaction. This is not so surprising since it is the operational tasks which appear to define nursing for the general and nursing populations. Doing these tasks – probably at the expense of other tasks perceived to be less central – is associated with satisfaction. Organizing tasks are perceived as least demanding, especially external functional contacts (e.g. contact with other wards in the hospital). Supportive tasks (e.g. reporting, registering and administrative work) are seen as least satisfying.

The correlations between the demands score and the satisfaction score for each of the categories of tasks vary between 0.41 (operational tasks) and 0.71 (supportive tasks). So, for each individual category of tasks it was found that the more demanding the respective category is perceived, the more satisfying the performance of tasks belonging to this category is for ICU nurses. Only for the subcategory "internal functional contacts" (contacts with the head nurse, physicians, colleagues, or secretarial staff) was a low correlation (0.05) between the demands score and the satisfaction score found. This subcategory of tasks is evaluated as fairly undemanding but at the same time fairly satisfying. In Appendix C, the mean demands score and the mean satisfaction score for each individual task are presented.

Next, the main results are summarized for each of the four categories of tasks.

Operational Tasks

The tasks "psychologically supporting patients" and "activating patients" are perceived as most demanding. However, "providing for the safety and comfort of a patient" is also perceived as most satisfying. The task "assisting colleagues" is seen as least demanding, whereas "lifting/weighing patients" is perceived as least satisfying.

Organizing Tasks

The tasks "hand-over meetings" and "contact with physicians" are seen as most demanding. The task "contact with another ICU in the hospital" is perceived as least demanding, but also as least satisfying. Moreover, "contact with the hospital management" is also perceived as not very satisfying. Finally, "contact with colleagues from own team" is perceived as most satisfying.

Preparatory Tasks

The tasks "admission of new patients" and "transport of patients to and from the ICU" are perceived as most demanding. However, "admission of new patients" is also perceived as most satisfying. The task "making time tables" (planning) is seen as least demanding and least satisfying.

Supportive Tasks

The task "supporting a patient's direct relatives after death of a patient" is perceived as most demanding, while "recruitment and selection of new colleagues" is perceived as least demanding. However, the latter is also perceived as least satisfying. The tasks "training when implementing new equipment" and "improving one's expertise by following courses" are perceived as most satisfying.

In general, it can be concluded that the above results are in line with common sense ideas of taxing and rewarding aspects of ICU nurses' jobs. In general, psychological aspects of patient care (such as emotionally supporting patients or supporting the family after the death of a patient) as well as tasks related to communication with other disciplines are perceived as demanding. In addition, communication with the hospital management and/or with other ICUs in the hospital is perceived as fairly dissatisfying. These results can probably be attributed to the fact that most training programs for ICU nurses are more strongly oriented towards technical nursing skills than towards psychological or communicative ones. Despite the (emotional) demands associated with it, nurses do enjoy psychosocial care of patients, which is clearly not the case for administrative tasks (e.g. making time tables). Contact with colleagues from their own team is perceived as very satisfying, probably because they are an important source of work-related social support. Finally, ICU nurses' are eager to maintain their expertise, as training and following courses are perceived as fairly satisfying.

Task Mix

Next, nurses were asked to estimate the percentage of time they spend on performing each particular category of tasks. The results are presented in Table 62. From this table, we can conclude that ICU nurses perform activities from all of the four categories of tasks. Of course, they spend most of their working time on operational tasks (56%). The lowest percentage of time is found for preparatory tasks (10%). The figures presented in Table 62 correspond quite well to the results of an earlier time sampling study among Dutch ICU nurses [8], in which it was found that nurses spend about 55% of their working time on operational tasks and about 25% on a combination of preparatory and supportive tasks. So, the fact

Table 62. Mean percentage of time spent on performing each of the categories of tasks ($n = 1954$)

	Percentage of time (0%–100%; Mean ± SD)
Category of tasks	
Operational tasks	56 ± 19
Organizing tasks	23 ± 9
Internal functional tasks	10 ± 7
External functional tasks	5 ± 5
Meetings	8 ± 6
Preparatory tasks	10 ± 8
Supportive tasks	12 ± 9

that the nurses' own reports on their usage of time yield results that are quite identical to those obtained by objective assessments lends support to the validity of these self-reports.

Problem Situations and Autonomy

In the third and last part of the WEBIC questionnaire, the frequency of occurrence of ICU-specific problem situations was inventoried, as was the level of autonomy to solve these problem situations. For each of the different categories of problem situations, the mean frequency and the mean level of autonomy are presented (Table 63).

Overall, the frequency of problem situations is quite low: the highest frequency is found for problem situations related to norms (e.g. unclear instructions). However, nurses' level of autonomy in solving problems related to norms is quite high too, which also applies to the levels of autonomy related to the other categories of problem situations. The lowest level of autonomy is found for problem

Table 63. Mean frequency scores and mean autonomy scores for each of the categories of problem situations ($n = 1954$)

	Frequency: 1–5 (Mean ± SD)	Autonomy: 1–5 (Mean ± SD)	Correlation: Frequency × autonomy
Situation category			
Norms	2.03 (0.60)	3.26 (0.50)	–0.19**
Patients	1.61 (0.75)	3.01 (0.75)	–0.05
Materials	1.68 (0.66)	2.98 (0.57)	–0.17**
Personal condition	1.81 (0.58)	3.34 (0.48)	–0.23**
Information	1.75 (0.86)	2.63 (0.62)	–0.18**
Planning	1.50 (0.76)	2.56 (0.70)	–0.25**

situations related to planning, which is probably due to the relatively low predictability of work flow in ICUs. In general, it can be concluded that in this sample the stressfulness of ICU nurses' jobs is rather low, as the frequency of ICU-specific problem situations is low and the level of autonomy to solve these problems is quite high.

The correlation between the frequency score and the autonomy score for each of the categories of problem situations varies between −0.05 (patients) and −0.25 (planning). These negative correlations can easily be explained by the fact that for each of these categories the frequency of occurrence of problem situations is low, whereas the level of autonomy in solving these problems is rather high. Only for the subcategory "patients", dealing with the variation and complexity of nursing, was a nonsignificant correlation (−0.05) between the frequency score and the autonomy score found. In Appendix D, the mean frequency score and the mean autonomy score for each individual problem situation are presented.

Next, the main results are summarized for each of the six problem situations.

Norms

The most frequent problem situations related to norms are "having to do too many things simultaneously" and "unexpected job activities interrupting the work schedule. However, mean levels of autonomy in solving these problems are high (3.16–3.43).

Patients

Problem situations related to patients are infrequent (1.59 and 1.64), and mean levels of autonomy in solving them are moderate (2.86 and 3.10 respectively).

Materials and Equipment

Problem situations related to materials are also infrequent (1.50–1.81), and again mean levels of autonomy in solving them are moderate (2.68–3.14).

Condition

The most frequent problem situation related to nurses' personal condition is "the idea that you are responsible for the life of your patients". Mean levels of autonomy in solving these problem situations are high (3.04–3.74).

Information

Problem situations related to information are infrequent (1.46–2.04), and mean levels of autonomy in solving them are moderate (2.32–2.84).

Planning

Again, problem situations related to planning are infrequent (1.10–2.00); however, mean levels of autonomy in solving them are relatively low (2.43–2.64).

In Tables 64 and 65, ICU nurses' opinion on feedback and their working environment is presented. Most of the complaints with respect to feedback about

Table 64. Feedback ($n = 1954$)

	... you do not get (%)	... yoll get too late (%)	... is not complete (%)	... is unreliable (%)
Feedback you would like to get from your direct superior ...	28	10	29	5
Feedback you would like to get from your colleagues ...	18	9	32	8
Feedback you would like to get from the physicians ...	39	8	23	5

Table 65. Work environment ($n = 1954$).

	Climate (%)	Lighting (%)	Interior design (%)	Lack of space (%)	Noise and bustle (%)
Ward	47	35	31	66	42
Location for taking a break	30	18	35	46	25

one's performance deal with completeness. Especially feedback from the direct superior (28%) and from colleagues (32%) is considered incomplete. Moreover, 28% of the nurses indicates that they do not get the feedback they would like to have from their direct superior, whereas 39% indicate that they do not get the feedback they would like to have from physicians.

Overall, nurses report quite a lot of problem factors with respect to their work site. The major complaints with respect to the work site relate to lack of space in the ward (66%) and in the location for taking a break (46%). Other major complaints with respect to the ward deal with climate (47%) and with noise and bustle (42%).

Identification of Risk Factors

To identify risk factors for ICU performance we compared the 25% best performing with the 25% worst performing ICUs. As objective performance indicators, the ICU's logits of mortality at two levels of severity of illness (measured by SAPS-II) were used (see "Psychometric Properties of the Work and Well-Being Scales"). The best and worst performing ICUs were compared (by means of *t* tests and ANOVAs) in four aspects:

1. Demands (the mean demands score for each of the categories of tasks)
2. Satisfaction (the mean satisfaction score for each of the categories of tasks)
3. Problem situations (the mean frequency of occurrence of each of the categories of problem situations)
4. Autonomy (the mean level of autonomy in solving each category of problem-situations)

Table 66. Comparison of the 25% best performing vs the 25% worst performing ICUs

	B20 Worst	B20 Best	B80 Worst	B80 Best
Risk factor				
Demands				Operational tasks Organizing tasks
Satisfaction		Operational tasks	Operational tasks Organizing tasks	
Frequent occurring problem situations	Norms Materials Information Planning	Personal condition	Materials Information Planning	
Lack of autonomy in problem situations	Materials Information		Norms Personal condition	

All of these analyses were performed twice: first for the 25% worst performing vs the 25% best performing ICUs on B20 and then for the 25% worst performing vs the 25% best performing ICUs on B80. The results are summarized in Table 66.

The 25% Worst Performing vs 25% Best Performing ICUs (B20)

First of all, we did not find any significant differences between the two groups with respect to their mean demands scores for each of the categories of tasks. Quite surprisingly, operational tasks are perceived as more satisfying ($t=2.59$; $p=0.010$) by nurses in the worst performing units compared to nurses in the best performing units. With the exception of problem situations related to patients, the worst performing units significantly differ from the best performing units in all categories of problem situations. In the worst performing units, the frequency of occurrence of problem situations related to norms ($t=3.47$; $p=0.001$), materials ($t=2.48$; $p=0.044$), information ($t=1.98$; $p=0.048$) and planning ($t=2.73$; $p=0.007$) is significantly higher than in the best performing units. However, in the worst performing units, the frequency of occurrence of problem situations related to nurses' personal condition is significantly lower ($t=-4.54$; $p=0.000$) than in the best performing units. Finally, in the worst performing ICUs, a significantly lower level of autonomy is found in solving situations related to materials ($t=-2.39$; $p=0.017$) and problems related to information ($t=-2.34$; $p=0.020$) than in the best performing units.

The 25% Best Performing vs 25% Worst Performing ICUs (B80)

First of all, we found significant differences between the two groups with respect to their mean demands scores for two of the categories of tasks. Operational tasks ($t=-4.48$; $p=0.000$) and organizing tasks ($t=-4.91$; $p=0.000$) are perceived as more demanding by nurses in the best performing units compared to nurses in the worst performing units. However, nurses in the best performing units also perceive operational tasks ($t=-3.24$; $p=0.001$) and organizing tasks ($t=-3.69$; $p=0.000$) as more satisfying compared to nurses in the worst performing units.

A higher frequency of problem situations related to materials ($t=7.58$; $p=0.000$), information ($t=3.51$; $p=0.000$) and planning ($t=5.70$; $p=0.000$) is found in the group of worst performing ICUs than in the group of best performing ICUs. In the worst performing ICUs, a significantly lower level of autonomy in solving situations related to norms ($t=-2.61$; $p=0.009$) and personal condition ($t=-2.65$; $p=0.008$) is found compared to the best performing units.

In general, the above results indicate that the number of risk factors is higher in the worst performing units than in the best performing ones (B20 and B80). Whereas some categories of tasks are perceived as more demanding in the best performing units compared to the worst performing units (B80), they are also perceived as more satisfying. Apparently, having to work very hard is rewarding for ICU nurses, a result that was also found in an earlier study among Dutch ICU nurses (De Rijk et al., submitted). When looking at the results with respect to problem situations, it can be concluded that in the worst performing units (B20 and B80) problems with respect to resources (materials, information and planning) occur more frequently. Moreover, both for B20 and B80 it was found that a lack of autonomy in solving problem situations is associated with a poorer objective performance.

Results: Work and Well-Being Questionnaire

Identification of High-Risk Groups

To identify high-risk groups with respect to workload and its negative consequences (burnout, dissatisfaction, poor morale), we performed *t* tests and ANOVAs for the following subgroups, based on:

- Gender (men vs women)
- Type of contract (part-time vs full-time)
- Age (quartiles): <27 years, 27–31 years, 31–37 years, >37 years
- Work experience (quartiles): <2.33 years, 2.33–5 years, 5–9.33 years, >9.33 years

The analyses were performed for all variables in the research model that reflect the perception of workload, its consequences (stress reactions) and individual resources to cope with (the consequences of) a high workload (efficacy and conscientiousness). Note that situational coping resources are not considered here, since they are not relevant for identifying high risk groups.

Workload

Perceived Quantitative Job Demands. Perceived quantitative job demands are higher for women than for men ($t=-3.3$; $p=0.001$) and for full-time workers than for part-time workers ($t=-8.8$; $p=0.000$). Perceived quantitative job demands are highest in the age category <27 years and are lowest in the age category 31–37 years ($F=7.3$; $p=0.000$).

Imbalance Patients/Imbalance Team. Full-time workers experience their relationships with patients as more imbalanced than do part-time workers ($t = -2.7$; $p = 0.007$). The same applies to the relationships with colleagues ($t = -2.2$; $p = 0.025$).

Stress Reactions

Burnout: Emotional Exhaustion. Emotional exhaustion is more prominent among women than among men ($t = -2.2$; $p = 0.028$) and among full-time workers than among part-time workers ($t = -4.7$; $p = 0.000$). Feelings of emotional exhaustion are highest in the age category 31–37 years and are lowest in the age category >37 years ($F = 2.6$; $p = 0.05$). Feelings of emotional exhaustion are highest in the category <2.33 years of ICU experience and are lowest in the category >9.33 years of ICU experience ($F = 4.5$; $p = 0.004$).

Burnout: Depersonalization. Depersonalization is more prominent among men than among women ($t = 3.9$; $p = 0.000$) and among full-time workers than among part-time workers ($t = -3.7$; $p = 0.000$). Feelings of depersonalization are highest in the age category 31–37 years and are lowest in the age category >37 years ($F = 6.0$; $p = 0.000$). Feelings of depersonalization are highest in the category 5–9.33 years of ICU experience and are lowest in the category >9.33 years of ICU experience ($F = 7.0$; $p = 0.000$)

Burnout: Reduced Personal Accomplishment. Feelings of personal accomplishment are higher among full-time workers than among part-time workers ($t = -4.0$; $p = 0.000$). Feelings of accomplishment are highest in the category <2.33 years of ICU experience and are lowest in the category 5–9.33 years of ICU experience ($F = 4.8$; $p = 0.003$).

Job dissatisfacton. Dissatisfaction is lower among women than among men ($t = -2.1$; $p = 0.032$). Job dissatisfaction is lowest in the category <2.33 years of ICU experience and is highest in the category 5–9.33 years of ICU experience ($F = 5.0$; $p = 0.002$).

Perceived Unit Performance. Nurses' opinions on the performance of their unit are more positive for part-time workers than for full-time workers ($t = -2.1$; $p = 0.037$). The highest evaluation of ICU performance is made in the category >9.33 years of ICU experience and the lowest evaluation is made in the category <2.33 years of ICU experience ($F = 3.2$; $p = 0.021$).

Personal Coping Resources

Efficacy. Feelings of efficacy are higher among men than among women ($t = 5.0$; $p = 0.000$). Feelings of efficacy are lowest in the age category <27 years and are highest in the age category >37 years ($F = 17.6$; $p = 0.000$). Feelings of efficacy are lowest in the category <2.33 years of ICU experience, whereas they are highest in the category >9.33 years of ICU experience ($F = 14.4$; $p = 0.000$).

Conscientiousness. Feelings of conscientiousness are higher among women than among men ($t = -2.5$; $p = 0.012$). Feelings of conscientiousness are lowest in the age category <27 years, and are highest in the age category >37 years ($F = 6.8$; $p = 0.000$). Feelings of conscientiousness are lowest in the category <2.33 years of ICU experience, whereas they are highest in the category >9.33 years of ICU experience ($F = 5.1$; $p = 0.002$).

Involvement/Commitment

Job Involvement. The level of job involvement is higher among women than among men ($t = -3.0$; $p = 0.003$) and among full-time workers than among part-time workers ($t = -8.1$; $p = 0.000$). The level of job involvement is lowest in the age category 31–37 years and is highest in the category <27 years ($F = 9.3$; $p = 0.000$). The level of job involvement is lowest in the category 5–9.33 years of ICU experience, whereas it is highest in the category <2.33 years of ICU experience ($F = 6.5$; $p = 0.0002$).

Organizational Commitment. The level of commitment to the ICU is lowest in the category <2.33 years of ICU experience and highest in the category >9.33 years of ICU experience ($F = 5.1$; $p = 0.002$).

Inspection of the research literature on the relationship between these sociodemographic characteristics and each of the variables in our research model yields quite inconsistent results. Therefore, it is difficult to compare the results of this study to earlier findings. In the following, some possible explanations for the above findings will be offered. With respect to gender differences, it can be concluded that women are more at risk regarding some aspects (perceived demands, emotional exhaustion and low efficacy), whereas men are more at risk regarding others (depersonalization, dissatisfaction, low conscientiousness and low involvement). As far as burnout is concerned, it is generally found that women experience more emotional exhaustion, whereas men are more likely to depersonalize patients or clients [44]. These gender differences can be interpreted in terms of masculine and feminine sex roles, i.e. women are expected to be more nurturing, sociable and sensitive to other people's feelings, whereas men are considered to be "tougher" and less emotional. In addition, it is quite likely that gender differences in self-efficacy also boil down to differences in the upbringing of men and women, i.e. men are expected to be more self-confident and self-reliant.

With respect to differences between full- and part-time workers it can be concluded that overall part-timers are less at risk than full-timers (imbalance, emotional exhaustion, depersonalization, reduced personal accomplishment and poor perceived unit performance). This finding can probably be explained by the fact that part-timers have a reduced exposure to stress-inducing factors at work. When looking at differences between the four age categories, two groups seem to be especially at risk, those <27 years (perceived quantitative job demands, low efficacy and low conscientiousness) and 31–37 years (emotional exhaustion, depersonalization and low job involvement). Nonetheless, nurses who are <27 years show the highest level of job involvement. It is quite remarkable that for the youngest age category problems are mainly related to (coping with) demands, whereas for the second age category burnout plays a more prominent role. Probably, nurses who start to work in an ICU feel overwhelmed by demands, whereas the second category feels worn out from the prolonged exposure to these same demands. Finally, nurses who are >37 years show the lowest levels of emotional exhaustion and depersonalization. This probably reflects a selection effect ("survival of the fittest" or the so-called healthy worker effect), i.e. only nurses who have developed adequate coping strategies will survive and stay healthy in a highly demanding working environment. This is also reflected by the fact that these nurses show the highest levels of efficacy and conscientiousness.

The results with respect to the four different categories of work experience are quite identical to those for the different age categories. This is not surprising, since age and work experience are highly correlated ($r=0.63$). Again two groups are at risk, those with <2.33 years of ICU experience (emotional exhaustion, perceived unit performance, efficacy, conscientiousness and commitment) and those with 5–9.33 years of ICU experience (depersonalization, personal accomplishment, satisfaction and involvement). Nurses with >9 years of ICU experience show the lowest levels of emotional exhaustion and depersonalization and the highest levels of efficacy and conscientiousness. Moreover, they have the highest score on measures of morale, such as perceived unit performance and commitment. Finally, nurses with <2 years of ICU experience again show the highest levels of job involvement.

Results: The Basic and Extended Research Models

Multilevel Analyses

Before testing the basic and the extended research model, multilevel analyses were performed for each of the variables in the research model. In multi-level analysis the total amount of variance in each variable is partitioned into the amount of variance that can be accounted for on the individual, the ICU, and the area levels. The results of these analyses are presented in Table 67.

For all variables there is a significant amount of variance to be explained on each of the three levels. As we are dealing with individual perceptions on work and well-being, percentages of variance are of course highest at the individual level. At the ICU level, especially high percentages of variance are found for perceived quantitative job demands, perceived unit effectiveness, task-oriented as well as social-emotional leadership and commitment to the ICU. This is to be expected, as all of these variables are more or less unit-related. At the area level, percentages of variance are high for perceived quantitative job demands, emotional exhaustion, self-efficacy and job involvement. Obviously, cross-national or cultural differences play a role here. Since the amount of variance that is explained at ICU level is statistically significant – albeit small – it makes sense to aggregate data on the ICU level. The rationale behind aggregating data on unit level is that scores on a particular variable reflect a common unit characteristic, at least to

Table 67. Partitioning of variance for the variables in the research model – multilevel analyses ($n = 2090$)

	Variance individual level (%)	Variance ICU level (%)	Variance area level (%)
Variable			
Perceived job demand	66	14	20
Investment patients	88	3	9
Outcomes patients	85	8	7
Investment team	92	2	6
Outcomes team	92	5	3
Emotional exhaustion	78	9	13
Depersonalization	94	4	2
Personal accomplishment	91	3	6
Perceived unit effectiveness	74	17	9
Self-efficacy	87	2	11
Autonomy	90	2	8
Task-oriented leadership	73	18	9
Social-emotional leadership	65	34	1
Job involvement	85	5	10
Organizational commitment	85	12	2

some extent. The results of the multilevel analysis support this rationale and hence provide a justification for testing the research model at unit level as well.

In analyzing the data pertaining to our research models, a stepwise approach was used. First, the basic research model (Fig. 5) was tested. In the second step, coping resources and involvement were added to the model (Fig. 6).

The Basic Research Model

The basic research model was tested using a so-called linear structural modeling technique with the EQS computer program [16]. This technique enables one to test how well a hypothesized model fits current empirical data. The basic model was tested on two levels, namely on the individual, or subjective, level (relating burnout to workload and unit performance as perceived by the ICU nurses themselves) and on the ICU, or objective, level (relating burnout to the objective indicators of workload and ICU performance). Because of the conceptual overlap between the burnout dimension personal accomplishment and the effect variable performance, it was decided to exclude this burnout dimension from the basic model. This overlap was demonstrated empirically by the fact that personal accomplishment loaded on the same component, termed morale, as perceived unit performance, whereas both other burnout dimensions constitute a separate component or factor (see Table 58). An additional reason is that recently the validity of personal accomplishment as an indicator of burnout has been questioned somewhat by some authors (e.g. [47, 33, 36]). These authors state that job stres-

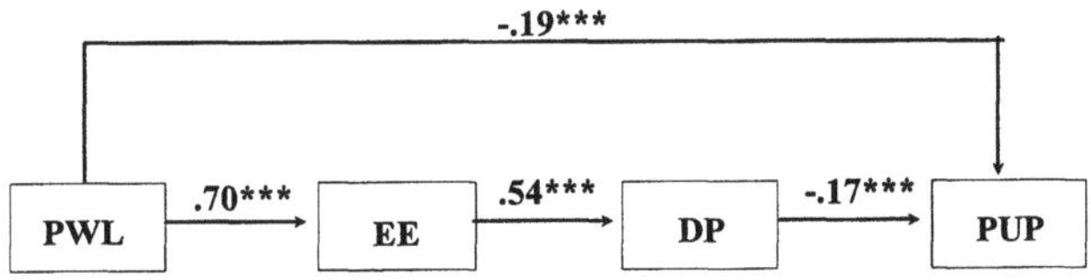

Fig. 8. Workload, burnout and performance (individual level) ($n = 2090$)

sors (such as job demands) lead to emotional exhaustion, which in turn brings about depersonalization, suggesting that care providers attempt to gain emotional distance from recipients as a way of coping with their feelings of exhaustion. Reduced personal accomplishment, however, seems not directly related to both other burnout dimensions, but instead develops in parallel with emotional exhaustion and depersonalization.

Model Test at the Individual Level

The results of the model test at the individual level are presented in Fig. 8. The model is made up of four latent variables that are measured by two (emotional exhaustion, depersonalization, perceived unit performance) or three (perceived workload) manifest variables. For emotional exhaustion, depersonalization and perceived unit performance, the items of the respective scale were randomly assigned to one of the manifest variables. The three subjective indicators of workload (i.e. perceived quantitative job demands, imbalance patients and imbalance team) are significantly intercorrelated (see Table 56), therefore they are represented in the model by one latent variable (perceived workload).

The EQS program indicated that our model fit quite well to the empirical data (CFI = 0.95). Fit indices such as the comparative fit index (CFI) should exceed 0.90 [16] in order to indicate a proper model fit. The numbers that are printed in Fig. 8 are so-called standardized path coefficients. The higher the value of these coefficients, the stronger the association that is indicated by the respective arrow. Path coefficients range from -1.0 to $+1.0$. The results with respect to our model test can be summarized as follows: The higher the perceived workload, the poorer the performance of the ICU is evaluated by the nurses. Second, a higher perceived workload is also strongly, positively associated with emotional exhaustion: the higher the workload, the higher the level of exhaustion. As expected, high levels of exhaustion lead to depersonalization. These in turn lead to a more negative evaluation of unit performance. Thus, the subjective experience of high workload is both directly and indirectly related to poor perceived unit performance.

Model Test at the Unit (ICU) Level

On this level, the model was tested twice: once for B20 (Fig. 9) and once for B80 (Fig. 10). As indicated before, data with respect to burnout (emotional exhaustion and depersonalization) were aggregated at unit level, i.e. for each ICU a mean unit score on each of these variables was calculated.

The EQS program again indicated that the model fit quite well to the data ($CFI_{B20} = 0.97$ and $CFI_{B80} = 0.97$). Though all relationships in the model are again

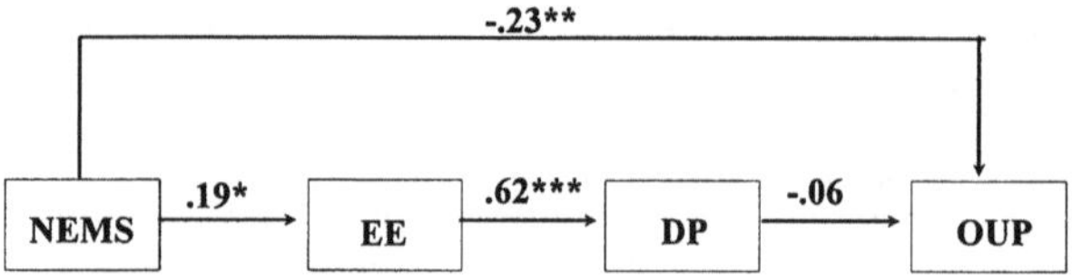

Fig. 9. Workload, burnout and performance (less severe patients; B20) at unit level ($n = 80$)

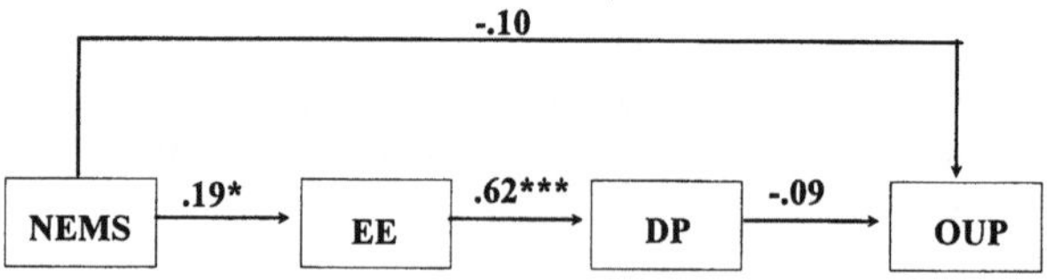

Fig. 10. Workload, burnout and performance (more severe patients; B80) at unit level ($n = 80$). *NEMS*, Nine Equivalents Manpower Use Score; *EE*, emotional exhaustion; *DP*, depersonalization; *OUP*, objective unit performance (B80 reversed)

in the expected direction, not all of them reach significance. This lack of significance is most probably due to the small sample size (i.e. 80 units), which reduces the statistical power of the significance test. First, objective workload turned out to be significantly, negatively related to objective performance for B20, but not for B80. Thus, for the less severe patients a higher objective workload is related to a poorer objective unit performance. Second, the higher the objective workload, the higher the mean level of emotional exhaustion in an ICU. Higher mean levels of emotional exhaustion are associated with higher mean levels of depersonalization. Finally, higher mean levels of depersonalization are negatively, but not significantly, related to objective unit performance (B20 and B80). Accordingly, contrary to expectations, the relationship between objective workload and objective unit performance is not mediated by burnout. However, a higher objective workload is indeed significantly, positively related to emotional exhaustion.

The Extended Research Model

Due to the nature of the variables that were added to the basic model (i.e. coping resources and involvement), the extended model can only be tested on the individual level. To test the possible moderating effects of: (a) coping resources on the workload-burnout relationship and (b) involvement on the burnout-performance relationship, hierarchical multiple regression analyses were performed (Tables 68, 69). As we found significant differences between specific subgroups in our sample with respect to workload, stress reactions, perceived unit performance and coping resources (see "Identification of High-Risk Groups"), we controlled for gender, type of assignment, area and years of ICU experience in the first step of these analyses. It should be noted that testing the effects of the different moderators in separate analyses increases the risk of chance capitalization.

Table 68. Hierarchical multiple regression analyses of job demands and: (a) job autonomy; (b) task-oriented leadership; (c) social-emotional leadership; (d) self-efficacy, and (e) conscientiousness on burnout, after controlling for gender, type of assignment, area and years of ICU experience ($n = 2090$)

Burnout dimension	EE					DP					PA				
Moderator	JA	SE	TL	SL	CO	JA	SE	TL	SL	CO	JA	SE	TL	SL	CO
Job demands	+	+	+	+	+	+	+	+	+	+	+	+	+	+	+
Moderator	–	–	ns	–	–	–	–	ns	–	–	+	+	+	+	+
Demands* moderator	ns	ns	ns	ns	ns	ns	ns	ns	ns	ns	ns	ns	ns	ns	+
R^2 (including control variances)	0.24	0.23	0.23	0 .25	0.24	0.05	0.05	0.05	0.07	0.09	0.15	0.16	0.10	0.10	0.16

+ significant positive relationship ($p \leq 0.5$); – significant negative relationship ($p \leq 0.5$); ns, nonsignificant relationship; EE, emotional exhaustion; DP, depersonalization; PA, personal accomplishment; JA, job autonomy; SE, self-efficacy; TL, task-oriented leadership; SL, social-emotional leadership; CO, conscientiousness.

Table 69. Hierarchical multiple regression analyses of two burnout dimensions (emotional exhaustion and depersonalization) and: (a) job involvement; (b) organizational commitment on perceived unit performane, after controlling for gender, type of assignment, area and years of ICU experience ($n = 2090$)

Burnout dimension	EE		DP	
Moderator	INV	COM	INV	COM
Burnout dimension	–	–	–	–
Moderator	+	+	+	+
Demands moderator	ns	ns	ns	ns
R^2 (including control variances)	0.20	0.33	0.20	0.33

Unfortunately, very little support was found for the hypothesized moderating role of coping resources and involvement. Only in one case was a significant effect of coping resources on the relationship between job demands and burnout found, i.e. the relationship between job demands and personal accomplishment is moderated by nurses' level of conscientiousness (i.e. their level of accuracy, efficiency and skillfulness). The interaction effect of quantitative job demands and conscientiousness on personal accomplishment is graphically represented in Fig. 11.

From the figure it can be concluded that, overall, nurses scoring high in conscientiousness have stronger feelings of personal accomplishment than nurses scoring low in conscientiousness. Whereas for nurses low in conscientiousness there is no significant relationship between job demands and feelings of personal accomplishment, this relationship is positive for nurses high in conscientious-

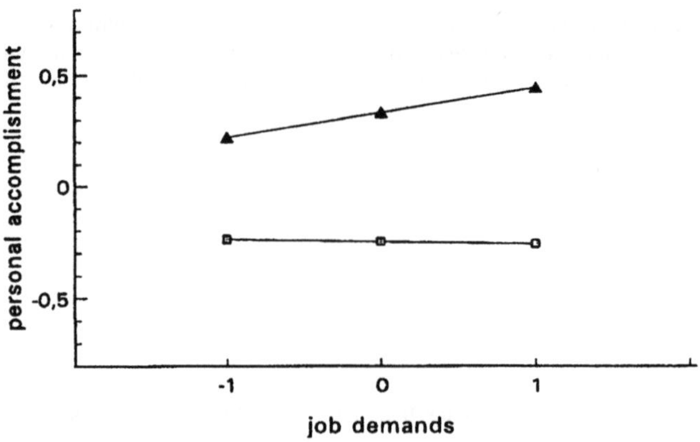

Fig. 11. The interaction effect of quantitative job demands and conscientiousness on personal accomplishment. Conscientiousness: *open squares*, high (−1 SD); *closed triangles*, low (+1 SD)

ness, i.e. higher demands are associated with stronger feelings of accomplishment. This positive relationship can probably be explained by the fact that, due to their high level of conscientiousness, these nurses are able to function properly even in situations with high demands, which in turn will boost their feelings of accomplishment. In addition, no significant influence of either job involvement or organizational commitment on the relationship between burnout and performance was found. However, it should be noted that some significant direct effects of coping resources as well as involvement were found (see Tables 68, 69). First, with the exception of the nonsignificant relationship between task-oriented leadership, and emotional exhaustion and depersonalization, each of the five coping resources is negatively related to emotional exhaustion and depersonalization and positively related to personal accomplishment. Thus, the more coping resources ICU nurses have at their disposal, the less burnout symptoms they report. Second, both job involvement and organizational commitment are significantly, positively related to perceived unit performance: the higher the level of psychological identification with the job and/or with the ICU, the better the performance of the ICU is evaluated by nurses.

Conclusions

To summarize, the aim of the EURICUS-I *Personnel* substudy was twofold:

1. To perform a detailed job analysis of ICU nursesand to identify risk factors for their well-being at work as well as to identify high-risk groups
2. To test a model of the relationship between ICU nurses' workload, their stress reactions (burnout and dissatisfaction) and the performance of their ICU

For this purpose, two questionnaires were distributed among the nursing staff of the 89 ICUs participating in the EURICUS-I project, i.e. the WEBIC questionnaire and the Work and Well-Being questionnaire. Response rates were 67% and 72%, respectively.

The job analysis revealed that, in general, having to work hard is rewarding for ICU nurses, as they consistently evaluate more demanding tasks as also being more satisfying. This applies in particular to operational tasks (nursing and medical care of patients). It was pointed out that the most central (i.e. operational) tasks are also the most satisfying ones since these define nursing. Thus, although the operational tasks are considered the most demanding, they are at the same time the most rewarding since they lay at the core of what nursing is all about. Alternatively, this finding may represent a selection effect, i.e. the decision to work in an ICU already implies a preference for demanding working situations. Looking more closely at the demands- and satisfaction scores within each of the different categories of tasks makes clear that special attention has to be paid to psychosocial aspects of patient care (including contact with relatives) and to (interdisciplinary and external) communication, as these tasks are perceived as either quite demanding or fairly dissatisfying.

With respect to ICU nurses' task mix, it was found that nurses perform activities from all of the four categories of tasks. They spend the most time on operational tasks (50%), and the least time on preparatory tasks (10%). The validity of nurses' self-reports about their usage of time was supported by the fact that similar results were obtained in a Dutch study that used an objective method (time-sampling) to asses nurses' activities.

Results with respect to ICU-specific problem situations showed that, at least in this sample, the stressfulness of ICU nurses' jobs is low, as illustrated by the low frequency of ICU-specific problem situations and the high level of autonomy to solve these problems. The most frequently occurring problems have to do with norms, and more specifically with ICU nurses' workload. This might be somewhat surprising given the generally held belief that ICU nursing is quite stressful (see [37]. However, despite these claims, that nursing in ICUs is particularly stressful and might thus cause stress reactions such as burnout or dissatisfaction, comparisons with other hospitals wards are inconclusive. Harris [24] reviewed 23 studies that compared ICUs and non-ICUs on several stress-related outcomes (e.g. job dissatisfaction, burnout, turnover, alienation, and diminished organizational commitment) that were measured with self-reports. Fifteen studies found no differences between ICUs and non-ICUs, three studies reported fewer stress reactions in ICUs, and only five studies indicated higher stress-related outcomes in ICUs. Perhaps, the fact that nurses in ICUs have a relatively high level of autonomy might explain why they do not experience their jobs as being particularly stressful.

To identify risk factors for ICU nurses' performance, the 25% worst performing units and the 25% best performing units were compared based on objective performance assesment using the SAPS-II score. Results indicated that the number of risk factors is indeed higher in the worst performing units than in the best performing ones. Especially, problems with respect to (a lack of) resources (materials, information etc.) occur more frequently in the worst performing units. Moreover, it is found that a lack of autonomy in solving problem situations is associated with a poorer objective performance. Thus, particular risk factors are more prominent in poor performing than in well performing ICUs.

To identify high-risk groups, specific subgroups were compared. Comparison by gender made clear that women were found to be more at risk on some work-related aspects, whereas men were more at risk on others. Overall, part-timer workers were less at risk than full-time workers, which is probably due to their lower exposure to stress-inducing factors at work. The results with respect to different age categories and length of work experience were quite identical and showed that two groups were especially at risk with respect to workload and burnout symptoms: the youngest/least experienced group < 27 years/ < 2.33 years of ICU experience) and the middle group (31–37 years/5–9.33 years of ICU experience). Whereas the first group probably has to develop a repertoire in order to cope adequately with the stresses of intensive care nursing, the coping resources of the second group are likely to be depleted by the prolonged exposure to demanding working situations. Psychologically, two mechanisms might be at work here: the young and inexperienced group is going through a period of work socialization, whereas the older and more experienced group is going through a process of wearing out or erosion of their coping repertoire. Probably, the latter is also related to the more stressful off-job situation of the somewhat older group. It is reasonable to assume that many of the ICU nurses in the older age group between 31 and 37 have small children they have to care for, which adds to the demands they face on the job.

The second part of the analysis dealt with the testing of both the basic and the extended research model. The basic research model was supported at the individual level, but not at the unit level: burnout mediates the relationship between perceived workload and perceived unit performance, but this is not the case for the relationship between objective workload and objective unit performance. Whereas ICU nurses' objective workload turns out to be significantly, positively related to burnout, burnout is not significantly related to objective unit performance. Moreover, almost no support was found for the extended research model, i.e. for the moderating role of coping resources and involvement on the relationship between workload and burnout, and burnout and performance. Instead, situational and personal coping resources have a direct effect on levels of burnout; that is, self-efficacy, conscientiousness, autonomy, and social-emotional leadership are associated with low levels of burnout (emotional exhaustion, depersonalization, and reduced personal accomplishment). In addition, direct effects of involvement and commitment are observed on nurses' perceived unit performance; the more involved and committed, the higher their performance.

Finally, some limitations of this study deserve attention. First, though the way of presenting the results may suggest causality, the cross-sectional design of this study does not permit causal inferences on the relationships between the variables in the research models. Second, in the previous analyses no distinction was made between different types of ICUs (small vs large; university vs nonuniversity, etc.) or between different areas. It cannot be excluded that results may look different for various subsamples. However, for reasons of economy, in this section a more general picture was drawn that can be used as a starting point as well as a background for more detailed analysis in particular subgroups.

The major strength of the present *Personnel* substudy is the combination of subjective questionnaire data and objective workload and performance data. As in most other studies subjective and objective indicators are relatively weakly intercorrelated. As Frese and Zapf [19] state in discussing this methodological issue:"...the use of objective judgements of work stressors leads to an underestimate of the 'true' correlation'." Despite the fact that the model that assumed that burnout plays an intermediate role between objective workload and objective unit performance was not confirmed, a positive association was found at unit level between a high objective workload and burnout (i.e. emotional exhaustion). This important result is corroborated by a similar finding in a study among 20 Dutch ICUs. Schaufeli et al. [43] showed that objectively assessed workload, as measured by the percentage of patients who were mechanically ventilated, was significantly and positively related to nurses' burnout at unit level.

Appendix A. Definition of variables in the extended research model

Workload

Nurses' workload is assessed both subjectively (by means of self-reports) and objectively (by scoring nursing activities performed during the previous 24 h). This yields the following two measures of workload:

1. Perceived quantitative job demands (subjective workload): nurses' perception of their workload in terms of the quantity of work they have to perform
2. Qualitative job demands (objective workload): measured with NEMS (Nine Equivalents of Nursing Manpower Use Score), a validated, simplified version of TISS (Therapeutic Intervention Scoring System)

Burnout

Burnout was selected as an indicator of ICU nurses' level of chronic stress. It can be considered a long-term stress reaction, reflecting a "wearing out" from prolonged exposure to the stresses of contact-intensive occupations, such as nursing. Burnout is assessed by means of self-reports and is characterized by three symptoms:

1. Emotional exhaustion: feeling "emotionally drained' from your work
2. Depersonalization: a callous and cynical attitude towards patients
3. Reduced personal accomplishment: feeling "incompetent" in your job

Performance

Performance is assessed both subjectively (by means of self-reports) and objectively (by means of clinical outcome data).

1. Perceived unit performance: nurses' judgement on the performance of their ICU
2. Objective unit performance: the ratio of observed vs predicted mortality at the ICU (i.e. the Standardized Mortality Ratio) at P20 of SAPS-II and P80 of SAPS-II

Coping Resources

1. Situational coping resources:
   - Autonomy: nurses' freedom of action in performing their work
   - Leadership: nurses' judgement on the head nurse's leadership behavior, measured with two different scales: (1) Social emotional leadership, i.e. the degree to which the head nurse is friendly and pays attention to her/his subordinates; (2) task-oriented leadership, i.e. the degree to which tasks are specified and monitored in detail by the head nurse
2. Individual coping resources
   - Self-efficacy: nurses' judgement on their personal abilities to attain goals and to overcome potential problems
   - Conscientiousness: nurses' judgement on their own level of conscientiousness

Job Involvement

1. Job involvement: the degree to which work plays a central part in nurses' life
2. Organizational commitment: nurses' level of identification with and involvement in the ICU

Appendix B. Correlations between variables in the extended research model

	DEM	IOp	IOt	EE	DP	RPA	Dsat	Pup	Aut	SEL	TOL	Sef	Con	Inv	Com
DEM	1.0000	0.1706**	0.1170**	0.4000**	0.1020**	−0.0928**	0.1937**	−0.0516*	0.1839**	−0.1382**	0.1110**	−0.0320	0.0373	0.1551**	−0.0876**
IOp	0.1706**	1.0000	0.2434**	0.1647**	0.0967**	0.0518*	0.1218**	−0.1449**	−0.0119	−0.0707**	−0.0633**	0.0281	0.0329	−0.0257	−0.0917**
IOt	0.1170**	0.2434**	1.0000	0.1423**	0.0034	0.0287	0.1356**	−0.1454**	−0.0087	−0.1033**	−0.0113	0.0199	0.0431	0.0339	−0.4112**
EE	0.4000**	0.1647**	0.1423**	1.0000	0.4345**	0.1325**	0.4733**	−0.1782**	−0.0142	−0.1961**	0.0247	−0.1264**	−0.1081**	−0.0377	−0.3131**
DP	0.1020**	0.0967**	0.0034	0.4345**	1.0000	0.2387**	0.2851**	−0.1662**	−0.0765**	−0.1292**	−0.0418	−0.0666**	−0.1082**	−0.0970**	−0.1813**
RPA	−0.0928**	0.0518*	0.0287	0.1325**	0.2387**	1.0000	0.3389**	−0.2110**	−0.2836**	−0.1375**	−0.0759**	−0.2803**	−0.2830**	−0.2670**	−0.2419**
Dsat	0.1937**	0.1218**	0.1356**	0.4733**	0.2851**	0.3389**	1.0000	−0.3411**	−0.2174**	−0.3053**	−0.0823**	−0.1840**	−0.1519**	−0.2644**	−0.4368**
Pup	−0.0146	−0.1449**	−0.1454**	−0.1782**	−0.1662**	−0.2110**	−0.3411**	1.0000	0.2110**	0.2094**	0.2070**	0.4120**	0.1195**	0.1940**	0.4721**
Aut	0.1839**	−0.0119	−0.0087	−0.0142	−0.0765**	−0.2836**	−0.2174**	0.2110**	1.0000	0.1019**	−0.0530*	0.1742**	0.1365**	0.1828**	0.2834**
SEL	−0.1382**	−0.0707**	−0.1033**	−0.1961**	−0.1292**	−0.1375**	−0.3053**	0.2094**	0.1019**	1.0000	0.1178**	0.1117**	0.0662**	0.1580**	0.3105**
TOL	0.1110**	−0.0633**	−0.0113	0.0247	−0.0418	−0.0759**	−0.0823**	0.2070**	−0.0530*	0.1178**	1.0000	−0.0329	0.0423	0.2012**	0.1561**
Sef	−0.0320	0.0281	0.0199	−0.1264**	−0.0666**	−0.2803**	−0.1840**	0.1420**	0.1742**	0.1117**	−0.0329	1.0000	0.4143**	0.0919**	0.1411**
Con	0.0373	0.0329	0.0431	−0.1081**	−0.1802**	−0.2830**	−0.1519**	0.1195**	0.1365**	0.0662**	0.0423	0.4143**	1.0000	0.1069**	0.1153**
Inv	0.1551**	−0.0257	0.0339	−0.0377	−0.0970**	−0.2670**	−0.2644**	0.1940**	0.1828**	0.1580**	0.2012**	0.0919**	0.1069**	1.0000	0.3277**
Com	−0.0876**	−0.0917**	−0.1442**	−0.3131**	−0.1813**	−0.2419**	−0.4368**	0.4721**	0.2834**	0.3105**	0.1561**	0.1411**	0.1153**	0.3277**	1.0000

*Significant ≤0.05; **Significant ≤0.01 (2-tailed).

Legend

DEM: quantitative job demands; IOp: imbalance patients; IOt: imbalance team; EE: emotional exhaustion; DP: depersonalization; RPA: reduced personal accomplishment; Dsat: job satisfaction; Pup: perceived unit performance; Aut: autonomy; SEL: social emotional leadership; TOL: task oriented leadership; Sef: generalized self-efficacy; Con: conscientiousness; Inv: job involvement; Com: organizational commitment

Appendix C. Mean demands score and mean satisfaction score for each of the WEBIC tasks

Operational tasks: demands

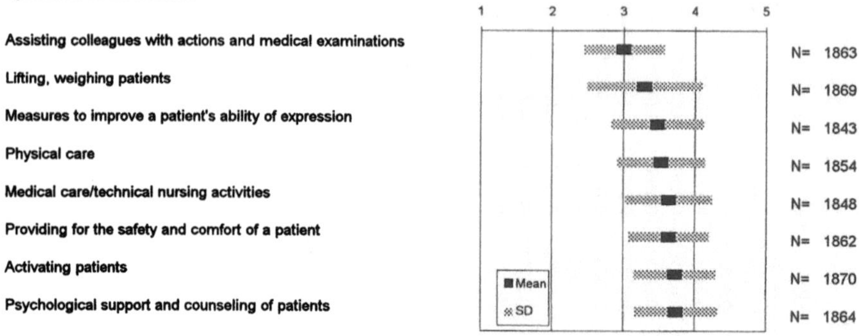

Operational tasks: satisfaction

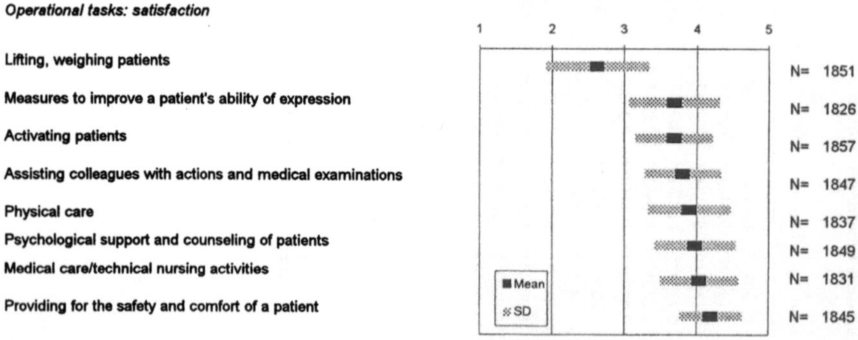

Organising tasks: demands

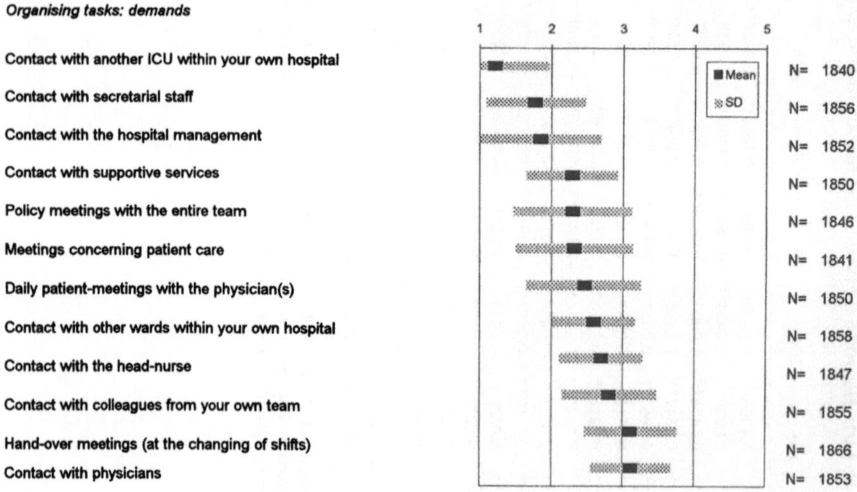

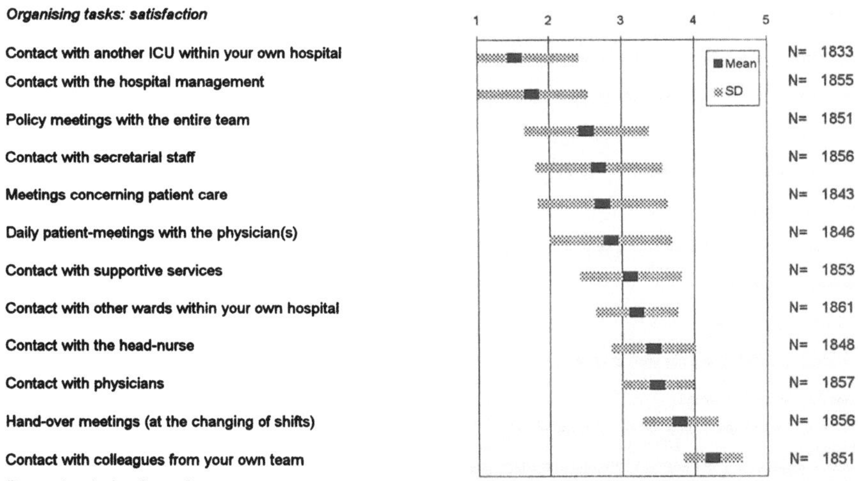
Organising tasks: satisfaction
1 2 3 4 5
Mean
SD
Contact with another ICU within your own hospital N= 1833
Contact with the hospital management N= 1855
Policy meetings with the entire team N= 1851
Contact with secretarial staff N= 1856
Meetings concerning patient care N= 1843
Daily patient-meetings with the physician(s) N= 1846
Contact with supportive services N= 1853
Contact with other wards within your own hospital N= 1861
Contact with the head-nurse N= 1848
Contact with physicians N= 1857
Hand-over meetings (at the changing of shifts) N= 1856
Contact with colleagues from your own team N= 1851

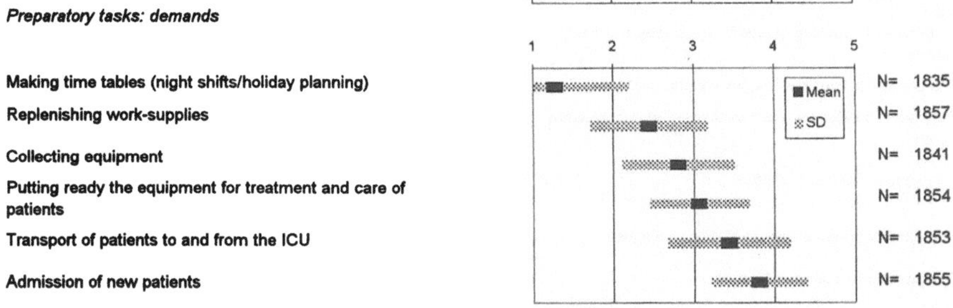
Preparatory tasks: demands
1 2 3 4 5
Mean
SD
Making time tables (night shifts/holiday planning) N= 1835
Replenishing work-supplies N= 1857
Collecting equipment N= 1841
Putting ready the equipment for treatment and care of patients N= 1854
Transport of patients to and from the ICU N= 1853
Admission of new patients N= 1855

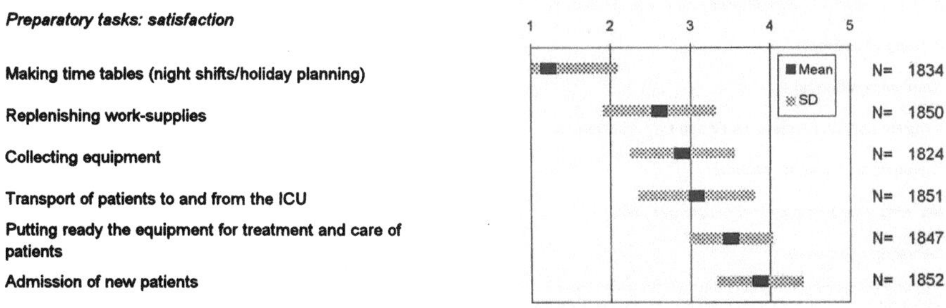
Preparatory tasks: satisfaction
1 2 3 4 5
Mean
SD
Making time tables (night shifts/holiday planning) N= 1834
Replenishing work-supplies N= 1850
Collecting equipment N= 1824
Transport of patients to and from the ICU N= 1851
Putting ready the equipment for treatment and care of patients N= 1847
Admission of new patients N= 1852

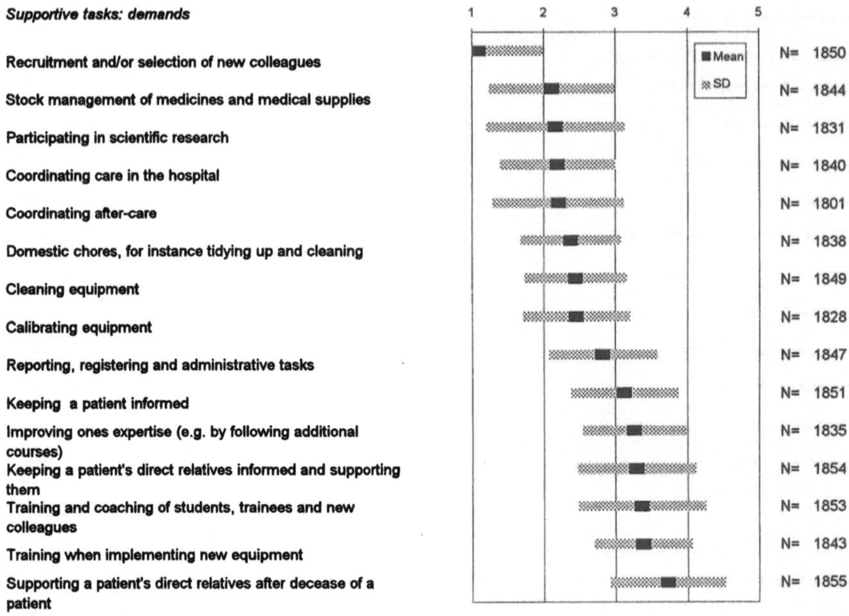
Supportive tasks: demands
1
2
3
4
5
Mean
SD
Recruitment and/or selection of new colleagues N= 1850
Stock management of medicines and medical supplies N= 1844
Participating in scientific research N= 1831
Coordinating care in the hospital N= 1840
Coordinating after-care N= 1801
Domestic chores, for instance tidying up and cleaning N= 1838
Cleaning equipment N= 1849
Calibrating equipment N= 1828
Reporting, registering and administrative tasks N= 1847
Keeping a patient informed N= 1851
Improving ones expertise (e.g. by following additional courses) N= 1835
Keeping a patient's direct relatives informed and supporting them N= 1854
Training and coaching of students, trainees and new colleagues N= 1853
Training when implementing new equipment N= 1843
Supporting a patient's direct relatives after decease of a patient N= 1855

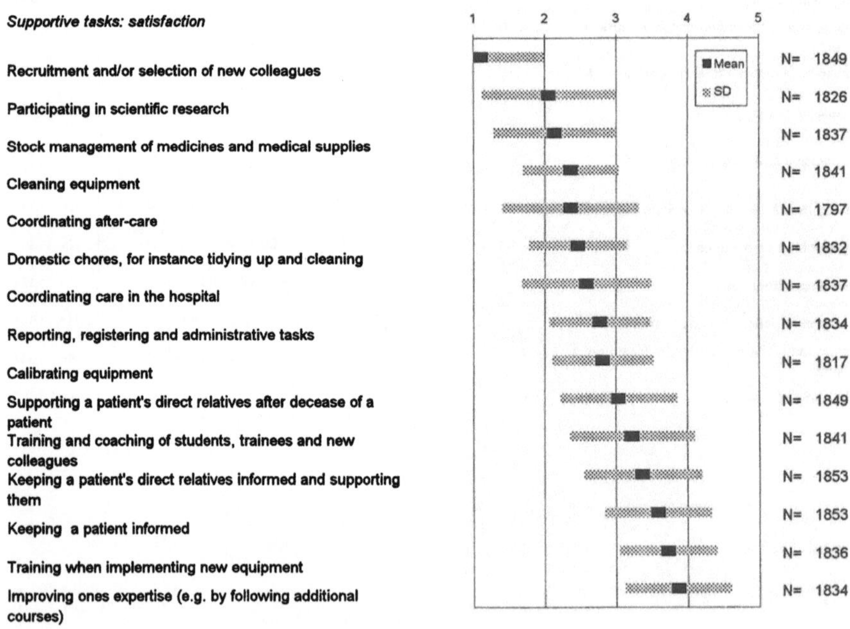
Supportive tasks: satisfaction
1
2
3
4
5
Mean
SD
Recruitment and/or selection of new colleagues N= 1849
Participating in scientific research N= 1826
Stock management of medicines and medical supplies N= 1837
Cleaning equipment N= 1841
Coordinating after-care N= 1797
Domestic chores, for instance tidying up and cleaning N= 1832
Coordinating care in the hospital N= 1837
Reporting, registering and administrative tasks N= 1834
Calibrating equipment N= 1817
Supporting a patient's direct relatives after decease of a patient N= 1849
Training and coaching of students, trainees and new colleagues N= 1841
Keeping a patient's direct relatives informed and supporting them N= 1853
Keeping a patient informed N= 1853
Training when implementing new equipment N= 1836
Improving ones expertise (e.g. by following additional courses) N= 1834

Appendix D. Mean frequency score and mean autonomy score for each of the WEBIC problem situation

Norms: frequency

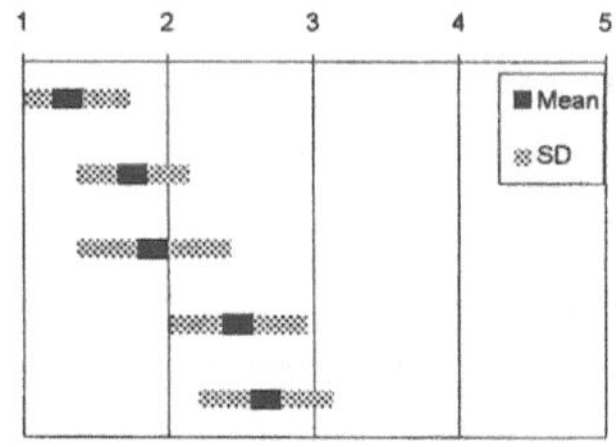

Instructions of the head-nurse are unclear	N= 1811
Instructions of the physicians are unclear	N= 1848
Paper work disturbing your work-schedule	N= 1842
Unexpected job activities interrupting your work-schedule	N= 1854
Having to do too many things simultaneously	N= 1857

Norms: autonomy

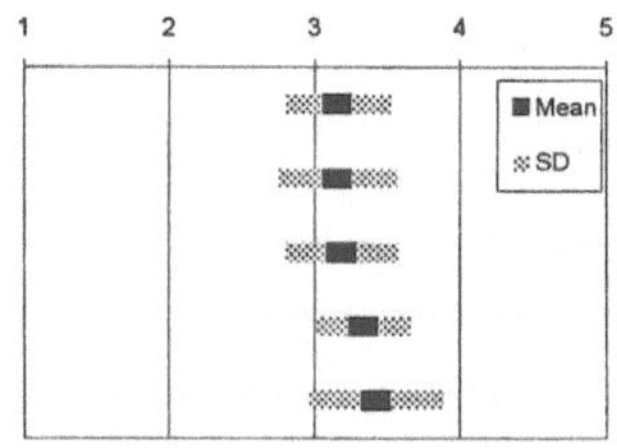

Having to do too many things simultaneously	N= 1794
Unexpected job activities interrupting your work-schedule	N= 1781
Instructions of the head-nurse are unclear	N= 1484
Instructions of the physicians are unclear	N= 1726
Paper work disturbing your work-schedule	N= 1630

Patients: frequency

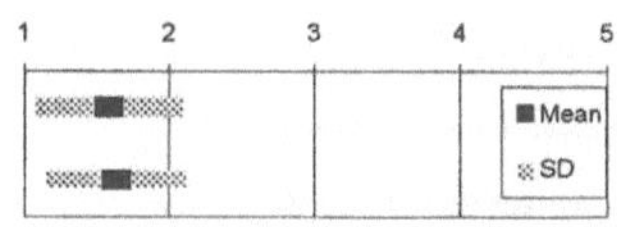

Too little variation in the nursing of patients	N= 1833
The nursing of patients is too complex	N= 1816

Patients: autonomy

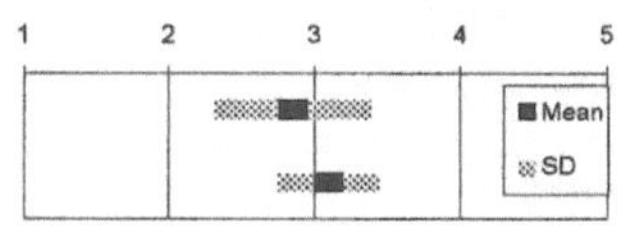

The nursing of patients is too complex	N= 1503
Too little variation in the nursing of patients	N= 1529

Materials: frequency

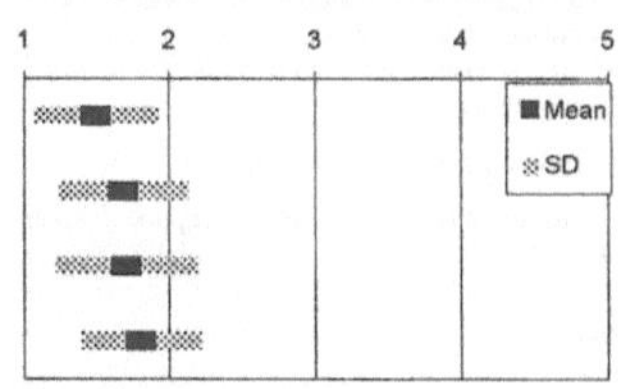

Insufficient quality of materials	N= 1846
Materials/equipment are not available at the ICU	N= 1851
Materials or equipment are not at the place agreed upon	N= 1852
Equipment which does not function properly or has broken down	N= 1852

Materials: autonomy

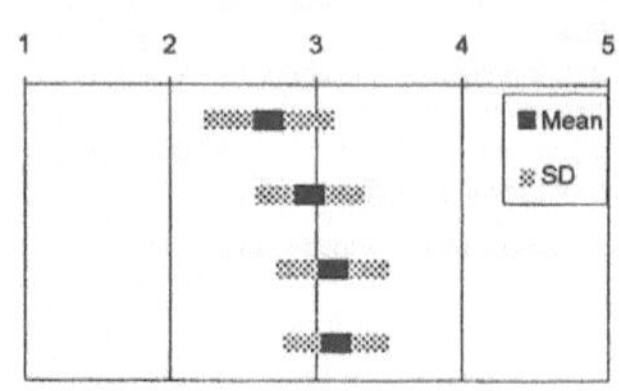

Insufficient quality of materials	N= 1643
Equipment which does not function properly or has broken down	N= 1760
Materials/equipment are not available at the ICU	N= 1723
Materials or equipment are not at the place agreed upon	N= 1692

Condition: frequency

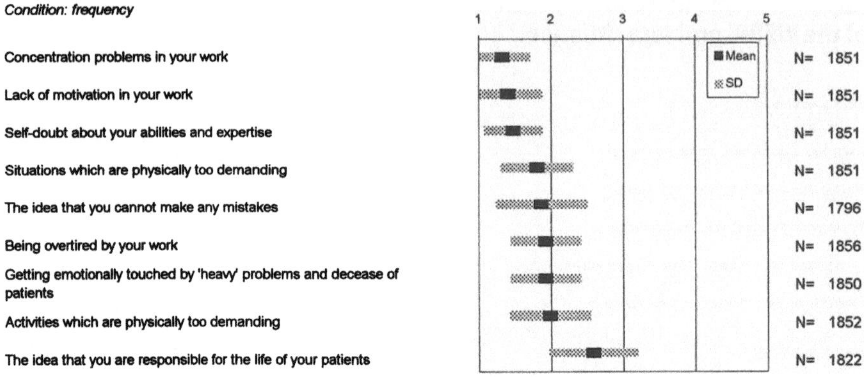

Condition: autonomy

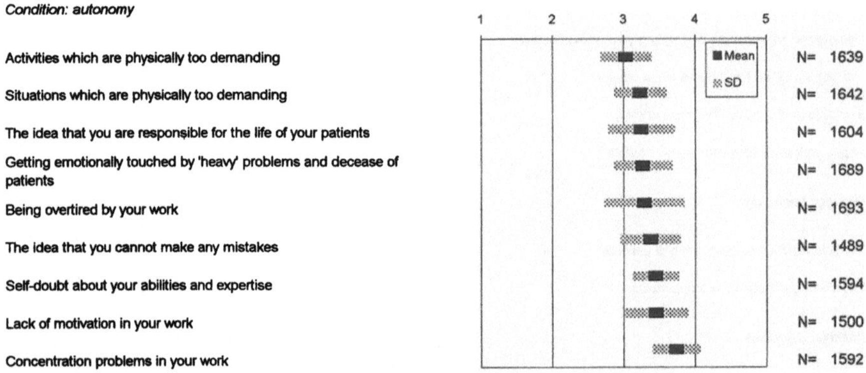

Information: frequency

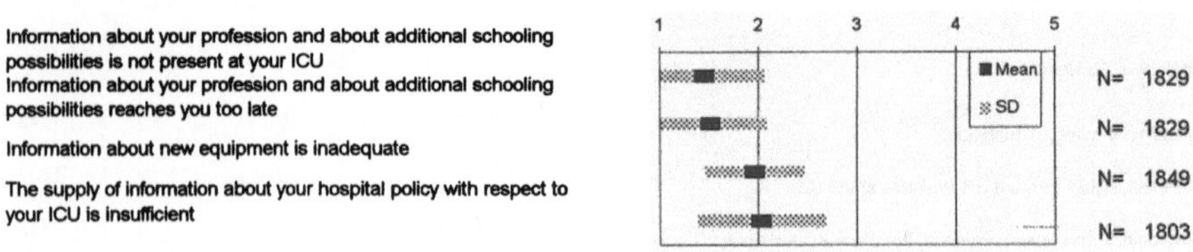

Information: autonomy

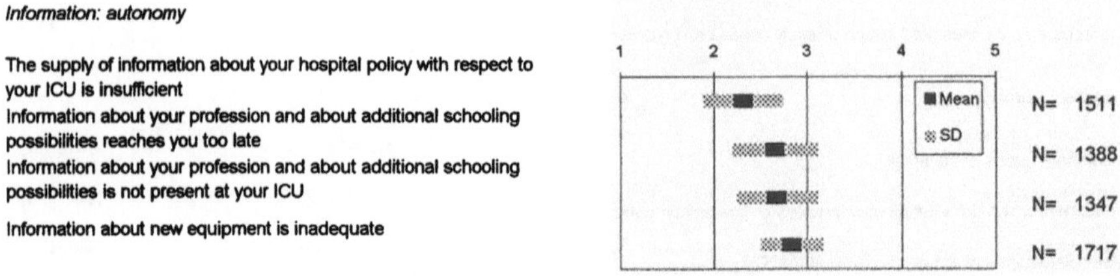

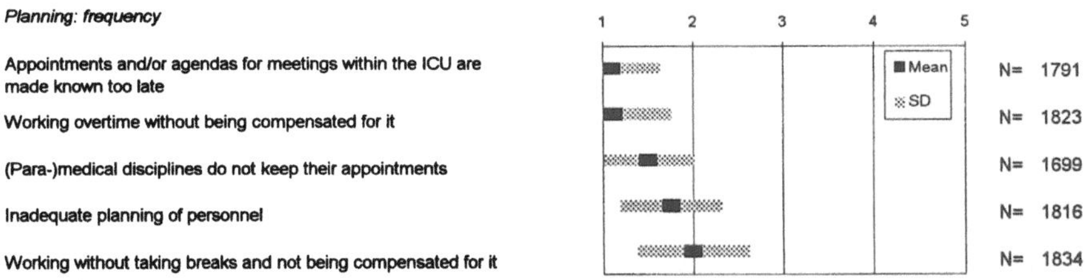
Planning: frequency
1
2
3
4
5
Mean
SD
Appointments and/or agendas for meetings within the ICU are made known too late
N= 1791
Working overtime without being compensated for it
N= 1823
(Para-)medical disciplines do not keep their appointments
N= 1699
Inadequate planning of personnel
N= 1816
Working without taking breaks and not being compensated for it
N= 1834

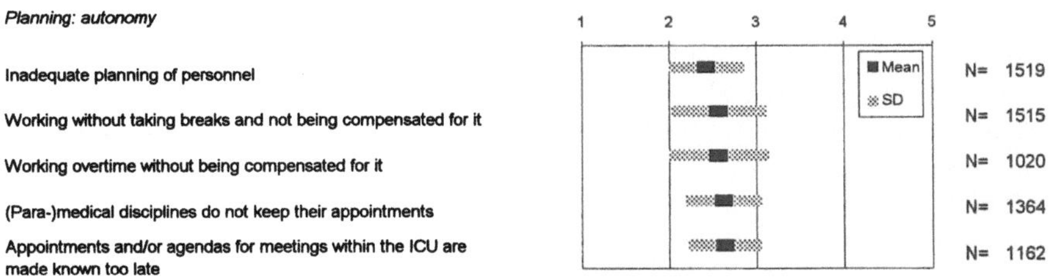
Planning: autonomy
1
2
3
4
5
Mean
SD
Inadequate planning of personnel
N= 1519
Working without taking breaks and not being compensated for it
N= 1515
Working overtime without being compensated for it
N= 1020
(Para-)medical disciplines do not keep their appointments
N= 1364
Appointments and/or agendas for meetings within the ICU are made known too late
N= 1162

Cultures in ICUs

G. Sanders and J. van der Veen

Introduction

In this section, the results of the *Culture* substudy will be presented. This comparative culture study is, as far as we know, the first of its kind in the field of ICUs in Europe. The *Culture* substudy is based on insights and experience gained in previous studies into the differences between national cultures [51] and the differences between the cultures of organizations [52]. In this report, the following topics will be dealt with:

- The definition of culture and the forms of cultural expression
- Measuring the culture of organizations: including a description of the six previously recorded dimensions of organizational culture
- The design of the comparative study of the ICUs
- The most important findings of the study

Definition of Organizational Culture

Our working definition of culture is: *The collective programming of the mind which distinguishes the members of one category of people from another.* This applies to organizations as well as to nations, regions, professions and generations. In the case of organizations, the "members" include not only employees and managers, but also various types of stakeholders: customers, interest groups, authorities. Our definition stresses that culture is: (1) something collective and not a characteristic of individuals; (2) mental "software", therefore invisible and intangible as such; and (3) only interesting to the extent that it differentiates among categories of people, that is, it is expressed in characteristics which some have and others do not. Some people may raise the objection that culture is not only in people's minds (the software), but also in the "hardware" produced by these people themselves or by their cultural ancestors: in the case of organizations, this hardware includes tangibles such as buildings, uniforms, company cars and the like. However, we believe that the essence of culture is not the hardware as such, but the meaning attached to it by the members of the culture.

Manifestations of culture are classified into four categories: symbols, heroes, rituals and values. They can be conceived as the successive layers of an onion: from shallow, superficial symbols to deeper rituals. Symbols are words, gestures, pictures or objects that carry a particular meaning within a culture. Symbols are at a fairly superficial level of mental programming, in the sense that it is relatively easy to introduce new symbols or abolish old ones. At a somewhat deeper level, a culture has its heroes. Heroes are persons, alive or dead, real or imaginary, who possess characteristics highly prized in the culture and who thus serve as role models to be followed. Rituals are collective activities which are technically superfluous but are socially essential within a culture. They are, therefore, carried out for their own sake, as when one pays respect to another member of the culture, or when ceremonial meetings take place; their liturgies and meanings to the insiders are, again, culture-specific. Symbols, heroes and rituals can be subsumed under the term "practices", because they are visible to an observer, although their cultural meaning lies in the way they are perceived by insiders. The core of culture is formed by values, in the sense of broad, nonspecific feelings of good and evil, beautiful and ugly, normal and abnormal, rational and irrational – feelings that are often unconscious and rarely discussible, which cannot be observed as such but which are manifested in behavior.

Measuring Organizational Cultures

Unless one is able to measure it, studying and talking about organizational culture has no meaning. The approach to measuring organizational culture has been developed in a large field research project of organizational cultures, managed by Sanders [52]. The project covered 20 different organizational units or departments in ten different organizations in Denmark and the Netherlands. Two steps can be distinguished: in-depth open interviews with nine members of each unit, followed by a paper-and-pencil survey of 60 members of each unit – 20 managers, 20 professional and 20 nonprofessional employees. The interview checklist contained questions such as: What are special terms here that only insiders understand? (to identify organizational symbols); What kind of people are most likely to make a fast career here? (to identify organizational heroes); Which events are celebrated in this organization? (to identify organizational rituals); and What things do people very much like to see happening here? What is the biggest mistake one can make? (to identify organizational values). The interviews were used to create a qualitative, empathic description of the culture of each of the 20 cases. In the standardized survey questionnaire, the items covered both organizational practices and the respondents' values related to the work and the organization.

The factor analysis of the survey results revealed that the 20 units differed mainly in the ways in which members perceived the daily practices. The practices (P) within the 20 units varied along six statistically independent dimensions:

1. Dimension P1: Process-oriented vs results-oriented
2. Dimension P2: Employee-oriented vs job-oriented
3. Dimension P3: Parochial vs professional
4. Dimension P4: Open system vs closed system
5. Dimension P5: Loose control vs tight control
6. Dimension P6: Pragmatic vs normative

Dimension P1 refers to a concern with either means (process-oriented) or goals (results-oriented). The key items selected show that, in process-oriented cultures, people perceive themselves as avoiding risks and as devoting only a limited amount of effort to their jobs; each day is pretty much the same. In results-oriented cultures, people perceive themselves as being comfortable in unfamiliar situations and as applying a maximum amount of effort; each day is felt to bring new challenges.

Dimension P2 refers to a concern for people (employee-oriented) or a concern for completing the job (job-oriented). The three key items show that, in employee-oriented cultures, people feel that their personal problems are taken into account, that the organization takes a responsibility for employee welfare and that groups or committees tend to make the important decisions. In the job-oriented units, people experience a strong pressure to complete the job, they perceive the organization as being only interested in the work that the employees do, not in their personal and family welfare; and they report that the important decisions tend to be made by individuals.

Dimension P3 contrasts units whose employees derive their identity largely from the organization (parochial) with units in which people identify with their type of job (professional). The key items show that members of parochial cultures feel that the organization's norms cover their behavior at home as well as on the job; they feel that, in hiring employees, the company takes their social and family background into account as much as their job competence. The responses also indicate that the employees do not look far into the future (they probably assume the organization will do this for them). By contrast, members of professional cultures consider their private lives their own business, they feel the organization hires on the basis of competence alone, and they do think far ahead.

Dimension P4 contrasts open systems with closed systems. The key items show that, in the open system units, members consider both the organization and its people to be open to newcomers and outsiders; almost anyone would fit into the organization and new employees require only a few days to feel at home. In the closed system units, the organization and its people are felt to be closed and secretive, even by insiders; only very special people fit into the organization and new employees need more than a year to feel at home (in the most closed unit, one member of the managing board confessed that he still felt an outsider after 22 years).

Dimension P5 refers to the amount of internal structuring in the organization. According to the key responses, people in loosely controlled units feel that no one thinks of costs, meeting times are only approximately adhered to, and jokes about the company and the job are frequent. People in tightly controlled units describe their work environment as cost-conscious, meeting times are punctually kept, and jokes about the company and/or the job are rare.

Dimension P6 deals with the popular notion of customer orientation. Pragmatic units are market-driven, whereas normative units perceive their task, regarding the outside world, as the implementation of rules given. The key items show that, in the normative units, the major emphasis is on correctly following organizational procedures, which are more important than results; in matters of business ethics and honesty, the units standards are felt to be high. In the pragmatic units, there is a major emphasis on meeting the customer's needs, results are more important than correct procedures and, in matters of business ethics, a pragmatic rather than a dogmatic attitude prevails.

In addition to the practices, the respondents' values were also measured, but they were more dependent on a person's educational level, sex, age and nationality than on organization membership as such. The following dimensions emerged from the research:

1. Dimension V1 refers to the need for security, that is, the degree to which security is valued by the employees in the organization. In most social systems, a balance exists between the ambiguities and uncertainties a system tolerates and the ambiguities and uncertainties it rejects. This balance differs between organizations. The Need for Security Scale deals with this balance: the extent to which a social system rejects ambiguous and uncertain situations. The need for security, as measured by this scale, refers to a value or motive people have: the value of security, the value of living in clear, well-defined circumstances. The questions pertinent to this scale relate to subjects such as the importance of variety and adventure in work, the importance of fringe benefits, the importance of one's career and the meaning of authority. At the high need for security extreme, we find organizations in which the behavior of people is directed at creating and keeping clear and well-defined circumstances in their organization. At the other extreme, we find organizations with a low need for security.
2. Dimension V2 deals with work centrality, that is, the extent to which, for most people in the system, work takes a central place in their total life pattern.
3. Dimension V3 contrasts a high need for authority with a low need for authority. A high need for authority goes together with the acceptance of inequality among ranks in the system.

Design of the Comparative Study of the ICUs

The Survey Questionnaire

In this study of culture, only written question lists were used. This contrasts with the previously implemented Danish-Dutch study in which in-depth interviews with the respondents were carried out. The questionnaire was aimed at collecting information on the four types of manifestations of culture: symbols, heroes, rituals and values. The first three are subsumed under the common label "practices" (Fig. 12). Practice items deal with what the respondent feels actually "is", whereas value items describe what the respondent feels "should be".

- Practices: Fifty-four questions assessed perceived practices in the respondent's work situation. We then cast all responses into a bipolar format under the general heading "Where I work ..." and used 5-point scales for which, e.g. 1 = "meeting times are kept very punctually" and 5 = "meeting times are only kept approximately". These 54 questions covered mostly symbols and rituals.
- Values: Twenty-two questions assessed work goals: the characteristics of an ideal job, such as "has an opportunity for high earnings" or "has security of employment", were each rated on a 5-point scale of importance. These were

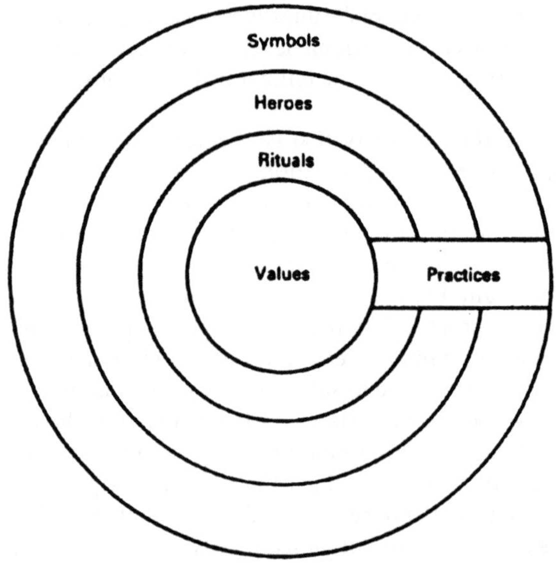

Fig. 12. Manifestations of culture from shallow to deep

taken from Hofstede and coworkers' previous cross-national research project [52] and from later extensions of it. Twenty-eight questions assessed general beliefs, such as "competition between employees usually does more harm than good", each rated on a 5-point scale from "strongly agree" to "strongly disagree". Twenty-five of these originated from previous cross-national research, mostly from Hofstede IBM studies [52] and from Laurent [53].

The Participating ICUs

The survey questionnaires were distributed across 90 ICUs in 12 countries. They were handed out to nursing personnel, doctors and support staff. All but one of the ICUs returned the questionnaires, producing a total of 2848. Approximately 8% of the questionnaires returned were blank or considered as being blank (less than 50% of the questions answered), leaving 2632 questionnaires. Item response was regarded as good: only 5% of the items were missed by more than 3% of the respondents.

Results

Introduction

The five important questions on which this study is based are:

1. Which dimensions in the field of practices and values that emerged from the comparative Danish-Dutch culture study seem to be significant for the description of ICU cultures?

2. What are the features of ICU cultures compared to other organizations, as established in the Danish-Dutch study?
3. What is the correspondence between the effectiveness of ICUs and their cultural features?
4. Which relationships exist between the cultural variables and those from the *Personnel* substudy?
5. Which relationships exist between the cultural variables and the characteristics of organization and management?

Dimensions of ICU Culture

The following scales, as previously found in the Danish-Dutch study, also appear to be present in the ICU study:

1. Dimension P1: Process-oriented vs results-oriented
2. Dimension P2: Employee-oriented vs job-oriented
3. Dimension P4: Open system vs closed system
4. Dimension V1: High vs low need for security

The reliability of the scales in this study was assessed. Cronbach α was computed (a measure for internal consistency) for each of the scales of unit scores. In this substudy, we used an α of at least 0.60 as a criterion, considering the broad categories measured. Table 70 shows the scales that met this criterion, with the associated reliability. Analysis of correlations between scales gives insight into the interdependence of the scales. Table 71 below lists the correlations ($N=78$).

Table 70. Cronbach α for each of the scales on unit scores ($n=78$)

	Scale	Cronbach α
P1	Process-oriented vs results-oriented	0.74
P2	Employee-oriented vs job-oriented	0.62
P4	Open system vs closed system	0.68
V1	Need for security	0.79

Table 71. Relationship between organization models and the culture scales

	Process vs results orientation P1	Employee vs job orientation P2	Open vs closed system P4	Need for security V1
P1	1.00*			
P2	−0.40*	1.00*		
P4	0.03	0.46*	1.00*	
V1	0.65*	−0.36*	0.07	1.00*

* Marks correlations significant at $p<0.01$.

Inspection of the correlations shows that between most scales they are high. P4 seems to be the least correlated or most unique scale. The correlation between the process/results orientation and the Need for Security Scale indicates a strong association between process orientation and the need for security in this study. In order to find out the significance of the dimensions in the ICU context, we conducted an in-depth interview with the project leader of the EURICUS-I project, who made site visits to all participating ICUs in the course of the research. In the context of the ICUs, these dimensions can be typified as follows:

- Dimension P1 (process-oriented vs results-oriented): For ICUs tending towards a process-oriented approach, working duties appear to be divided into fixed tasks. There is mention of standardization, in which there is little autonomy for the nursing staff. Given the fact that there is a clear allocation of tasks between doctors and nursing personnel, the nursing staff feel themselves to be dependent on the doctors. Procedures are followed on account of the procedures. The emphasis on protocols is related to the inclination to protect oneself against risks. In ICUs tending towards a results-oriented approach, the tasks of the doctors and the nursing personnel are more geared towards the realization of the goals formulated for each patient. There is mention of doctors and nursing staff cooperating in teams: for both the doctors and the nursing staff, there is a certain amount of autonomy and mutual independence. Nursing staff often have the full responsibility of looking after the patients assigned to them: they take charge of all the necessary executive and coordinating tasks. The maintenance of protocols has to do with achieving the specified goals.
- Dimension P2 (employee-oriented vs job-oriented): In the more employee-oriented ICUs, there is a caring attitude towards the people working there. The staff are regarded as the most important asset of the organization. There is mention of comradely and respectful contact between doctors and nursing staff. The latter have the idea that they are able to introduce topics for discussion which are important to them during meetings and at other occasions. The staff members are able to appreciate one another's position. The findings concerning contact between the doctors and the nursing staff also apply to contact that the doctors and nursing staff have with the patients and their families. In the more job-oriented ICUs, there is more an attitude of "every man for himself". The work that has to be done is the central issue. One assumes that the personal welfare of the staff is of secondary importance. There is little or no mutual support or attunement. Time will show where and when people are getting bogged down in their work.
- Dimension P4 (open system vs closed system): In ICUs which are regarded as being more open, the personnel tend to see their department as being an integrated component of the hospital. In general, new staff members feel at home reasonably quickly in these units. More closed ICUs are inclined to regard themselves as being a more isolated department within the hospital. People admit that newcomers have to endure a strict selection procedure and that it generally takes a long time before new employees feel at home in the unit. This originates from the idea that only exceptional people fit into the unit.

- Dimension V1 (high vs low need for security): Personnel in ICUs with a high need for security seek a high degree of certainty. They look for – and feel comfortable in – predictable situations. Personnel with low need for security require a lower degree of certainty: they look for – and feel comfortable in – unpredictable situations.

The Results of the ICU Study Compared to the Results of the Danish-Dutch Study

Using the database with culture diagnoses, the culture scores of ICUs can be compared to other work organizations in our database. The database consists of 20 culture diagnoses for a varied group of organizations in Denmark and the Netherlands. Due to the differences found between the various European areas, the comparison was restricted to Danish and Dutch ICUs.

Figure 13 displays, for all four scales (V1, P1, P2 and P4), the ranges for the scores of the Dutch and Danish ICUs (light bars) plotted against the scores of the organizations in the database (dark bars). The bars represent the range, from the lowest to the highest scoring units.

- Process-oriented vs results-oriented: The ICUs in this sample are found to be on the results-oriented side in the database ($p \leq 0.007$) (see Fig. 13). This finding indicates that personnel in ICUs see themselves as being comfortable in unfamiliar situations and as putting in maximum effort; each day is felt to bring new challenges.
- Employee-oriented vs job-oriented: The employee-oriented vs job-oriented opposition found in ICUs displays a small shift ($p \leq 0.007$) towards the job-oriented side of the scale. The general impression, however, is that the scores of the ICUs are grouped around the center of the scores in the database.
- Open vs closed system: The open vs closed system scores for the Danish and Dutch ICUs are grouped around the center of the organizational units in the database ($p = 0.418$).
- Need for security: In our database this is chiefly related to national differences. Danish organizations show a lower need for security than Dutch ICUs. Figu-

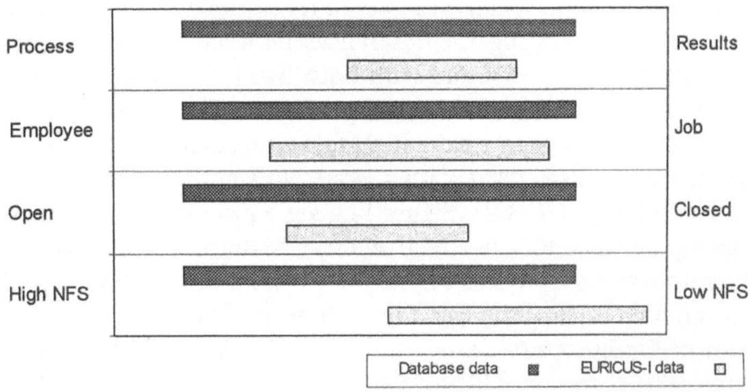

Fig. 13. Position of ICU's on the culture scales compared to organizations in the database. For explanation, see text

re 13 shows that Dutch and Danish ICUs are found at the low need for security side of this scale ($p=0.019$) (high score on V1). The low need for security indicates that security is not a strong value in ICUs and that ambiguities and uncertainties are allowed in ICUs to a greater extent than in other organizations. The association with low need for security may be indicative of the character of the work and the ambiguities and uncertainties involved. Being a value dimension (stable characteristic of people), this can indicate that people with low need for security values are selected to work in ICUs, in the sense that people with high need for security will not be hired or will leave the organization. Additional analysis shows that all Danish ICUs have a lower need for security than the Dutch ICU with the lowest need for security. This result is a replication of the differences found in previous research [45]. Separate analysis of the Dutch and Danish sample showed that the three organizational units with the lowest scores in each of the countries were ICUs.

In summary: Danish and Dutch ICUs were compared to (Danish and Dutch) organizations in the database. The differences found concern two scales: process-oriented vs results-oriented and need for security. In ICUs, a comparatively high degree of results orientation is found and a comparatively low need for security are found.

The Relation Between Effectiveness of ICUs and Cultural Features

The EURICUS-I project is directed towards identifying nonmedical factors which influence the effectiveness of ICUs. Effectiveness, in this study, is measured by mortality corrected for severity of illness. B20 represents the effectiveness in patients with a low severity of illness, and B80 represents the effectiveness in patients with a high severity of illness. In this section, the relationship between the culture scales (V1, P1, P2 and P4) and measures of the effectiveness of the ICUs is analyzed. In a first analysis, correlations between the four culture scales and B20 and B80 were computed. The results showed no significant correlations between effectiveness and culture. A second analysis was performed; this time, the differences between European areas were first eliminated. In this analysis (analysis of covariance) accounting for differences between European areas, a significant correlation of P1 was found with both B20 ($\beta=-0.41$; $SE=0.0075$; $p=0.029$) and B80 ($\beta=-0.59$; $SE=0.0048$; $p=0.002$). The amount of variance in B20, explained by European areas and P1 taken together, is 32% (R^2adj = 18%); for B80 the amount is also 32% (R^2adj = 18%). No significant relationships were found with scales P2, P4 and V1. Figure 14 gives a graphical representation of the relationship between P1 and effectiveness. The dotted lines show the trend between effectiveness and process-oriented vs results-oriented, for all of the 78 ICUs. The solid lines show the trend in each of the European areas. As can be seen, in most of the European areas, results-oriented ICUs (high score on P1) perform better (low scores on B20 and B80). This is the case for nine of 12 distinguished European areas in terms of B20, and for ten of the 12 European areas in terms of B80.

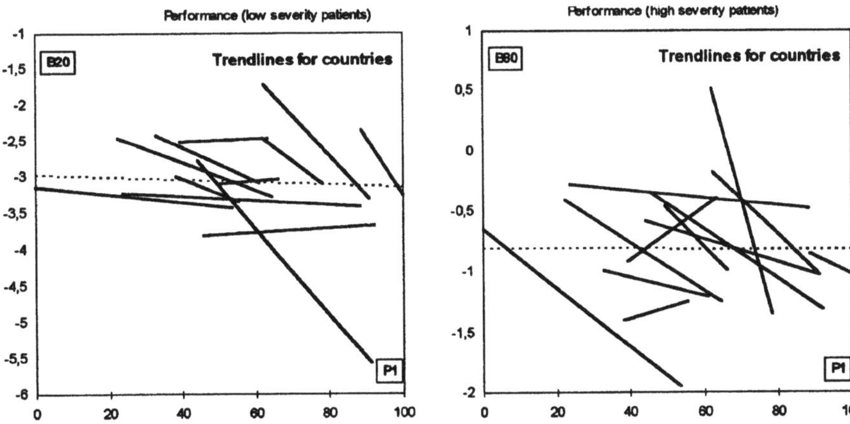

Fig. 14. Relationship between performance and process vs results orientation by European area

These analyses indicate that, within European areas, mortality ratios, corrected for severity of illness, are higher in the more process-oriented ICUs than in the more results-oriented ICUs.

The Relationship Between the Cultural Features and Variables from the *Personnel* Substudy

The following variables from the *Personnel* substudy were linked to the cultural features:

- Burnout: This factor reflects subjective stress complaints and is made up of the scales Emotional Exhaustion and Depersonalization.
- Morale: This factor reflects the motivational/attitudinal component of ICU nurses' well-being at work and is made up of three scales, Job Involvement, Organizational Commitment and Personal Accomplishment.
- Satisfaction: Nurses' overall satisfaction with their job is measured with a one-item rating which is scored on a 5-point faces measure.

The burnout and morale variables correspond to the factors found in the second-order factor analysis concerning the human resources outcomes variables in the *Personnel* substudy.

The following correspondences have all been calculated by means of a regression analysis. It appears that burnout corresponds to European area, job orientation and the imbalance team variables from the *Personnel* substudy (explained variance 54%). Morale appears to correspond to the Europeans area, results orientation and employee-orientation (explained variance 59%). Satisfaction is connected to a high P/N ratio, results orientation and employee orientation (explained variance 51%).

Table 72. Relationship between organization models and the culture scales

	Processk vs results orientation	Employee vs job orientation	Open vs closed system	Need for security
Model I				
Model II		0.40**		−0.28*
Model III				0.37**

The Relation Between Cultural Features and Characteristics of Management and Organization

An analysis was made of the relationship between the culture scales and characteristics of the organization. The scales were related to characteristics of the formal organization as described in the site visits (Table 72).

The results show that a high need for security is associated with organizational model II. In this model, the strategic apex lies outside the unit. Low need for security is found in ICUs with organizational model III. Here, the strategic apex lies within the ICU. External and internal standards may be the key factors here. Orientation towards external demands may require an organization to limit ambiguity and uncertainty within the organization. In model III types of ICUs, the internal strategic apex forms a buffer between external demands and the ICU, whereas, in model II ICUs, the strategic apex itself is external to the ICU, reducing the distance between the ICU workers and the outside world. No significant correlations were found between process orientation vs results orientation and the organizational characteristics. Organizational model II is significantly correlated with job orientation. Here, the strategic apex is outside the ICU. This result matches the result found in our previous research, in which operating against external standards was associated with job orientation, whereas operating against internal standards was associated with employee orientation [52].

Conclusion and Implications

The research has indicated a relationship between the results orientation and the effectiveness of the ICUs, for both high-risk and the low-risk patients. These findings conform to the correspondence previously found [14] between organizational practices (team-oriented cultures, supportive leadership, effective coordination, timely communication and collaborative, open problem-solving approaches), and outcomes of ICUs (lower risk-adjusted LOS). At the same time, the research also shows a relationship between results orientation, and morale and satisfaction. In this, the results-oriented vs process-oriented dimension fulfils a central role with regard to the (effectiveness of) the functioning of ICUs. Which implications can be deduced for the growth of more result-oriented ICUs? Which management commitments are linked to these? Some interesting indications concerning these can be found in Sherwood's article, "Creating Work Cultures with Competitive Advantage" [55]. In his view, cultures like these can also be referred to as "high-performance, high-commitment work cultures". The characteristics of a high-performance, high-commitment work culture are:

1. Delegation: giving responsibility for decisions and actions to the people who have the most relevant and timely information or the most appropriate skills.
2. Teamwork across boundaries: involving the right people at the right time. Everyone in the organization must be integrated into service of the product and the customer, rather than being focused mainly on his/her function or discipline.
3. Empowered people: by providing opportunities and valuing contributions. Everyone is expected to accept and exercise the responsibility necessary to get his/her job done, in addition to helping others accomplish tasks.
4. People integrated with technology: the ability to exercise initiative and creativity on the work floor. Such people are in charge of the technology.
5. A shared sense of purpose: sharing a vision that is based on a clear set of values describing both the organization's mission (purpose) and the methods for realizing it.

A feature of these five characteristics is the pattern of internal control [54]. At the individual level, internal control means that a person assumes that, in the long run, he/she will receive what he/she has earned. At the organizational level, internal control refers to organizations which function according to the perspective they themselves have chosen. If this is applied to ICU leadership, then there is a whole arsenal of conceivable instruments to encourage ICUs to develop in a more results-oriented way. The point of departure here is that there must be a clear vision regarding the way in which the ICU should function. It is evident that personnel management can be used as a lever in order to bring about this type of desired development. This process can be influenced by factors such as recruitment and selection, promotion policies and education, and professionalization.

Summary

A comparative culture study took place in 89 ICUs in 12 European countries. In this study, use was made of scales previously developed by Hofstede et al. [52] for research into 20 organizations in Denmark and the Netherlands. In the ICU study, the following scales were distinguished: process orientation vs results orientation, employee orientation vs job orientation, open system vs closed system, high need for security vs low need for security. If the scores for the ICUs are compared to those for the 20 organizations, the ICUs appear, on average, to be more results-oriented and the staff members of the ICUs have a relatively low need for security. In almost every country, there seems to be a correspondence between results orientation and the effectiveness of the ICUs, for both high risk and low risk patients. A number of implications can be deduced with regard to ICU management. These refer to the development of a more results-oriented attitude.

Finances

M. Jegers

Introduction

Nonclinical management of an ICU is a quite novel topic on the research agenda. An excellent state of the art review can be found by Reis Miranda et al. [69], from which it is clear that hardly any systematic knowledge, even descriptive accounts, exist in this particular field. This observation is even more pronounced in the financial management of ICUs[1]. The purpose of the substudy is to shed some light on the costing, budgeting and cost-accounting procedures of ICUs in 12 European countries.

Data

The data collection involved country coordinators selecting ICUs in their countries in a nonrandom way. Therefore, our descriptive data, obtained by a written questionnaire distributed and collected by the country coordinators, is by no means to be considered as representative. Nevertheless, the findings are interesting in their own right and will, at least in our view, contribute to a first impression of costing, budgeting and cost-accounting practices in ICUs.

The Cost Structure of European ICUs

The Concept of ICU Costs

The importance of costs is not found in the fact that cost accountants love to calculate them, but in their potential to reflect the underlying resource use or input during a predetermined period of time at a predetermined level of analysis. This level can be the hospital, the hospital unit or even the patient. In the present discussion, we will confine ourselves to the unit level[2]. Therefore, we define direct costs as costs exclusively attributable to the ICU, and indirect[3] or overhead costs

[1] An exception, at the hospital level, is Pettersen [66], who found evidence of a systematic decoupling of budgets and performance in Norwegian governmental hospitals. In this author's view the budgetary procedures are more a set of ritual rhetorics vis à vis the political world than an instrument of managerial control. Scholarly papers on hospital cost accounting are also rare. Exceptions are [59] and [65].

[2] For an example of ICU costing at the patient level, see [70].

[3] Confusingly, in health economic texts, the term "indirect cost" is also used in a different way, namely costs due to lost earnings, lost product or lost income due to a specific medical treatment [64]. For another, at least nonconventional, definition of direct costs (costs that can be directly measured) see [56].

as costs borne at the hospital level for the benefit of more than one unit. Examples of such overheads are general management and administration, taxes, heating, and catering. When calculating the cost of an ICU, one should decide whether to include direct costs or not. The answer depends on the research question at hand. There seems to be a consensus in the literature that in cases in which ICU management or ICU outcome is the focal point of the research, or in cases in which the costs of different ICUs are compared, only direct costs are relevant [56, 57, 62, 71]. Direct costs can be both fixed or variable. This distinction is contingent on the reference time span one takes into consideration. If this is very long, say 20 years, then nearly all costs are variable. If this is very short, say 1 day, they are mostly fixed. Traditionally, 1 year is taken. In such a situation, the direct costs of an ICU are a mix of fixed and variable costs, and therefore influenced by the level of activity or output[4]. Clearly, an assessment of resource use in an ICU should take into consideration output, however measured[5]. But in a first stage, the level of the costs themselves should be determined. For ICUs, collecting the necessary data is "exceedingly time consuming ..., very labor intensive and ... not free from difficulties" [61]. This might be the reason that, in the review by Gyldmark [62], 13 ICU cost studies out of the 20 studies reviewed were based on charges, and four others on the cost of an average bed day at the hospital level[6]. Although a number of these studies were published in very highly reputed academic journals, it goes without saying that this is a completely inappropriate way of measuring ICU costs.

A Standardized ICU Cost Model

The interpretation of differences in resource use or costs between ICUs should be made taking into consideration at least the following elements [62]:
- Differences in technology
- Differences in capacity
- Differences in medical policies
- Differences in research and training activities
- Differences in costing methods

Obviously, the first four elements reflect "real" differences, whereas the last one is only "virtual", obscuring analysis of the ICUs managerial and medical policies. A natural way to cope with this problem is to develop a "standardized cost model ... to avoid misleading results and to enable comparison of study results" [62]. This

[4] which can include training and research

[5] ICU output is clearly a multidimensional concept. At least four dimensions can be distinguished: care and cure, research, education and also available capacity. The fact that these dimensions are not independent from one another makes measurement of ICU output a difficult task.

[6] In Rapoport et al. [68] resource use is measured by a weighted number of hospital days, in which weights were set more or less arbitrarily.

Table 73. General structure of periodic, total direct ICU costs

Tangibles	*Current costs*
Depreciation	Wages
Rents	Other current costs
Leases	
Maintenance	

Table 74. Subdivision of tangibles

Medical equipment
Nonmedical equipment
Beds and mattresses
Other

Table 75. Categories of staff

Medical director
Medical codirectors
Physicians
Head nurse
Nurse
Others

is exactly what we intend to do here. Dependent on the purpose of the study and the availability of data, numerous authors have presented ICU costing formulas[7]. These were combined with the answers of the EURICUS-I respondents to arrive at a proposal for a standardized model of total periodic (e.g. 1 year) direct ICU costs (Table 73).

The main distinction is that between costs related to tangibles and current costs. An important category of current costs are the wages. In Table 74 a further subdivision of the tangibles is presented. Wages should be subdivided according to the categories of staff; Table 75 shows a possible subdivision. A number of other current costs are also relevant for an ICU; Table 76 shows the most important ones. Theoretically, the cost of storable products consists not only of the amount consumed, but also of the costs of the funds tied up in their inventories. When inventories are kept at the ICU level, this (financial) cost[8] is a direct cost and can be, at least in principle, determined.

[7] Examples are the papers cited in the previous sections, the papers reviewed by Gyldmark [62] and, for the Netherlands, the studies by Hilgeman et al.[63] or Reis Miranda and Spangenberg [2].

[8] "Opportunity cost" in economics jargon.

Table 76. Important current costs in an ICU, except wages

Pharmaceuticals
Disposables
Blood products (including human albumin)
Tests
X-ray/CT scans
Dialyses
Physiotherapy
Hotel, linen, clothing
Administration
Other

Assumptions

In order to arrive at a more or less standardized way of measuring the different ICU costs components, we propose to use uniform valuation rules accross the countries involved in our sample. In our view, this will allow us to reflect more accurately real differences in resource use. To determine the cost of nonrented or leased tangibles we use a linear depreciation scheme, and assume 10 years to be a reasonable estimation of the tangibles' useful life span[9]. This implies that we did not take into consideration the cost of tangibles older than 10 years. Although 10 years seems a rather high estimation from a practical point of view leading to rather low cost figures, various ICUs in the sample reported older equipment being in use. Some of the maxima are reported in Table 77.

In order to cope with the radically different remuneration systems, we used a set of standardized wages per FTE. These are reported in Table 78 (in ECU[10]): To

Table 77. Maximum age of some tangibles in use in EURICUS I

Type	Age (years)
Ventilator	24
Defibrillator	19
Pacemaker	19
Pumps	19
Monitor	18
Module	14
Analyzer	14
Humidifier	12
Bronchoscope	12

[9] No residual value is assumed.

[10] All figures are expressed in European Currency Units (ECU). The USD/ECU exchange rate was 1.12 on December 31, 1993 (International Monetary fund 1995, which is the source for all exchange rates used).

Tabe 78. Wages applied (ECU 1993)

Category	Wage
ICU director	90 000
ICU codirector	80 500
Physician	69 000
Head nurse	32 200
Nurse	29 900
Other	27 600

Table 79. Standard price per laboratory test (ECU 1993)

Category of tests	Price
Clinical/chemical	1.0
Haematological	1.4
Bacteriological	6.9
Parasitological	1.4
Virological	6.9
Other	3.5

determine the cost per laboratory test, two sources were consulted. Raes [67] for Belgium and the Vereniging Klinisch Chemici Noord [72] for the Netherlands. Based on their calculations and a (subjective) assessment of the frequency of the different tests, we arrived at the standards of Table 79. Based on the cost study by Walravens et al. [73] for Belgium, we use a unit cost of 23 ECU and 46 ECU for X-rays and CT scans, respectively. Gheyle et al. [60] determine a cost of 184 ECU for dialysis without erythropoietin (EPO), and 207 ECU for a dialysis with EPO. Finally, the hourly rate for physiotherapy was set at 18.4 ECU.

Results

We recall the fact that our sample is not appropriate to generate data representative for all European ICUs. In the EURICUS-I sample we selected those ICUs which provided the necessary data to enable us to estimate their 1993 cost according to the aforementioned methodology. Twenty-five ICUs met these requirements[11]. In Table 80 the total cost and the cost/patient per day in ECU are presented for these 25 units. Cost differences can be explained by different possible

[11] Eight from Spain, 5 from Finland and Denmark, 2 from Italy and 1 from Germany, The Netherlands, France, Luxembourg and the United Kingdom. For 15 ICUs the maintenance cost had to be estimated based on the available data. We used 18% of depreciation costs. Also in 15 cases the equivalent FTE number of nurses was derived from the actual number of nurses. Here a rate of 84% was applied.

Table 80. Summary cost data (ECU)

Number of beds	Occupancy rate (%)	Total cost (ECU)	Cost/patient/day (ECU)
4	94	957 971	693
5[b]	79	841 555	583
5[b]	81	1 165 202	788
5[a]	76	1 100 256	793
6	102	2 966 893	1328
6[b]	65	703 623	494
6[a]	79	2 028 086	1172
6[ab]	91	973 063	488
7[a]	56	1 396 949	976
8	109	1 036 013	325
8[a]	82	2 799 757	1169
8[a]	90	1 798 829	684
8[ab]	64	1 706 993	913
8[ab]	110	1 043 397	324
9[b]	68	1 520 701	681
9[ab]	68	1 865 629	835
10[b]	65	5 031 147	2120
10[b]	75	1 948 182	712
10[a]	96	2 425 948	692
11[b]	89	1 695 063	474
11[ab]	91	2 486 422	681
12[ab]	82	2 435 401	678
14[ab]	83	2 617 924	617
22[ab]	68	5 247 294	961
33[a]	95	8 084 288	706

[a] Maintenance cost estimated,
[b] FTE nurses estimated

reasons, of which case mix is one of the most important. We think that our data do not allow a systematic analysis of this or other relationships. The cost structure in the 25 ICUs is shown in Table 81.

Notwithstanding important differences between the sampled ICUs, some clear conclusions emerge from Table 81: labor is the most important component of total cost, almost always between 50% and 80% of total cost. Tangibles (if not too old) and pharmaceuticals are next in line. The other cost components are mostly marginal, with the exception of the cost of disposables and, sometimes, blood products and laboratory tests.

Table 81. Cost structure of ICUs (%)

Beds	Tangibles	Labor	Pharmaceuticals	Disposables	Blood	Test 0	Radiology	Dialysis	Physical therapy	Other
4	12	67	8	6	1	2	3	0	0	0
5[b]	1	84	2	1	6	2	4	0	0	0
5[b]	2	73	8	7	1	8	1	0	0	0
5[a]	19	56	7	4	6	3	3	0	0	1
6	23	52	7	4	10	2	2	1	1	0
6[b]	4	74	12	4	0	1	5	0	0	0
6[a]	5	64	13	9	5	0	2	0	1	0
6[ab]	3	78	7	6	1	3	3	0	0	0
7[a]	14	48	6	5	3	2	2	19	0	0
8	2	96	2	0	0	0	0	0	0	0
8[a]	2	67	16	3	5	4	2	0	1	0
8[a]	8	69	14	4	3	2	1	0	0	0
8[ab]	7	56	9	7	3	2	2	1	1	12
8[ab]	3	72	18	6	0	0	2	0	0	0
9[b]	2	68	14	9	1	1	4	0	1	0
9[ab]	5	73	11	11	0	0	0	0	0	0
10[b]	2	27	42	7	21	0	1	0	0	0
10[b]	16	55	17	3	6	2	1	0	0	0
10[a]	1	62	26	5	1	3	2	0	0	0
11[b]	6	79	5	7	1	0	2	0	0	0
11[ab]	3	63	19	7	3	0	3	1	0	0
12[ab]	15	44	15	20	0	0	4	0	2	0
14[ab]	2	51	4	5	4	32	3	0	0	0
22[ab]	2	51	13	6	6	18	3	0	1	0
33[a]	1	69	15	7	3	2	3	0	0	0

[a] Maintenance cost estimated,
[b] Full time equivalent nurses estimated

Budgeting Procedure

In the questionnaire protocol budgeting was defined as a decision by hospital authorities concerning allowable expenses for every unit in the hospital during a given period. Theoretically, a distinction between expenses and investments should be made. An investment is a payment for the acquisition of an asset that is expected to be in use for more than 1 year, e.g. equipment, computers, furniture, software. Expenses are the other payments. It is of note that we have not considered the revenue budgets of ICUs.

Drawing Up of the ICU Budget

In a relatively large number of cases, ICU managers stated that no specific ICU budget existed. This was especially the case in Belgium (at least for current expenses), Italy, Spain (two hospitals were in an "experimental" stage of establishing budgets) and Portugal. In at least one English hospital of our sample, an ICU budget does not exist, although it "has been repeatedly requested". When present, the ICU budget mostly consists of at least one of the following components, be it separate or combined: (a) current wage expenses; (b) other current expenses; (c) investments. As can be seen from Table 82, specific investment budgets for ICU are not frequently met.

The budgeting procedures described by our respondents mostly contain both formal and informal elements. Three generic categories of procedures can be discerned[12]: (1) bottom-up; (2) top-down; (3) just top.

Table 82. Presence of an investment budget

	Yes	No	No answer
European area			
Belgium	3	1	2
Denmark	1	5	0
England	1	7	0
Finland	5	0	0
France	2	2	0
Germany	1	2	0
Italy	1	5	1
Netherlands	4	2	0
Poland	1	4	3
Portugal	1	2	2
Spain	8	18	3
Overall	29	48	11

[12] One hospital in England intended to implement in the near future a zero base budgeting system.

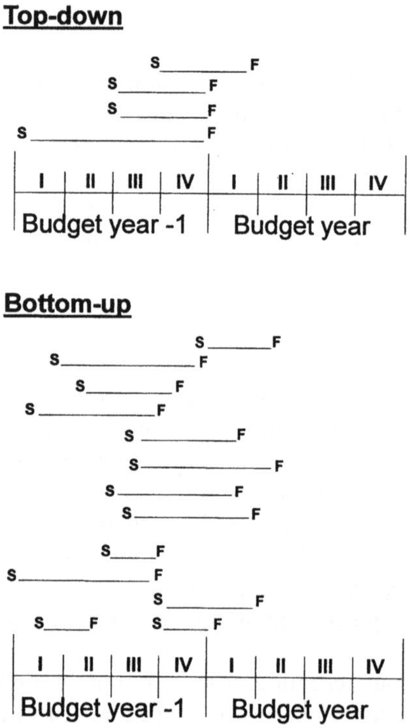

Fig. 15. Timing of budgeting procedures

In the just top procedure, a given authority, be it the director, a board or a counsel, decides on the ICU budget without any participation by ICU members (e.g. in some Polish hospitals). In some cases, this procedure is disguised as an objective rule: the budget is based on last year's budget, possibly with some allowance for inflation (e.g. in Denmark, England or France), or a fixed percentage of the hospital budget (e.g. 4% in an English hospital). In the case of a top-down procedure or a bottom-up procedure the ICUs medical director is always consulted. This is not always the case for the head nurse. The timing of the procedural steps substantially differ across countries and across hospitals within the same country. In Fig. 15 some examples are presented.

On the horizontal axis two consecutive years are represented, subdivided in quarters of a year. The last year is the year in which the budget applies. The points labeled "S" mark the start of the formal budgeting procedure, the points "F" the final, formal budget decision. In almost all cases the procedure starts in the year preceding the budget year. In a number of cases the procedure comes to a formal end in the first or even second quarter of the budget year itself.

Budgetary Flexibility

Once the budget has been approved, it can be implemented in different ways. One important characteristic is budgetary flexibility: the possibility of transfering

Table 83. Perception of presence of budgetary flexibility

	Presence	Absence	No answer
European area			
Belgium	1	3	2
Denmark	3	3	0
England	7	1	0
Finland	5	0	0
France	3	1	0
Germany	2	0	1
Italy	2	1	4
Netherlands	3	3	0
Poland	0	4	4
Portugal	2	1	2
Spain	9	16	4
Overall	38	33	17

budgeted amounts from one part of the ICU budget to another, without having to seek approval by the hospital management, and/or the possibility to exceed budgeted amounts without approval by the hospital management. The evaluation of flexibility is clearly a matter of perception. In Table 83 the perception of the presence or absence of budgetary flexibility is presented.

Not taking into account the nonrespondents, we observe a small majority of our sample to perceive some budgetary flexibility. In countries such as Poland we did not find any perceived flexibility, whereas all English and Finnish ICUs of our sample mentioned the presence of perceived flexibility in their situations. As an (albeit extreme) illustration of existing flexibility the following question was included in the questionnaire: "A sudden crisis can only be solved by hiring unbudgeted staff for your unit. Do you have the authority to do this ?" The answers are shown in Table 84: As could be expected, the answer in most cases is "No". Striking exceptions are the English ICUs in our sample (8 Yes) and the Finnish ones (4 Yes vs 1 No). A related, but different question, is whether ICU managers would like to enjoy more flexibility than presently attributed to them. Table 85 shows that the answer here is a clear "yes":

Only in the case of our German, Italian[13] (and Luxemburg) respondents, did ICU managers who were happy with their perceived flexibility outnumber the others. Those who would like more flexibility were asked in which respect. More investment flexibility (both for new equipment as for replacements) seems to be frequently desired, as is more flexibility in transfering amounts of money within the budget. Less frequently mentioned items are staffing, rewarding policies and drug expenses.

[13] When not taking non-respondents into account.

Table 84. Authority to hire unbudgeted staff due to a sudden crisis

	Yes	No	No answer
European area			
Belgium	0	5	1
Denmark	3	3	0
England	8	0	0
Finland	4	1	0
France	1	3	0
Germany	1	2	0
Italy	0	5	2
Netherlands	2	4	0
Poland	0	4	4
Portugal	2	3	0
Spain	1	17	1
Overall	22	58	8

Table 85. Wish for more budgetary flexibility

	Yes	No	No answer
European area			
Belgium	4	0	2
Denmark	5	1	0
England	5	3	0
Finland	3	2	0
France	2	1	1
Germany	0	2	1
Italy	0	2	5
Netherlands	5	1	0
Poland	4	0	4
Portugal	2	0	3
Spain	19	3	7
Overall	49	16	23

Budget Control

The concept of budget control was defined in the questionnaire protocol as a formal procedure by which hospital management verifies whether the diverse units do keep their expenses and investments within the budgeted amounts. The presence of such a control procedure at the ICU level is reflected in Table 86.

No clear picture emerges, suggesting that the implementation of a budget control system is initiated by the hospital management itself and not by regulatory obligations. One element of budget control is the need to seek approval for some

Table 86. Presence of budget control procedure at ICU level

	Yes	No	No answer
European area			
Belgium	1	4	1
Denmark	3	3	0
England	6	2	0
Finland	4	1	0
France	3	1	0
Germany	1	2	0
Italy	2	4	1
Netherlands	3	3	0
Poland	2	2	4
Portugal	1	4	0
Spain	11	18	0
Overall	37	45	6

categories of expenses or investments. In a number of hospitals (especially but not only in Poland, Italy and Spain.) all ICU expenses and investments need to be authorized by higher levels. In some cases (e.g. in Belgium) only investments cannot be made without approval. In others all expenses exceeding a certain value are to be approved. These critical values widely diverge. In Denmark, for example, limits between 5000 and 25000 DKK are reported; in Finland between 15000 and 200000 FIM, in the Netherlands between 500 and 2000 NLG,

Table 87. Presence of a budget control system within the ICU

	Yes	No	No answer
European area			
Belgium	0	5	1
Denmark	1	5	0
England	4	3	1
Finland	2	3	0
France	0	4	0
Germany	0	3	0
Italy	0	4	3
Netherlands	3	3	0
Poland	1	3	4
Portugal	0	3	2
Spain	3	23	3
Overall	14	60	14

Table 88. Presence of evaluation of budgetary performance

	Yes	No	No answer
European area			
Belgium	0	4	2
Denmark	5	1	0
England	6	2	0
Finland	4	1	0
France	3	1	0
Germany	1	2	0
Italy	2	2	3
Netherlands	4	2	0
Poland	2	1	5
Portugal	1	3	1
Spain	11	16	2
Overall	40	35	13

in the UK between 4000 and 5000 GBP. ICU management could consider running its own budget control system, be it a stand alone system or a system integrated into a comprehensive decentralized hospital budget control system. Table 87 proves that such a situation is seldom met. The differences between the numbers of "yes" answers in Tables 86 and 87 suggest that in many hospitals in which budgetary controls are in place, these controls are run at the hospital level and not at the unit level. An essential element in a comprehensive budgetary system is the presence of a budgetary evaluation at the unit level. In most countries, with Belgium, and to a lesser extent Spain and Portugal, as notable exceptions, such an evaluation is found, although not in all the hospitals in our sample (Table 88).

Perceived Effect on Managerial Efficiency

In most countries there is a quite unanimous perception of the effect of budgetary procedures on the efficiency of ICU management. In Belgium, England, Finland, Italy and the Netherlands our respondents seem to perceive a positive effect. In Denmark, Poland and Spain an opposite conclusion can be reached (Table 89).

Cost Accounting in ICUs

Presence of a Cost Accounting System on the ICU

In the protocol of the questionnaire a cost-accounting system was defined as a "method by which the ICU calculates the cost of its activities, globally (for the

Table 89. Perception of effect of budgetary procedures on managerial efficiency

	Yes	No	No answer
European area			
Belgium	3	1	2
Denmark	2	4	0
England	6	2	0
Finland	5	0	0
France	2	2	0
Germany	1	1	1
Italy	4	0	3
Netherlands	5	1	0
Poland	1	4	3
Portugal	1	2	2
Spain	4	21	4
Overall	35	38	15

unit) or per unit of activity (e.g. days, treatment, patient, TISS point)". Table 90 shows that such a system is absent in most of the ICUs of our sample.

Costing systems used are very diversely, even for the 14 cases in our sample. A very detailed system has been developed by Edbrooke et al. [58]. In this system direct and indirect costs are distinguished, direct costs being costs defined as attributable to individual patients. Examples of direct costs are drug costs, disposable equipment costs, direct staff costs, procedure costs. All relevant data are registered automatically through an automated patient data management system. Indirect costs include ICU equipment maintenance and depreciation, in-

Table 90. Presence of cost accounting system within the ICU

	Yes	No	No answer
European area			
Belgium	0	5	1
Denmark	0	6	0
England	4	4	0
Finland	4	1	0
France	0	4	0
Germany	0	3	0
Italy	1	4	2
Netherlands	2	4	0
Poland	3	2	3
Portugal	0	4	1
Spain	0	28	1
Overall	14	66	8

direct staff costs (at the ICU level), and building maintenance and depreciation. All the data required to calculate indirect costs are available in the hospital's management information system. Indirect costs are then expressed in monetary units/patient-bed hours and allocated to specific patients' direct costs taking his/her individual number of bed-hours into consideration. Notice that overhead costs at the hospital level (e.g. human resources department costs, financial costs) are not taken into consideration. Other, less sophisticated, systems are also in use in our sample. Examples of the most simple ones are: only the cost of disposables and pharmaceuticals, only the cost of materials used and depreciation of equipment, a predetermined cost per TISS point, based on quarterly data in one case, and set at 38 GBP in another case. Most Finnish hospitals in our sample apply a standard linear cost function for the cost of a patient day: Fixed cost per day + [cost per TISS point] x TISS points.

Clearly, the number of TISS points is considered to be a good activity measure. Examples of fixed costs observed are 4300 FIM, 210 FIM or 28 ECU. Examples of variable costs per TISS point observed are, respectively, 72 FIM, 500 FIM and 175 ECU. In one case, costs of scheduled patients and unscheduled patients are differentiated.

Knowledge of the Cost/Bed Per Day

Table 91 describes whether at the ICU level any knowledge, however obtained, exists on the cost/bed per day. In almost half the cases the answer is "yes". As estimates of this cost can be obtained from data collected and processed at the hospital level, this result does not contradict the figures presented in Table 90. Unfortunately for comparative purposes almost every hospital in our sample uses a different cost definition. In some cases, the cost/bed per day is even approximated by a hospital average, unaffected by resource consumption differences be-

Table 91. Knowledge of cost/bed/day

	Yes	No	No answer
European area			
Belgium	0	5	1
Denmark	2	3	1
England	6	2	0
Finland	5	0	0
France	3	1	0
Germany	1	2	0
Italy	1	2	4
Netherlands	2	4	0
Poland	3	2	3
Portugal	2	3	0
Spain	13	16	0
Overall	38	41	9

Table 92. Reported minimal and maximal cost/bed/day per country, in US $ (end 1994)[a]

	Minimal	Maximal
European area		
Denmark	1576	3551
England	943	2473
Finland	908	1792
France	1048	1684
Netherlands	555	1256
Poland	492	2531
Portugal	566	767
Spain	24	1450

[a] Exchange rates collected from the IMF International financial statistics.

tween hospital units. Other sources of differences in cost calculations are, e.g., the treatment of overheads and indirect costs, physicians' wages, and depreciation schemes. In some cases the budgeted cost/bed per day is considered to be "the" cost/bed per day, in other cases the amount paid by health insurers. Therefore, wide ranges between cost figures not explained by differences in case mix, available staff and equipment exist within countries, casting doubt on their usefulness in economically rational decision-making at the ICU level. In Table 92 the range of costs are presented in US $ (end 1994). Of course, these figures are only of a documentary nature.

Conclusion

This outline presents budgetary and cost-accounting procedures in a nonrandom sample of ICUs in 12 European countries. The impression is of nonsystematic diversity[14]. Hospital management or ICU managers can initiate a more or less sophisticated budgetary control system, but this does not appear to be an obligation in most countries in our sample. We can conclude that cost calculation methods in a majority of ICUs studied are rather underdeveloped.

References

1. Reis Miranda D, Langrehr D (1990) National and regional organization. In: Reis Miranda D, Williams A, Loirat Ph (eds) Management of intensive care – guidelines for better resource use. Kluwer Academic, Dordrecht, The Netherlands, pp 83–102
2. Reis Miranda D, Spangenberg JFA (eds) (1992) Quality, efficiency and organization of intensive care units in The Netherlands. Van Denderen, Groningen, The Netherlands
3. Le Gall JR, Lemeshow S, Saulnier F (1993) A new simplified acute physiology score (SAPS II) based on an European/North American multicenter study. JAMA 270:2957–2963

[14] Attempts to relate components of the budgetary procedures to each other, to hospital size or ICU size proved to be in vain.

4. Knaus WA, Wagner DP, Draper EA, Zimmerman JE (1985) APACHE II: A severity of disease classification. Crit Care Med 13:818–829
5. Knaus WA, Wagner DP, Draper EA, et al (1991) The APACHE III prognostic system; risk prediction of hospital mortality for critically ill hospitalized adults. Chest 100:1619–1636
6. Lemeshow S, Teres D, Klar J et al (1993) Mortality probability models (MPM II) based on an international cohort of intensive care unit patients. JAMA 270:2478–2486
7. Cullen DJ, Civetta JM, Briggs BA, Ferrara LC (1974) Therapeutic Intervention Scoring System: A method for quantitative comparison of patient care. Crit Care Med 2:57–60
8. Reis Miranda D, De Rijk A, Schaufeli WB (1995) Simplified therapeutic intervention scoring system: The TISS-28 items: results from a multicenter study. Crit Care Med 24, 64–73
9. Reis Miranda D, Iapichino G, Moreno R (1996) NEMS: Nine Equivalents of nursing Manpower use Score. Intensive Care Med 22, S296
10. Jones J and Rowan K (1995) Is there a relationship between the volume of work carried out in Intensive Care and its outcome? Int J Technol Assess Health Care 11, 762–769
11. Georgopoulos BS (1986) Organizational structure, problem solving and effectiveness: a comparative study of hospital emergency services. Jossey-Bass, San Francisco
12. Comstock DE and Scott WR (1987) Technology and the Structure of Hospital Subunits: Distinguishing Individual and Workgroup Effects'. In: Flood AB and Scott WR (eds.) Hospital structure and performance. Johns Hopkins University, Baltimore
13. Zimmerman JE, Shortell SM, Rousseau DM et al (1993) Improving intensive care: Observations based on organizational case studies in nine intensive care units: A prospective, multicenter study. Crit Care Med 21:1443–1451
14. Shortell SM, Zimmerman JE, Rousseau DM, Gillies RR, Wagner DP, Draper EA, Knaus, WA, Duffy J (1994) The performance of intensive care units: does good management make a difference? Med Care 32:508–524
15. Bandura A (1977) Self-efficay: Toward a unifying theory of behavioral change. Psychol Rev 84:191–215
16. Bentler PM (1992) EQS: Structural equations program manual. Cork: BMDP Statistical Software
17. Byrne BM (1993) The Maslach burnout inventory: testing for factorial validity and invariance across elementary, intermediate and secondary teachers. J Occup Organiz Psychol, 66:197–212
18. Dunham RB, Herman JB (1975) Development of a female faces scale for measuring job satisfaction. J Appl Psychol 60:629–632
19. Frese M, Zapf D (1988) Methodological issues in the study of work stress: objective versus subjective measurement of work stress and the question of longitudinal studies. In: Cooper CL, Payne R (eds) Causes, coping and consequences of stress at work. John Wiley, Chichester, pp 375–411
20. Furda J (1995) Werk, persoon en welzijn [Work, person and well-being]. Utrecht, Universiteit Utrecht
21. Furda J, Meyman TF, Schreurs PJG, Castermans C (1993) Copingstijl, sociale isolatie en regelmogelijkheden [Coping behaviour, social isolation and decision latitude]. In: Gaillard AWK, Kompier MAJ (eds). Werkstress en Arbeidsongeschiktheid: Preventie en Interventie. MAKLU, Antwerpen/Apeldoorn, pp 67–82
22. Furda J, Jonge J de, Le Blanc PM, Meijman TF, Scheenen J (1994) Het Demand-Control-Support model in relatie tot gezondheidsklachten en herstelklachten: een longitudinale studie [The demand-control-support model in relation to health complaints and recovery complaints: a longitudinal study]. Gedrag andOrganisatie 7:225–238
23. Goldberg LR (1990) An alternative 'description of personality': The big-five factor structure. J Pers Soc Psych 59:1216–1229
24. Harris RB (1989) Reviewing nursing stress according to a proposed coping-adaptation framework. Adv Nurs Sci 11:12–28
25. Hobfoll SE, Freedy J (1993) Conservation of resources: A general stress theory applied to burnout. In: Schaufeli WB, Maslach C, Marek T (eds) Professional burnout: Recent developments in theory and research. Taylor andFrancis, New York, pp 115–134

26. Jamal M (1985) Relationship of job stress to job performance: a study of managers and blue collar workers. Hum Rel 38:409–424
27. Jerusalem M, Schwarzer R (1986) Selbstwirksamkeit. In: Schwarzer R (ed) Skalen zur Befindlichkeit und Persönlichkeit. Institut für Psychologie, Freie Universität Berlin, pp 3–14
28. Jong RD de, Eck H van, Bosch K van den (1993) Big five personality factors, leadership and military functioning. In: Raad B de , Hofstee W, Van Heck G (eds) Personality psychology in Europe. Tilburg University, Tilburg, 5:216–221
29. Jonge J de, Landeweerd JA, Nijhuis FJN (1993) Constructie en validering van de vragenlijst ten behoeve van het project 'Autonomie in het werk' [Construction and validation of the questionnaire for the research project XXXJob autonomyXXX]. Studies Bedrijfsgezondheidszorg no. 9. Maastricht: Rijksuniversiteit Limburg
30. Karasek RA (1985) Job content instrument: questionnaire and users guide, Revision 1.1, University of Southern California, LA
31. Karasek R, Theorell T (1990) Healthy work: Stress, productivity and the reconstruction of working life. Basic Books, NY
32. Keijsers GJ, Schaufeli WB, Weterings M (1992) Organisatie en management [Organization and management]. In: Reis Miranda D, Spangenberg JFA, Kwaliteit, doelmatigheid en organisatie van intensive care units in Nederland. FRICE, Groningen, pp 79–98
33. Koeske GF, Koeske RD (1989) Construct validity of the Maslach Burnout Inventory: A critical review and reconceptualization. J Appl Behav Sci 25:131–144
34. Kunin T (1955) The construction of a new type of attitude measure. Personnel Psychol 8:65–78
35. Ladewich BH, White PN (1984) Dual earner marriages: The family social environment and dyadic adjustment. J Fam Issues 5:343–362
36. Leiter MP (1993) Burnout as developmental process: Consideration of models. In: Schaufeli WB, Maslach C, Marek T (eds.), Professional burnout: Recent developments in theory and research. Taylor and Francis, NY pp 237–250
37. Lewandowski LA, Kositski AM (1983) Research priorities for critical care nursing: a study by the American Association of Critical Care Nurses. Heart and Lung 12:35–44
38. Maslach C, Jackson SE (1986) MBI: Maslach Burnout Inventory; manual research edition. Consulting Psychologists, University of California, Palo Alto
39. Mathieu JE, Zajac DH (1990) A review and meta-analysis of the antecedents, correlates and consequences of organizational commitment. Psychol Bull 108:171–194
40. Mulder M, Ritsema van Eck JR, Jong RD de (1971) An organization in crisis and noncrisis situations. Hum Rel 24:19–41
41. Nunnaly JC (1978) Psychometric theory. McGraw-Hill, NY, pp
42. Schaufeli WB, Enzmann DU, Girault N (1993) Measurement of burnout: a review. In: Schaufeli WB, Maslach C, Marek T (eds.) Professional burnout: Recent developments in theory and research. Taylor and Francis, NY, pp 199–215
43. Schaufeli WB, Keijsers GJ, Reis Miranda D (1995) Burnout, technology use and ICU performance. In: Sauter SL, Murphy LR (eds) Organizational risk factors for job-stress. American Psychologic Association, Washington DC, pp 259–271
44. Schaufeli WB, Buunk AP (1996) Professional burnout. In: Schabracq MJ, Winnubst JAM, Cooper CL (eds) Handbook of work and health psychology. Wiley, Chichester, pp 311–346
45. Schaufeli WB, Van Dierendonck D, Van Gorp K (1996) Burnout and reciprocity: towards a dual level social exchange model. Work and Stress 10:225–237
46. Sitter LU de (1989) Moderne sociotechniek [Modern sociotechnics]. Gedrag en Organisatie, 4:222–251
47. Shirom A (1989) Burnout in work organizations. In: Cooper CL, Robertson I (eds) International review of industrial and organizational psychology Wiley, Chichester pp. 25–48
48. Shortell SM, Rousseau DM, Gillies RR, Devers KJ, Simons TL (1991) Organizational assessment in intensive care units (ICUs): Construct development, reliability and validity of the ICU nurse-physician questionnaire. Med Care 29:709–727
49. Van Dierendonck D, Schaufeli WB, Sixma HJ (1994) Burnout among general practitioners: A perspective from equity theory. Journal of Social and Clin Psychol 13:86–100

50. Vaas S, Dhondt S, Peeters MHH, Middendorp J (1995) De WEBA-methode [The WEBA-method]. Alphen aan den Rijn: Samson
51. Hofstede G (1991) Cultures and organizations: Intercultural cooperation and its importance for survival. Harper-Collins, London
52. Hofstede G, Neuijen J, Ohayv D, Sanders GJEM (1990) Measuring organizational cultures: a qualitative and quantitative study across twenty cases. Admin Sci Q 35:286–316
53. Laurent A (1983) The cultural diversity of western conceptions of management. international studies of management and organization 13:75–96
54. Rotter JB (1966) Generalized expectancies for internal versus external control of reinforcement. Psychol Monographs vol. 80
55. Sherwood J (1988) creating work cultures with competitive advantage. Organizational Dynamics pp 5–27
56. Chalfin DB, Cohen IL, Lambrinos J (1995) The economics and cost-effectiveness of critical care medicine. Intens Care Med 21:952–961
57. Durand-Zaleski I (1994) Estimating the cost of intensive care. Intens Care Med 20:538–539
58. Edbrooke DL, Wilson AJ, Gerrish SP, Mann AJ (1994) The Sheffield costing system for intensive care. Working Paper, Central Sheffield University Hospital
59. Eldenburg L, Kallapur S (1995) Changes in hospital service mix and cost allocations in response to changes in Medicare reimbursement schemes. University of Arizona. Working Paper
60. Gheyle D, Jegers M, Matthijs P (1994) Kostenvergelijking tussen twee vormen van nierfunctievervangende therapie: continue ambulante peritoneale dialyse en centrum-hemodialyse. Tijdschrift voor Geneeskunde 50:12
61. Gilbertson AA, Smith JM, Mostafa SM (1991) The cost of an intensive care unit: a prospective study. Intens Care Med 17:204–208
62. Gyldmark M (1995) A review of cost studies of intensive care units: problems with the cost concept. Crit Care Med 23:5
63. Hilgeman CN, Koopmanschap MA, Rutten FFH (1992) Kosten van intensive care in Nederland. Rotterdam, IMTA 92.17
64. Koopmanschap MA, Rutten FFH (1994) The impact of indirect costs on outcomes of health care programs. Health Econ 3:6
65. Noreen E, Soderstrom N (1994) Are overhead costs strictly proportional to activity? Evidence from hospital service departments. J Accounting Econ 17:255–278.
66. Pettersen IJ (1995) Budgetary control of hospitals: ritual rhetorics and rationalized myths? Financial Accountability and Management 11:207–211
67. Raes H (1993) De klinische biologie in cijfers, Tijdschrift van de BVLT 20:6
68. Rapoport J, Teres D, Lemeshow S, Gehlbach S (1994) A method for assessing the clinical performance and cost-effectiveness of intensive care units: a multicenter inception cohort study. Crit Care Med 22:9
69. Reis Miranda D, Williams A, Loirat Ph (eds.) (1990) Management of intensive care: guidelines for better use of resources, Kluwer Academic, Dordrecht, The Netherlands
70. Ridley S, Biggam M, Stone P (1991) Cost of intensive therapy: a description of methodology and initial results. Anaesthesia 46:523–530
71. Shiell AM, Griffiths RD, Short AI, Spiby J (1990) An evaluation of the costs and outcome of adult intensive care in two units in the UK. Working Paper, Centre for Health Economics, University of York, UK
72. Vereniging Klinisch Chemici Noord (1995), Verrekening laboratorium-diagnostiek, Heerenveen, Symposium KCN
73. Walravens C, Tielemans L, Beeckmans J, Matthijs P (1994) Kostenanalyse van de nomenclatuur der geneeskundige verstrekkingen, Brussel, DWTC

8 Highlights of the EURICUS-I Data

Data Handling and Analysis

R. Moreno, A. van Dort, K. Rowan, and G. Apolone

This report describes the various procedures performed concerning quality control of the clinical data (A-sheet, Fig. 1), including a discussion of how they were measured, and the NEMS data (B-sheet; Fig. 2) in the EURICUS-I project. The controls started immediately after the field research and were performed on the already received data. The numbers presented therefore differ from the final data used in the final analysis of EURICUS-I since was possible to retrieve a large part of the missing values.

First, the checks performed on the data entry are described. In the section "Random Data Entry Checks"inter-rater and intra-rater reliabilities are presented. In the following section checks on the completeness of the clinical data are described. Logical and consistency checks can be found in the section "Checks for Logical and Consistency Errors on the A-Sheet". For split-data analysis the database was split into two parts, as described in the section "Assessment of Severity of Illness Scoring". Finally the performance of the original SAPS-II model and the uniformity of fit across different stratifications were assessed. Analysis of the data concerning the MPM-II scoring system is not presented as this scoring system was not put to further use in the study analysis.

Random Data Entry Checks

The handling and data checks concerning the entry of data are summarized in Fig. 3.

Analysis of Reliability

Methods

For the first 20 patients admitted to each participating ICU after the start of the study, data were recollected for each patient by the same individual (intra-rater reliability check). On 12 separate days during the study, specified in advance by the investigators, a subset of the data (admission and discharge details) were recollected for each patient by a separate individual (inter-rater reliability check).

Patient code no.: □□□□□□□

day month year
Date of birth: ....../....../.......
If not known, estimated age in years: ....

EURICUS I
A - SHEET

ADMISSION DATA

	day month year	
Admission date hospital	.... / .... /199...	Patient was admitted to the ICU from:
Admission date ICU	.... / .... /199...	1 □ Operating theatre 2 □ Recovery room 3 □ Emergency room
Time of admission	......h.......m	4 □ ward 5 □ other ICU 6 □ other hospital 7 □ other

Is this a readmission?* YES / NO
Former code: ....

Type of admission* 1 □ surgical - unscheduled
2 □ surgical - scheduled
3 □ medical

Diagnosis*: ....
(on other side)

MPM$_0$ (AT ADMISSION) (circle <u>yes</u> or <u>no</u>)

PHYSIOLOGY
Coma/deep stupor at admission .... YES / NO
Systolic BP ≤ 90 mmHg .... YES / NO
Heart rate ≥ 150 beats/minute .... YES / NO

CHRONIC DIAGNOSES
Metastatic malignant neoplasm .... YES / NO
Cirrhosis .... YES / NO
Chronic renal compromise or insufficiency .... YES / NO

ACUTE DIAGNOSES
Intracranial mass effect .... YES / NO
Gastrointestinal bleeding .... YES / NO
Cardiac dysrhythmias .... YES / NO
Cerebrovascular incident .... YES / NO
Acute renal failure .... YES / NO

OTHER
On mechanical ventilation .... YES / NO
CPR prior to ICU admission .... YES / NO
Medical or unscheduled surgery admission .... YES / NO

SAPS II (worst values within the first 24 hours)

AIDS .... YES / NO
Metastatic cancer .... YES / NO
Hematologic malignancy .... YES / NO
Heart rate .... (rate/min)
Systolic BP .... (mmHg)
Temperature .... (oC)
FiO2 .... (%)
PaO2 .... (mmHg)
Leucocytes (WBC) .... (10E3/ml)
Bilirubin .... (mg/dL)
Urinary output .... (L/day)
Blood urea or blood urea nitrogen .... (mg/dL)
Serum K+ .... (mMol/L)
Serum Na+ .... (mMol/L)
Serum HCO3 .... (mMol/L)

GLASGOW COMA SCORE
Active eye-opening ....
Best motor response ....
Best verbal response ....
(on other side)

DISCHARGE DATA

Did the patient die in the ICU?	YES / NO	Patient was discharged from the ICU to:
Discharge date from ICU	.... / .... /199...	1 □ ward 5 □ home to die
Time of discharge from the ICU:	......h ....m	2 □ other ICU 6 □ other hospital
Did the patient die in the hospital?	YES / NO	3 □ High/Medium Care (intermediate care) 7 □ other
Discharge date from hospital:	.... / .... /199...	4 □ home
	day month year	

Fig. 1. A-sheet

Patient code no.: ☐☐☐☐☐☐☐

Scoring date: day month year ....../....../.......

Scoring time: ..... h ..... m

EURICUS I

B - SHEET

NEMS

Nine Equivalents of Nursing Manpower use Score

1 ☐ **Basic monitoring.** Hourly vital signs, regular record and calculation of fluid balance.

2 ☐ **Intravenous medication** Bolus or continuously, not including vaso-active drugs.

3 ☐ **Mechanical ventilatory support.** Any form of mechanical/assisted ventilation, with or without PEEP (e.g. CPAP), with or without muscle relaxants.

4 ☐ **Supplementary ventilatory care.** Breathing spontaneously through endotracheal tube; supplementary oxygen any method, except if 3) applies.

5 ☐ **Single vaso-active medication** Any vaso-active drug.

6 ☐ **Multiple vaso-active medication.** More than one vaso-active drug, disregarded type and dose.

7 ☐ **Dialysis techniques.** All.

8 ☐ **Specific interventions in the ICU.** Such as ET intubation, introduction of pacemaker, cardioversion, endoscopy, emergency operation in the past 24 hours, gastric lavage. Routine interventions such as X-rays, echocardiography, ECG, dressings, introduction of venous or arterial lines, are not included.

9 ☐ **Specific interventions outside the ICU.** Such as surgical intervention or diagnostic procedure. The intervention/ procedure is related with the severity of illness of the patient and makes an extra demand upon manpower efforts at the ICU.

Fig. 2. B-sheet

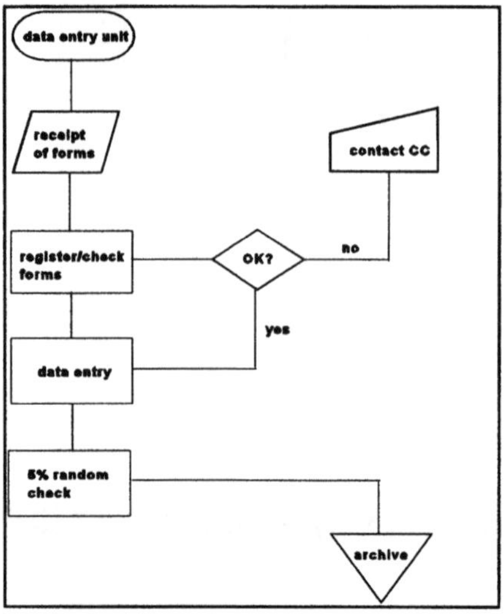

DATA-ENTRY RANDOM CHECKS

A-sheets N = 9,804 forms
Checked N = 761 forms (7.8%)

Total of 1,706 errors in 761 forms
Average of 2.2 errors per form
On 47 variables that means an error of 4.7%

Number of NEMS forms	N = 41,393
Checked	N = 3,982 (9.5%)

Total of 256 errors in 3,298 forms
Average of 0.07 errors per form
On 9 variables that means an error of 0.7%

Fig. 3 Data entry check system

Correlation coefficients were employed to describe the level of association for continuous data and κ statistics the level of agreement for categorical data.

Results

A total of 89 (86.4%) ICUs from those originally recruited completed the EURICUS-I study. Of these, 51 (57.3%) participated in the intra-rater reliability study. The level of association was high for continuous variables, with correlation coefficients greater than 0.8, and agreement was good for categorical variables, with values for κ statistics above 0.6, except for hospital discharge status (0.54). Agreement improved when missing values were excluded from the analyses; for example, the κ statistics for hospital discharge status improved to 0.93. A total of 48 (53.9%) ICUs participated in the inter-rater reliability study. Both continuous and categorical variables showed good levels of reliability with values of κ statistics for categorical variables greater than 0.6. Again, exclusion of missing data improved results.

Conclusion

This study showed that data collected as part of the formal reliability studies in the EURICUS-I study demonstrated good reliability. However, only a sample of the ICUs contributed data and, therefore, these results may reflect some volunteer bias. Nevertheless, the results show that a high level of accuracy is possible when collecting case mix and outcome data.

Checks for Completeness

These checks aimed at understanding whether the irregular and/or non-consecutive inclusion in the study of all patients admitted to the ICU during the research period could represent a bias of importance to the quality of the collected data.

Check at ICU Level

The ICUs were questioned as to whether all patients admitted to the ICU during the research period were included in the study. If this was not the case, the ICU was requested to indicate reasons for noninclusion and to state any used exclusion criteria. If patients were excluded, the ICUs were requested to give information concerning those patients regarding: (a) dates of admission at and discharge from the ICU; (b) age; (c) outcome. The answer was not provided by 29 ICUs. From the responding ICUs, 267 admissions were excluded from the study in seven units. One ICU was a mixed critical care unit (CCU)/ICU. From the 375 admissions to this unit during the research period, 122 patients entered the study including three patients to the ICU on October 3, 1994. The 256 exclusions concerned: admission diagnosis of suspicion of MI; elective cardioversion; pre/post-pacemaker insertion; post-arrest if admitted unintubated. The ICU provided a list with dates of admission, age, length of stay (LOS) and outcome regarding the excluded patients (21 of these patients died). Seven of the patients excluded at the other ICUs concerned admissions with "do not resuscitate" (DNR) orders (these patients died). For the exclusion of the other patients no exclusion criteria were provided. Figure 4 shows that the admission pattern remained constant during the study period, with a dip around Christmas 1994.

Check at Database Level

In Groningen the database was analyzed to see whether there was consecutiveness of patient code numbers at the ICU level. Lists of omissions were produced and presented to the respective ICUs via the country coordinators. Two sorts of

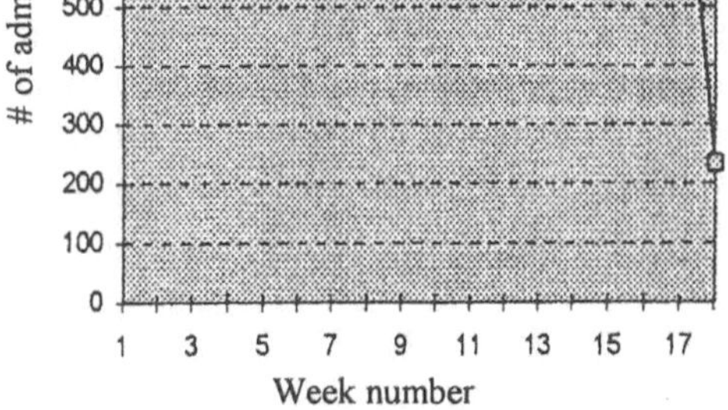

WEEK	# of admissions
1	815
2	863
3	846
4	873
5	857
6	881
7	897
8	906
9	894
10	874
11	880
12	894
13	753
14	788
15	844
16	885
17	863
18	232

Fig. 4. Admissions per week

answers were obtained: (a) the received code labels have been rendered useless/not utilized; (b) the respective patients were still in the hospital and therefore the data would be sent later.

Completeness at Item Level

Here we analyzed in the population the available data on readmission, location of admission, age, diagnosis, LOS in the ICU, type of admission, outcome in the ICU and in the hospital, and location of discharge, admissions/bed per year (ABY), and hospital size.

Readmission

Data on readmission are available for 14105 patients (missing: 1164 patients).

Admission From

Data on the place from where the patient was admitted are available for 14756 patients. Where the patient was admitted from was significantly related to death in the hospital: $\chi^2 = 2846$; df=14; $p < 0.001$).

Age

For age, data on 14979 patients are available. When the mean age of the patients who were discharged alive is comparef with that of patients who died in the hospital, there is a highly significant difference (two-tailed *t* test $p < 0.001$), with non-survivors 6.4 years older than survivors.

Diagnosis/Diagnostic Category of Admission

We analyzed the primary reason for ICU admission using 78 mutually exclusive disease categories. After data collection began, another category, "79 other postoperative diseases", was considered. Data on diagnosis is available for 14820 patients. If we exclude all patients with missing data regarding diagnostic category and outcome in the hospital, diagnostic category was significantly related to hospital outcome ($\chi^2 = 760.5$; df=18; $p < 0.001$).

Length of Stay in the ICU

Data on LOS in the ICU are available for 15267 patients.; however, in calculating this parameter some problems occurred. All patients with a discharge date equal to the admission date were considered to have a LOS of 0 days. Results must be analyzed with caution and eventually analysis needs tobe done again after correction of this abnormality. When we compare the mean LOS of the patients who were discharged alive with that of the patients who died in the hospital, there is a highly significant difference (two-tailed *t* test $p < 0.001$), with the LOS of non-survivors almost double that of survivors.

Type of Admission

Data on type of admission are available for 14817 patients (missing: 452 patients). Type of admission is strongly related to outcome ($\chi^2 = 3030$; df=6;

$p < 0.001$), with medical and unscheduled surgery patients having the worst prognosis.

Outcome in the ICU

Data on outcome in the ICU are available for 14746 patients (missing: 523 patients).

Outcome in the Hospital

Data on the outcome in the hospital are available for 13754 patients (missing: 1515 patients).

Site of Patient Discharge

Data on the site of discharge for the patients who survived ICU are available for 12099 patients.

Checks for Logical and Consistency Errors on the A-Sheet

A flow-chart (Fig. 5) of procedures was used for dealing with these checks:

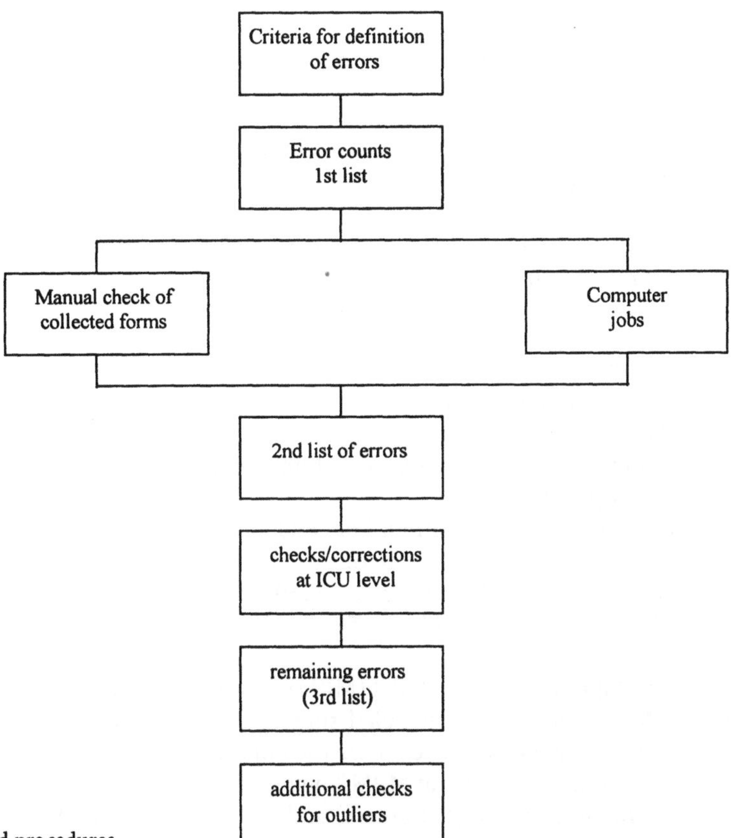

Fig. 5. Followed procedures

Criteria

The following types of errors were analyzed:

1. Date errors:
   - All dates which were not filled in
   - Hospital admission prior to date of birth
   - Hospital admission after research period
   - Hospital admission after ICU admission
   - Hospital admission after hospital discharge date
   - Hospital admission after ICU discharge date
   - ICU admission after ICU discharge date
2. Time errors:
   - Admission time after scoring time of first B-sheet
   - Admission time after discharge time
3. Readmission errors:
   - Different hospital admission date
   - Different date of birth
4. Diagnosis errors:
   - Postoperative is medical type of admission
   - Nonoperative is surgical type of admission
5. "Admitted from" errors:
   - Patients admitted from the operating theater or from the recovery room should have a "postoperative diagnosis" and a "surgical type" of admission
6. Died in the ICU errors:
   - When died in the ICU is checked and "not died" in the hospital, and/or "discharged to" is also checked.

Numerical checks were made on extreme deviations from the normal values for:

Heart rate >300 bpm
Systolic blood pressure >300 mm Hg
Temperature >-1 and <26 or $>44\,°C$
FiO_2 $>0\%$ and $<21\%$ or $>100\%$
PaO_2 $>0\%$ and $<2\%$ or $>50\%$
Leukocytes $>50\,000$/ml
Bilirubin >0 and <1 µmol/l or >1500 µmol/liter
Urine output >30 l/day
Blood urea >0 and <1 mmol/l or >70 mmol/l
Potassium >0 and <1 mmol/l or >9 mmol/l
Sodium >0 and <105 mmol/l or >180 mmol/l
HCO_3 >0 and <5 mmol/l or >50 mmol/l

Note: Mortality Prediction Model (MPM) and type of admission were compared for MPM "medical or unscheduled surgery admission" and type of admission "surgical scheduled". MPM data were compared with SAPS data and the first NEMS. It was anticipated that MPM "metastatic neoplasm" and SAPS "metastatic cancer" should coincide (121 errors) and that patients in MPM on "mechanical ventilation" should have item 3 or 4 scored on NEMS first day (84 errors). It was however decided not to include the comparison of data between MPM and SAPS because those scores may concern different times on the admission day: MPM registers data values observed at admission + 1 h and SAPS the worst values within the first 24 h. The score of nominal variables in MPM is based on information collected from the patient's record or on clinical judgement. It is therefore possible that, e.g., initial information/opinion regarding "metastatic cancer" is adjusted within the first 24 h, or that an initially diagnosed "chronic renal compromise or insufficiency" could not be confirmed by an abnormal BUN.

Results

The first list of errors found according to the above criteria was analyzed. In the 15041 A-sheets inspected, 5280 errors were detected on 4104 forms. The weekly incidence of errors decreased during the study period. However, this weekly decrease of errors is not significant (ANOVA) when indexed at ICU level.

Manual Checks and Computer Jobs

As at least 4.7% of the errors could be due to entry errors when transferring data from the forms to the computer (see above), all the forms with errors were manually revised and data entry corrected when appropriate. After this, the following computer jobs were devised and run:

1. Date errors:
   - For the A-sheets without ICU admission date, set admission date to the first NEMS date.
   - For the A-sheets without ICU discharge date, set the discharge date to last NEMS date.
2. Readmission errors:
   - If "readmission" in A-sheet is "yes", look at the previous admission; hospital admission dates must be equal on both admissions, otherwise it is not a readmission and the box is emptied.
3. Diagnosis errors:
   - Type of admission is more important than diagnosis. For the surgical type of admission with a nonoperative diagnosis, create a translation table for nonoperative diagnosis into postoperative diagnosis. For the medical type of admission and not coming from the operating theatre (1) or recovery room (2) with a postoperative diagnosis, create a translation table for postoperative diagnosis into nonoperative diagnosis.
4. "Admitted From" errors:
   - If "admitted from" is operating theatre (1), recovery room (2) or emergency room (3) and if type of admission is "surgical unscheduled", MPM medical/unscheduled surgery admission is "yes". If type of admission is "surgical scheduled" MPM medical /unscheduled surgery admission is "no".
5. ICU death errors:
   - If died in ICU is "yes", died in the hospital is also "yes"; if died in ICU is "yes", "discharge to" is set to 0.

Table 1 presents the data on errors, handled as described above.

Table 1. Errors found

Variable	Total number of errors	Remaining errors after mnning jobs
Date	1809	675
Readmission	183	0
Diagnosis	590	(112)
Admitted from	360	(198)
ICU dead	96	0
Heart rate	0	0
Blood pressure	2	2
Temperature	3	3
FiO_2	0	0
PaO_2	68	68
Leukocytes	35	35
Billrubin	3	3
Urinary output	4	4
Blood urea	237	237
Potassium	5	5
Sodium	5	5
Bicarbonate	52	52
Admission type	138	27
Overall	3590	1116

Control at ICU Level

After running the computer jobs and having controlled the typing errors (manual checks of records), 1024 errors still remained on 1002 A-sheets. These were mailed (faxed) to the ICUs (via country coordinators) for correction of possible errors after comparing with the ICU data. "Diagnosis errors" (65 of the 112 errors were missing diagnoses) and "Admitted from" errors (198) were not included in the questionnaires. The reason was the danger of obtaining a "correction" which was not a more correct alternative than an empty box. Checks from about 600 patients were retrieved and 699 (68.3%) "suspected errors" have been corrected/confirmed.

Additional Checks

Due to diversity in the units used for some variables (e.g. PaO_2, BUN, bilirubin) checks on the registered values at ICU level were performed (clinical judgement), controlling for the units of registration indicated by the respective ICUs:

- PaO_2: Some values were registered in units different than those indicated by the ICUs. Some values entered were clearly improbable/not credible and 14 values were excluded from the data; 20 were corrected into the appropriate units (kPa).

- BUN: The same as for PaO_2. Two values were eliminated from the database. According to the available ICU information, values were corrected to the given units on four ICUs.
- Bilirubin: The same as above. One value was excluded; 18 values were corrected according to information available.
- Potassium: Two values were excluded (12 and 21.5 mmol). Two others were corrected after control of the respective forms.
- Leukocytes: One value was excluded (-4.1).
- FiO_2: One value was corrected.
- Urinary output: Three values were excluded because they were excessively high (30; 30; 40 liters). Two values were corrected.

Five diagnoses and one admission date were corrected according to the respective forms. It was checked whether mortality did match between readmission and previous admission for those patients having more than one admission to the ICU. There were 20 cases of mismatched/incomplete information that were found and corrected.

Based on the information provided the following corrections were introduced in the database, after comparing/confirming the outlier values with the original forms: There were 59 FiO_2 values registered as 0 that were corrected as missing values; 14 temperature values were checked and nine were corrected according to the forms, two were accepted (26 and 45), three were given as missing values (60; two impossible to read); seven low systolic BPs were confirmed and two corrected; seven heart rate values were confirmed and two corrected; ten bilirubin values were corrected and one accepted; eight leukocytes values were given as missing values, two were corrected and five were accepted; two sodium values were corrected and two accepted; one potassium value was corrected and one accepted; two BUN values were corrected and one accepted; three bicarbonate values were accepted, and two given as missing values.

Assessment of Severity of Illness Scoring Systems

R. Moreno

Splitting of the Database

For analytic purposes the database was split in two halves. First we tried, for the whole file, to randomly select a fraction of two thirds per ICU as the development sample. Therefore the file was sorted by ICU identification and then the split file command was activated to split 0.66 per unit using SPSS for Windows version 6.1. This gave a very large and unacceptable variation in the numbers of cases per ICU for the development and validation samples. The second approach was to split the file into 89 files, one file per unit. The number of cases to sample was determined for every unit (number of patients *2/3). This number was rounded off to the nearest integer, so SPSS could exactly extract randomly these cases from the files. The 89 files were then merged together before extracting the development and validation samples. In the total A-sheet file the variable SAMPLE was marked with a "D" for the development cases and with a "V" for the validation cases. The file was then split physically into DEVELOP.DBF and VALIDAT.DBF. These files were used at a later stage for the development of new models.

Assessment of Original SAPS-II and MPM_0 Performance in the EURICUS-I Database

Introduction

The computation of SAPS-II and MPM_0 was done according to the original definitions [1, 2]. A problem appeared in the computation of the respiratory parameters (PaO_2/FiO_2 ratio), since no data were collected on the A-sheet regarding mechanical ventilation during the first 24 h in the ICU. It was decided to cross-tabulate data on mechanical ventilation at admission ± 1 h (MMECHAN) and data on mechanical ventilation during the first day in the ICU (from first day NEMS – B-sheet). We assumed that, if MMECHAN = yes *or* mechanical ventilation on first NEMS = yes, then the patient had been ventilated (6175 patients). In this case, we calculate PaO_2/FiO_2 ratio and scored SAPS according to this value. Otherwise, we assumed that the patient was not on the ventilator during the first 24 h and thus no score was assigned to PaO_2/FiO_2 ratio on SAPS-II.

Exclusion Criteria

The exclusion criteria were those expressed in the original guidelines: patients < 18 years of age, readmissions, acute coronary care patients, burns and patients in the postoperative period after coronary artery bypass surgery. To keep comparability between both systems, patients with a LOS in the ICU of < 8 h were also excluded. Four ICUs did not collect complete data on MPM_0 and were excluded. After applying the exclusion criteria described above, the data of 10027 patients were available to the study (8020 survivors and 2007 nonsurvivors).

Overall Goodness-of-Fit

Mortality on the ICU was 13.9% and hospital mortality was 20.0% in this sample. The mean scores aggregated at ICU level were largely different for both models, with medians ranging from 18 to 45 on the SAPS-II score; from 2.9 to 34.8 on the SAPS-II probability; and from 3.9 to 39.3 on the MPM_0 probability. Both severity scores (Table 2) were significantly related to mortality ($p < 0.001$). The predicted risk of dying in the hospital, as calculated by the two models, showed a highly significant correlation (multiple R: 0.741). However, although highly correlated, the results from the two models were widely dispersed, with a significant number of outliers, as already described in other studies. The models could explain only part of the variance across units, with SAPS-II explaining 69.2% of the variance and MPM_0 71.3%.

Table 2. The severity scores

	Global	Survivors	Nonsurvivors
SAPS-II score	31 (21–44)	28 (19–38)	50 (37–64)
SAPS-II probability of death	11.7 (4.2–32.6)	8.8 (3.3–21.3)	46.1 (19.6–75.3)
MPM probability of death	13.1 (5.8–33.0)	10.6 (4.9–23.2)	41.4 (17.0–72.3)

Results are presented as median (interquartile range); nonsurvivors presented higher scores than survivors ($p < 0\ 001$ for all).

Discrimination

For estimation of the discriminative power of the models, the area under the receiver operating characteristic (ROC) curve was used. The results were 0.822 (standard error 0.005) for SAPS-II and 0.785 (standard error 0.006) for MPM_0. The area for SAPS-II was similar to the area on the original SAPS-II model (0.8229); for MPM_0 it was significantly lower (0.824). Comparison of the SAPS-II and MPM_0 curves using the modification of the *Z* statistics proposed by Hanley and McNeil [3] showed a statistically significant difference (two-sided test, $p < 0.0001$), meaning that SAPS-II presented an overall true-positive rate relative to the false-positive rate much higher than MPM_0. Figure 6 shows the plots of the ROC curves of the two models. Table 3 shows the classification tables for SAPS-II and MPM_0. With a decision criterion of 10%, sensitivity, that is, the proportion of deaths predicted by the models, was similar (88.3% for SAPS-II and 88.1% for MPM_0); the false-positive rate was high for both systems (SAPS-II 44.7% and 52.0% on MPM_0); the overall correct classification was higher on SAPS-II (62.0%)

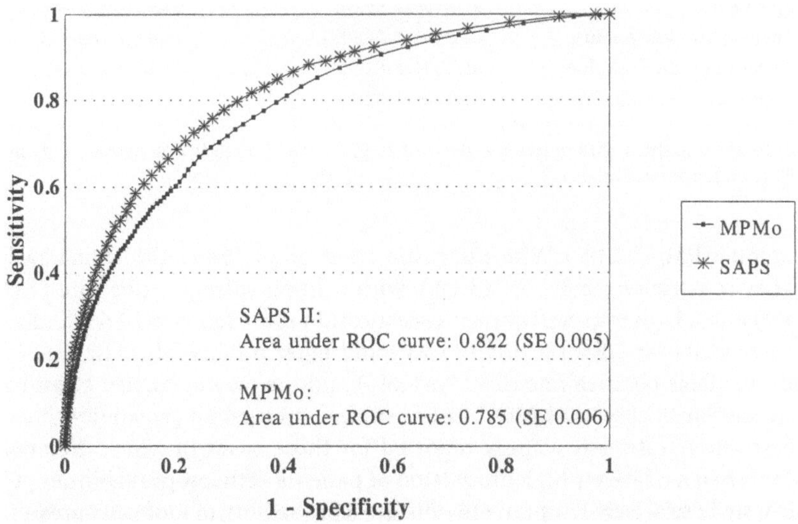

Fig. 6. Receiver operating characteristic (ROC) curves for SAPS-II and MPM_0. For both models the relationship between true positives (sensitivity) and false positives (1 − specificity) are presented

Table 3. Classification tables for SAPS II and MPMO

	SAPS-II		MPMo	
	Predicted to live	Predicted to die	Predicted to live	Predicted to die
Decision criteria 10%				
Observed survivors	4439	3581	3853	4167
Observed nonsurvivors	234	1773	238	1769
Sensitivity	88.3 (86.9–89.7)		88.1 (86.7–89.6)	
Specificity	55.4 (54.3–56.4)		48.0 (47.0–49.1)	
Positive predictive value	33.1 (31.9–34.4)		29.8 (28.6–31.0)	
Negative predictive value	95.0 (94.4–95.6)		94.2 (93.5– 94.9)	
Overall correct classification	62.0 (61.0–62.9)		56.1 (55.1– 57.0)	
Decision criteria 50%				
Observed survivors	7412	608	7269	751
Observed nonsurvivors	1078	929	1141	866
Sensitivity	46.3 (44.1–48.5)		43.2 (41.0–45.3)	
Specificity	92.4 (91.8–93.0)		90.6 (90.0–91.3)	
Positive predictive value	60.4 (58.0–62.9)		53.6 (51.1–56.0)	
Negative predictive value	87.3 (86.6–88.0)		86.4 (85.7–87.2)	
Overall correct classification	83.2 (82.5–83.9)		81.1 (80.4–81.9)	
Decision criteria 90 %				
Observedsurvivors	7979	41	7969	51
Observed nonsurvivors	1782	225	1850	157
Sensitivity	11.2 (9.8–12.6)		7.82 (6.65–9.0)	
Specificity	99.5 (99.3–99.6)		99.36 (99.19–99.5)	
Positive predictive value	84.6 (80.3–88.9)		75.48 (69.63–81.3)	
Negative predictive value	81.7 (81.0–82.5)		81.16 (80.39–81.9)	
Overall correct classification	81.8 (81.0–82.6)		81.04 (80.27–81.8)	

Results are presented with decision criteria of 10 %, 50% and 90 % In brackets are indicated the 95% confidence intervals.

than on MPM_0 (56.1%). With a decision criterion of 50%, SAPS-II had a slightly higher sensitivity (46.3% vs 43.2%), with a lower false-positive rate (7.6% vs 9.4%) and a higher overall correct classification rate (83.2% vs 81.1%). At a decision criterion of 90%, sensitivity was also higher on SAPS-II (11.2% vs 7.8%), both the false positive rate (0.5% vs 0.6%) and the overall correct classification were similar (81.8% vs 81.0%). The low values observed for sensitivity, that is, the true-positive rate, was already reported for those cases in which the analyzed sample had a relatively high proportion of patients with low probabilities of mortality, since relatively few patients will have a probability of mortality greater than the chosen decision criterion [4].

The cross-tabulation of the predictions by both models (SAPS-II and MPM_0) at a fixed decision criterion (50%) is presented in Table 4. The two methods predict-

Table 4. Comparison of the classification tables for SAPS-II and MPM_0 at a decision criteria of 50%

	MPM_0	
	Predicted to live	Predicted to die
Survivors: SAPS-II		
Predicted to live	6983 (87.1 %)	429 (5.4 %)
Predicted to die	286 (3.6 %)	322 (4.0 %)
Nonsurvivors: SAPS-II		
Predicted to live	851 (42.4 %)	227 (11.3 %)
Predicted to die	290 (14.5 %)	639 (31.8 %)

In brackets are indicated the percentages for each cell.

ed the same outcome in 8795 patients. For the survivors group the two methods predicted the same outcome in 7305 patients. Regarding the 715 patients for whom the predictions did not agree, SAPS-II predicted significantly (McNemar's test, $p<0.001$) more patients (429) than MPM_0 (286). For nonsurvivors the two methods predicted the same outcome for 1490 patients. Regarding the 517 patients for whom the predictions did not agree, SAPS-II predicted correctly 227 whereas MPM_0 predicted correctly 290 (McNemar's test, $p<0.005$).

Calibration

Figures 7 and 8 present the calibration curves of SAPS-II and MPM_0. These curves demonstrate that as the predicted risk of hospital mortality (either by SAPS-II or by MPM_0) increased the proportion of patients who died also increased. However, for SAPS-II-predicted risks >40%, the observed mortality within each risk group lay significantly below the diagonal line; in other words the model overestimates mortality in sicker patients. The same pattern is present regarding the MPM_0 model, with the shift becoming apparent around 30% predicted risk of death.

The Hosmer-Lemeshow goodness-of-fit test H is done by collapsing the table based on fixed values of the estimated probabilities and comparing the observed and expected number of patients in each of the 20 cells to determine whether the discrepancy is acceptably small. This test showed a significant discrepancy between predicted and observed outcomes for both models (Table 5). The Hosmer-Lemeshow goodness-of-fit test C is done by collapsing the table based on percentiles of the estimated probabilities and comparing the observed and expected number of patients in each of the 20 cells to determine whether the discrepancy is acceptably small; this test revealed a similar result (Table 6). The implication is that the models do not accurately predict the outcome of patients in the EURICUS-I sample.

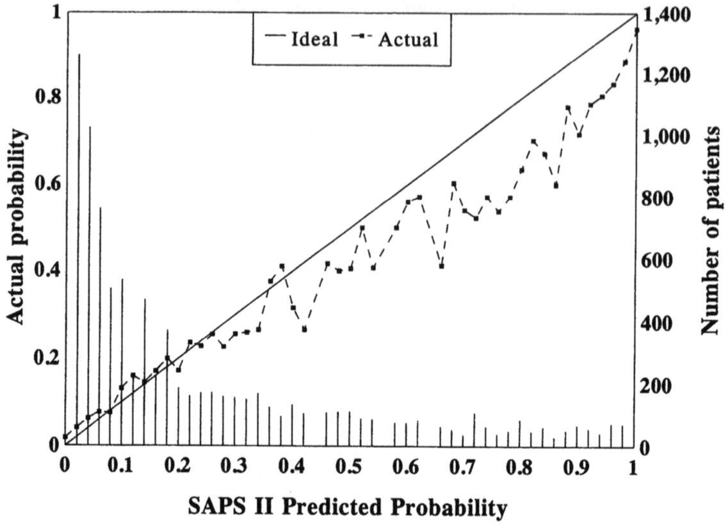

Fig. 7. SAPS-II calibration curve. The *solid line* represents perfect correspondence between actual and predicted risk of death; the *dotted line* the observed vs predicted risk of death. *Bars* provide the distribution of patients in the analyzed groups

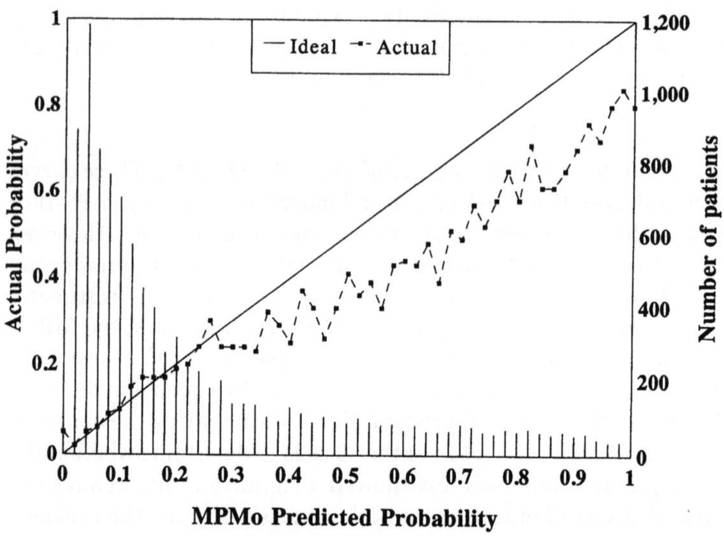

Fig. 8. MPM_0. The *solid line* represents perfect correspondence between actual and predicted risk of death; the *dotted line* the observed vs predicted risk of death. *Bars* provide the distribution of patients in the analyzed groups

Table 5. Hosmer-Lemeshow goodnes-of-fit test H for SAPS II and MPM_0

	Observed and expected frequencies by decile				Total
	Observed deaths	Expected deaths	Observed survivors	Expected survivors	
SAPS-II[a]					
Decile					
0.00–0.10	234	200.4	4439	4472.64	4673
>0.10–0.20	286	263.5	1531	1553.50	1817
>0.20–0.30	189	210.0	660	639.02	849
>0.30–0.40	210	238.8	485	456.17	695
>0.40–0.50	159	204.1	297	251.94	456
>0.50–0.60	204	239.0	232	196.97	436
>0.60–0.70	126	152.6	111	84.41	237
>0.70–0.80	195	256.6	148	86.36	343
>0.80–0.90	179	217.3	76	37.73	255
>0.90–1.00	225	252.0	41	13.97	266
Total	2007	2234.3	8020	7792.70	10027
MPM_0[b]					
Decile					
0.00–0.10	238	213.7	3853	3877.3	4091
>0.10–0.20	345	308.5	1833	1869.5	2178
>0.20–0.30	246	259.1	812	798.9	1058
>0.30–0.40	154	206.0	438	386.0	592
>0.40–0.50	158	220.0	333	271.1	491
>0.50–0.60	158	231.3	264	190.7	422
>0.60–0.70	157	222.0	185	120.0	342
>0.70–0.80	189	250.4	146	84.6	335
>0.80–0.90	205	262.6	105	47.5	310
>0.90–1.00	157	195.7	51	12.3	208
Total	2007	2369.2	8020	7657.8	10027

Tables were collapsed on fixed values of the estimated probabilities.
[a] χ^2: 218.2; df, 10; $p<0.0001$.
[b] χ^2: 437.1; df, 10; $p<0.0001$.

Uniformity of Fit

To evaluate the uniformity of fit, that is, the ability of the model to adjust between subgroups, we stratified patients using two different strategies: (1) patient-related criteria included in the models and for which we should expect that the models take them into account (age group and type of patient) and (2) patient-related criteria not included in the models (location in the hospital before ICU admission and diagnostic category). These strategies were chosen since they represent important characteristics of the patients present at ICU admission and do not depend on therapeutic aspects. Together with severity of illness, this set of variables comprises the baseline categories of patient characteristics. Afterwards, the performance of the models was evaluated in each of these mutually exclusive subgroups using formal tests of discrimination, calibration and observed/expected (O/E) mortality ratios as described above.

Table 6. Hosmer-Lemeshow goodnes-of-fit test C for SAPS-II and MPM_0

	Observed and expected frequencies by decile				Total
	Observed deaths	Expected deaths	Observed survivors	Expected survivors	
SAPS-II[a]					
Decile					
0.00–0.02	21	9.4	958	969.6	979
>0.02–0.03	38	23.2	939	953.8	977
>0.03–0.05	60	49.2	1098	1108.8	1158
>0.05–0.08	53	53.2	766	765.8	819
>0.08–0.12	96	93.2	906	908.8	1002
>0.12–0.17	178	166.0	1006	1018.0	1184
>0.17–0.27	183	188.5	706	700.5	889
>0.27–0.39	290	330.0	736	696.0	1026
>0.39–0.64	411	495.1	565	480.9	976
>0.64–0,1.0	677	826.5	340	190.5	1017
Total	2007	2234.3	8020	7792.7	10027
MPM_0[b]					
Decile					
0.00–0.03	26	23.3	983	985.7	1009
>0.03–0.05	55	38.2	941	957.8	996
>0.05–0.07	57	60.4	961	957.6	1018
>0.07–0.10	93	83.8	894	903.2	987
>0.10–0.13	129	113.6	874	889.4	1003
>0.13–0.18	167	154.6	836	848.5	1003
>0.18–0.27	224	220.6	779	782.4	1003
>0.27–0.42	264	335.1	739	667.9	1003
>0.42–0.65	373	530.1	630	472.9	1003
>0.65–1.00	619	809.7	383	192.3	1002
Total	2007	2369.2	8020	7657.8	10027

Tables were collapsed on deciles of the estimated probabilities.
[a] χ^2: 208.4; df, 10; $p<0.0001$.
[b] χ^2: 308.2; df, 10; $p<0.0001$.

Patient-Related Criteria Included in the Models

Stratification of patients according to these criteria was done by type of patient (unscheduled surgery, scheduled surgery and medical) and by age group (Table 7). When data were stratified by type of patient, discrimination was lower for both models in scheduled surgical patients. Hosmer-Lemeshow tests H and C revealed significant differences between observed and predicted mortality and the O/E mortality ratios were <1 in all groups, with a trend of less deviation for scheduled surgical patients. In other words, both models significantly overestimated mortality.

Stratification by age group showed a decreasing discriminative power of SAPS-II with increasing age; for MPM_0 the general trend was similar but the pattern was less clear. This was associated with significant discrepancies in Hosmer-Lemeshow statistics in higher age groups and with O/E mortality ratios that did

Table 7. Uniformity of fit of SAPS-II and MPM_0

Criteria	*N*	SAPS-II				MPM_0			
		ROC (SE)	H test	C test	O/E (95% CI)	ROC (SE)	H test	C test	O/E (95% CI)
Type of patient									
Uns. Surgery	1966	0.797 (0.012)	61.32 [a]	60.80	0.87 (0.82–0.93)	0.747 (0.012)	140.99	126.38 [a]	0.82 (0.77–0.88)
Sch. Surgery	2417	0.783 (0.019)	34.04 [a]	28.78 [a]	0 79 (0.68–0 90)	0.710 (0.021)	39.51 [a]	28.53 [a]	0.84 (0.73–0.96)
Medical	5563	0.808 (0.007)	167.32 [a]	154.22 [a]	0.92 (0.89–0.96)	0.770 (0.007)	291.57 [a]	256.28 [a]	0.85 (0.82–0.89)
Age group (years)									
18–24	454	0.981 (0.041)	19.79	22.43	0.59 (0.36–0.81)	0.788 (0.049)	19.69	23.99	0.56 (0.33–0.80)
25–34	757	0.859 (0.021)	17.22	8.18	0.95 (0.80–1.10)	0.784 (0.027)	34.61	16.52	0.83 (0.69–0.98)
35–44	901	0.837 (0.018)	21.26	19.61	0.93 (0.81–1.05)	0.784 (0.027)	54.52 [a]	48.31 [a]	0.89 (0.76–1.01)
45–54	1254	0.834 (0.015)	28.71	24.30	0.94 (0.84–1.03)	0.777 (0.022)	54.07	44.55	0.84 (0.75–0 93
55–64	2044	0.803 (0.013)	73.86	65.72	0.88 (0.81–0.95)	0.805 (0.016)	118.97	103.13	0.80 (0.73–0.86)
65–74	2735	0.809 (0.010)	71.48	67.33	0.88 (0.83–0.93)	0.775 (0.014)	103.49	115.67	0.85 (0.80–0.90)
75–84	1555	0.784 (0.013)	52.52	48.40	0.91 (0.85–0.97)	0.776 (0.011)	124.42	120.14	0.89 (0.83–0 95)
≥85	32	0.716 (0.031)	27.08	16.92	1.02 (0.88–1.15)	0.735 (0.014)	23.71	22.80	0.97 (0.84–1.10)

Stratification by patient-related criteria included in the models. Excluded from the analyses 81 patients with missing data on type of patient.
Uns. Surgery, unscheduled surgery; Sch. Surgery, scheduled surgery; *N*, number of patients; ROC, area under receiver operating characteristics; H test, Hosmer-Lemeshow goodness-of-fit test H; C test, Hosmer-Lemeshow goodness-of-fit test C; O/E ratio, observed/expected mortality ratio; CI, confidence interval; SE, standard error.
[a] $p < 0.001$.

not enclose 1.0 in patients 55 – 84 years for SAPS-II and 45 – 84 years for MPM_0. It should be noted that in very young patients (18 – 24 years), both models largely overestimated mortality (O/E mortality 0.59 for SAPS-II and 0.56 for MPM_0).

Patient-Related Criteria Not Included in the Models

Stratification of patients according to these criteria was done according to their location in the hospital before admission to the ICU (operative theatre/recovery room, emergency room, ward, and other ICU/other hospital) and by diagnostic category (Tables 8, 9). Regarding the location of the patient before admission to the ICU, both models presented a better discriminative power for patients admitted from the operative theatre/recovery room and emergency room. Hosmer-Lemeshow tests H and C were significant in all groups, though lower in patients admitted from the operative theatre/recovery room. Analyses of the O/E mortality showed that both models overestimated mortality in patients admitted from the operative theatre/recovery room and from the emergency room and underestimated mortality in patients admitted from the ward.

Stratification by diagnostic category also showed very large variations in discrimination and calibration. Both models overestimated mortality in nonoperative, cardiovascular and metabolic patients and underestimated mortality in nonoperative gastrointestinal (SAPS-II) and in septic (MPM_0) conditions; in post-operative patients overestimation of mortality was marked in the case of SAPS-II but also present for MPM_0.

Conclusions

Evaluation of the goodness-of-fit of a general outcome prediction model is a crucial step in its application to a new population. A recent consensus conference (RAND/UCLA/Harvard Center for Health Care Financing Policy Research, 1993) stated that "Mortality prediction models are almost always over specific for the patient samples upon which they were developed, and thus performance usually deteriorates when models are applied to different population samples.... For this reason, we recommend that mortality prediction models always be tested in patient samples distinct from those in which the models were developed". Our results show that, when evaluated in this independent, multicenter and international database, the discriminative power of SAPS-II was similar to that indicated in the original publication (lower for MPM_0). However, both models calibrate poorly, with very relevant and statistically significant differences between predicted and observed mortality. Most striking were results of the analyses between subgroups, with very large differences in the performance of the models. It should be pointed out that discriminative power, as measured by the area under the ROC curve was always >0.70 for both models in all analyzed subgroups. This is very important, since a marked decrease of the discriminative ability of a logistic model can hardly be corrected [5]. With respect to calibration, better predictive accuracy was achieved in scheduled surgery patients admitted from the operative theatre/recovery room, younger patients, patients with nonoperative

Table 8. Uniformity of fit of SAPS-II and MPM_0

Location	*N*	SAPS-II				MPM_0			
		ROC (SE)	H test	C test	O/E (95% CI)	ROC (SE)	H test	C test	O/E (95% CI)
OT/RR	3647	0.841 (0.010)	60.27 [a]	54.87 [a]	0.82 (0.76–0.88)	0.797 (0.011)	123.42 [a]	103.08 [a]	0.79 (0.73–0.85)
ER	2912	0.838 (0.011)	154.14 [a]	130.16 a	0.76 (0.71–0.81)	0.828 (0.010)	212.69 [a]	190.03 [a]	0.68 (0.63–0.73)
Ward	1822	0.767 (0.012)	152.33 [a]	142.35 [a]	1.13 (1.08–1.19)	0.707 (0.013)	209.01 [a]	210.65 [a]	1.13 (1.07–1.19)
Other	1516	0.794 (0.013)	63.62 [a]	62.91 [a]	0.95 (0.88–1.02)	0.759 (0.014)	102.22 [a]	90.97 [a]	0.87 (0.80–0.94)

Stratification by location of the patient before admission to the ICU (excluded from the analyses 130 patients with missing data on location before admission to ICU).

OT, operative theatre, RR, recovery room; ER, emergency room; *N*, number of patients; ROC, area under receiver operating characteristics; H test, Hosmer-Lemeshow goodness-of-fit test H; C test, Hosmer-Lemeshow goodness-of-fit test C; O/E ratio, observed/expected mortality ratio; CI, confidence interval; SE, standard error.

[a] $p<0.001$.

Table 9. Uniformity of fit of SAPS-II and MPM_0

Category	*N*	SAPS-II				MPM_0			
		ROC (SE)	H test	C test	O/E (95% CI)	ROC (SE)	H test	C test	O/E (95% CI)
Nonoperative									
Cardiovasc.	1890	0.833 (0.012)	89.19 [a]	75.84 [a]	0 79 (0.73–0.86)	0.829 (0.013)	147.59 [a]	128.03 [a]	0.71 (0.65–0.77)
Respiratory	1408	0.756 (0.014)	101.14 [a]	89.76 [a]	1.01 (0.94–1.08)	0.692 (0.016)	152.18 [a]	169.47 [a]	1.04 (0.96–1.11)
GI	324	0.757 (0.029)	45.48 [a]	42.36 [a]	1.31 (1.16–1.47)	0.714 (0.031)	28.48	30.44 [a]	1.04 (0.90–1.18)
Neurological	618	0.827 (0.018)	18.18	22.47	1.09 (0.99–1.18)	0.806 (0.019)	29.63 [a]	15.15	0.96 (0.86–1.05)
Sepsis	236	0 776 (0.031)	24.74	55.54 [a]	1.08 (0.95–1.20)	0.705 (0.034)	30.72	35.05	1.14 (1.01–1.28)
Trauma	327	0.855 (0.026)	5.55	5.01	1.02 (0.85–1.19)	0.803 (0.031)	24.77	12.30	0.88 (0.72–1.03)
Metabolic	515	0.831 (0.040)	116.71 [a]	96.66 [a]	0 33 (0.18–0.48)	0.792 (0.036)	148.09 [a]	134.50 [a]	0.27 (0.14–0.41)
Others	332	0.832 (0.026)	11.31	19.63	0.89 (0.74–1.03)	0.762 (0.030)	27.95	21.33	0.88 (0.73–1.03)
Postoperative									
Cardiovasc.	723	0.839 (0.023)	19.13	12.01	0.80 (0.65–0.94)	0.814 (0.025)	37.41 [a]	12.74	0.86 (0.70–1.01)
Respiratony	475	0.778 (0.031)	40.45 [a]	30.63 [a]	0 77 (0.58–0.97)	0.758 (0.036)	18.00	21.76	0.79 (0 59–1.00)
GI	1542	0.814 (0.013)	19.77	18.91	1.01 (0.93–1.09)	0.766 (0.014)	65.74 [a]	68.15 [a]	1.02 (0.94–1.10)
Neurological	580	0.877 (0.021)	11.65	27.16	0.82 (0.68–0.96)	0.828 (0.026)	36.04 [a]	39.86 [a]	0.66 (0.53–0.79)
Trauma	402	0.802 (0.029)	19.55	21.21	0.79 (0.65–0.94)	0.741 (0.032)	31.19 [a]	42.89 [a]	0 75 (0.61–0.89)
Others	575	0.771 (0.051)	79.98 [a]	45.11 [a]	0 35 (0.15–0.56)	0.738 (0.056)	62.00 [a]	45.53 [a]	0.34 (0.13–0.54)

Stratification by diagnostic category. Excluded from the analyses 80 patients with missing data on diagnostic category.
Cardiov., cardiovascular/vascular, GI, gastrointestinal; *N*, number of patients; ROC, area under receiver operating characteristics; H test, Hosmer-Lemeshow goodness-of-fit test H; C test, Hosmer-Lemeshow goodness-of-fit test C; O/E ratio, obsened/expected mortality ratio; CI, confidence intenval; SE, standard error.

[a] $p<0.001$.

neurological, septic or trauma diagnoses (or postoperative gastrointestinal, neurologic or trauma diagnoses). All of these characteristics appear to be associated in some way with a "true" lower severity of illness, and both models overestimated mortality in more severely ill patients. Can this be explained only by differences between the original reference population and EURICUS-I patients ? Our study was performed using models which are now almost 5 years old, and it may be that the relationship between the degree of physiologic derangement (measured directly in the case of MPM_0 or indirectly by SAPS-II score) and mortality has changed; that is, that for the same degree of dysfunction mortality is today lower, especially in the most severely affected patients. This point is probably more important than variations in case mix, since baseline characteristics and overall mortality rate are similar, except for a slightly higher proportion of medical patients (55.9% vs 48.4% in original database). We do not have however information on two factors that can have an important influence on outcome: previous location before admission to the ICU and diagnosis, and this can impair comparison of the populations. Assignment of all the differences between observed and predicted mortality to variations in the quality of care between the ICUs in EURICUS-I and those in ENAS/MPM_0, as suggested previously in the literature [6], seems abusive in this situation. Our database comprises 16060 patients (analyzed 10027 patients), collected in 12 European countries, with a sampling strategy for maximizing variance in clinical and nonclinical factors. The database can be viewed as reflecting a reference level of care in ICUs similar to that measured in databases used for development of the employed models.

At present we want to stress the following: (1) the importance of global performance evaluation of the general outcome prediction models before their use in independent populations, and (2) the need for better quantification of patient baseline characteristics and formal evaluation of application of the models to specific subgroups. Moreover, correct choosing of the adequate statistical method to compare intensive care populations appears to need more research.

Analysis of ICU Performance

Václav Fidler

ICU Performance

The primary objective of EURICUS-I was to examine the relationship between ICU performance and the substudy variables. One of the natural indicators of ICU performance is hospital mortality. For valid comparisons of ICUs with respect to this indicator an adjustment for differences in relevant case mix factors is needed. The adjustment can be accomplished with help of a suitable severity of illness scoring system. The EURICUS-I was designed to use the SAPS-II [1] and the MPM_0 [2] scoring systems.

The traditional use of severity of illness scoring systems for comparison of ICUs consists of predicting the number of deaths in each unit and calculation of standard mortality ratios (SMRs). In accordance with this, the original EURICUS-I protocol stipulated the use of the SMR as the dependent variable. The traditional SMR-based approach has, however, theoretical drawbacks which can be avoided by using a different method of analysis. Results presented here were obtained by this "new" method [8]. In the next three sections ("Direct and Indirect Standardization", "Logistic Regression and Standardization", "Methods of Hypothesis Testing"), the basics of this approach are explained. This is followed by "Results and "Conclusions".

Direct and Indirect Standardization

The problem of adjusting for differences in case mix (as defined by a severity of illness score) is in essence that of combining stratum-specific mortality rates with strata defined by the score. Classical epidemiology offers two methods, direct and indirect standardization. The indirect method uses stratum-specific mortality rates of a standard population (e.g. all ICUs in a study) for calculation of the expected mortality in each population (ICU). The total expected mortality is then compared to the observed one by computing the SMR, defined as the ratio of observed and expected mortalities. This SMR has a clear-cut interpretation as far as the comparison of a single ICU to the standard is concerned. In general, however, it is not possible to compare SMRs calculated for different ICUs: the difference in SMRs can be entirely due to differences in case mix (as defined by the scoring system) of different populations. The direct method uses stratum-specific mortality rates of each ICU for calculation of the expected mortality in each stratum of a standard population. Summing up these numbers yields – for each ICU – the directly adjusted mortality rate. This mortality rate would apply if the ICU in question would have the case mix composition of the standard population. Here it is perfectly valid to compare directly adjusted mortality rates of ICUs; the result may in general depend on the standard population used. In conclusion, the directly standardized mortality rates are suited for comparison of mortality in different ICUs, this in contrast to the SMRs (see also [7]).

Logistic Regression and Standardization

The relationship between the probability of death and a given scoring system is conveniently described by means of the logistic regression model. Let $P_{ij} = P(x_{ij})$ denote the death probability of the j-th patient ($j = 1, \ldots, J_i$) in the I-th ICU ($I = 1, \ldots, I$), where I is the number of ICUs, J_i is the number of patients of the I-th ICU, and let x_{ij} be the severity of illness score (e.g. the SAPS-II-score) of the patient. Logistic regression model assumes that $\text{logit}(P_{ij}) = \ln(P_{ij}/(1 - P_{ij}))$ is given by:

$$\text{logit}(P_{ij}) = \beta_{0i} + \beta_{1i}\, x_{ij} \qquad (1)$$

where $\beta_{01},\ldots,\beta_{0I}$ and $\beta_{11},\ldots,\beta_{1I}$ are model parameters. Under this model the dependence between the logit-mortality and the score in the I-th ICU is described by a line with β_{0i} as the intercept and β_{1i} as the slope. Note that the lines for different ICUs need not be parallel. It is possible that two lines cross: this means that their relative performance depends on the severity of illness score of a patient. The model can be used for calculation of directly standardized mortality rates. We just sum the I-th ICU probabilities calculated for all the x's, i.e. patients, in the standard population. Examples of standard populations are the total group of ICUs, an ICU with some chosen composition of patients (as defined by the score, or simply by a single value of the score). In the case of different slopes a reasonable option is to calculate the logit of mortality for low, median and high risk patients, defined as the 20th, 50th and 80th percentile of the distribution of the severity score, respectively, and use these variables – in the sequel denoted as B20, B50 and B80 – as the outcome variables.

As already indicated above, the ordering of the ICUs will depend on the population chosen as the standard one. The situation is simplified if the lines for all ICUs are parallel, that is if $\beta_{11}=\ldots=\beta_{1I}$. In that case we may confine our attention to the intercepts β_{0i}s as the outcome variable. The relationship of the above sketched approach to the traditional SMR approach is as follows. The SMR-based approach uses the model $\text{logit}(P_{ij})=\beta_0+\beta_1 x_{ij}$ with common intercept and slope for all ICUs. The probabilities P_{ij}s are viewed as mortality rates in a standard population and are used to calculate the expected number of deaths in each ICU and the corresponding SMR. Apart from the drawback of the indirect method of standardization, this common intercept approach has yet another drawback. Omitting ICU effects from the model (that is, setting all β_{0i} equal to β_0) may introduce a bias in β_1. (It is a well-known fact that omitting an important variable from logistic regression model induces confounding.) More generally, when constructing a severity of illness scoring system by means of logistic regression, simple pooling of ICUs may have a negative impact on the validity of the system. Note that all three mainstream scoring systems, APACHE, SAPS and MPM, were derived from pooled data without taking the possible differences between ICUs into account.

Method of Hypothesis Testing

Once we have the outcome variables, that is the variables B20, B50 and B80, or the intercept in case of parallel lines, we can carry out ordinary multiple regression to examine the effect of substudy variables and to test the EURICUS-I hypotheses. We refer to this analysis as the fixed-effects approach. While being quite straightforward, this approach has a minor drawback. It treats the response variable for different ICUs as independent. The responses are instead – due to the fact that they are based on the same data set – correlated. A more sophisticated approach is to directly model the effect of the ICU-specific explanatory variables on the mortality. This can be done as follows.

Firstly, we start with a model $\beta_0+\beta_1 x_{ij}+\gamma' w_i$, where $\gamma'=(\gamma_1,\ldots\gamma_K)$ are K parameters associated with ICU explanatory variables $w_i'=(w_{i1},\ldots w_{iK})$. This model includes K+2 parameters, typically much less than the 2·I parameters required for separate intercepts and slopes. As it is impossible to collect all relevant ICU information, this model cannot be expected to explain all the variability in mortality between ICUs. We expect less variability within units than between units, or, in another words, we expect positive correlation between outcomes of patients treated in the same ICU. A possible way to build in the within-unit dependence into our model is to add random effect terms, $\delta_1 U_{1i}$ and $\delta_2 U_{2i}$:

$$\text{logit}(P_{ij})=(\beta_0+\delta_1 U_{1i})+(\beta_1+\delta_2 U_2)xij+\gamma' w_i \quad (2)$$

where δ_1 and δ_2 are (scalar) parameters and U_{1i} and U_{2i} are random effect variables specific for the I-th unit. The pairs (U_{1i}, U_{2i}) are independent standard normal random variables. Inclusion of the random intercept effect term $\delta_1 U_{1i}$ simultaneously either increases ($\delta_1 U_{1i}>0$) or decreases ($\delta_1 U_{1i}<0$) the survival probability of all the patients treated in the I-th ICU. The random slope term $\delta_2 U_{2i}$ similarly increases ($\delta_2 U_{2i}>0$) or decreases ($\delta_2 U_{2i}<0$) the influence of the severity score on the survival probability in the I-th ICU. Models of the above type with random and fixed effects terms are known as random or mixed effects models, or as multilevel models with patients at level 1 and nested within level 2 units, the ICU's.

In summary, to study the relationship between ICU performance and the substudy variables, two related approaches are used:

1. The fixed effects approach consists of calculation of an (SAPS-II-corrected) index of ICU performance; the relationship of this index to the substudy variables is studied by means of multiple regression analysis.
2. The random effects approach examines the relationship between patient outcome (alive/dead) and the substudy variables and is studied by means of logistic regression analysis with random ICU effects.

Results

The analysis started with 9674 patients from 79 ICUs. The case mix of the total group is described by the following percentiles of the SAPS-II distribution: $P_{10}=13$, $P_{20}=18$, $P_{50}=30$, $P_{80}=46$, $P_{90}=57$. The logistic model with SAPS-II as the only explanatory variable did not fit well (one could argue that if it fitted well, there would be hardly any reason to try to explain differences between ICUs by substudy variables):

$$\text{logit}(\text{mortality})=-2.046(\pm 0.037)+0.0736(\pm 0.0019)\cdot(\text{SAPS-II-30}) \quad (3)$$

The deviance of this model was 7292.31 (df=9672), the goodness-of-fit tests indicated poor model fit (the deciles of risks test: $P=0.014$; the deciles of predicted death probability test: $P=0.002$). The model with separate intercepts for each ICU and with a common slope improved the fit and fitted reasonably well:

$$\text{logit (mortality)} = \beta_{ICU} + 0.0756\,(\pm 0.0020) \cdot (\text{SAPS-II-30}) \tag{4}$$

The deviance was 7001.24 (df=9594), the goodness-of-fit tests resulted in $P=0.08$ (the deciles of risks test) and $P=0.13$ (the deciles of predicted death probability test). Comparison of the deviances of the two models (the likelihood ratio, LR, test of the H_0: "β_{ICU}s are equal", LR=7292.31 − 7001.24=291.07, df=78, $P<0.001$) shows that allowing for separate intercepts improves the model. The assumption that differences between ICUs are constant on the logistic scale of probabilities of death irrespective of the SAPS-II score can be tested by fitting the model which allows the SAPS-II slopes to be different:

$$\text{logit (mortality)} = \beta_{1,ICU} + \beta_{2,ICU} \cdot (\text{SAPS-II-30}) \tag{5}$$

The deviance of this model was 6850.89 (df=9516); the model fit was good ($P=0.45$ by the deciles of risks test and $P=0.81$ by the deciles of predicted death probability test). The LR test of the H_0: "β_{2ICU}s are equal", LR=7001.24 − 6850.89=150.35, df=78, $P<0.001$ rejected the hypothesis of common SAPS-II slopes. The rejection of the hypothesis of parallel lines necessitates separate analyses of ICU performance indicators B20, B50 and B80. Figure 9 shows that these indicators lead to a different ranking of ICUs than the traditionally computed SMRs, in particular for low risk patients (B20). Normal probability plots of B20, B50 and B80 suggested that the distribution of these SAPS-II-corrected indices is well approximated by a Gaussian distribution. There were, however, two ICUs with rather very good performances (i.e. low values). In the course of further analysis it became clear that these ICUs had to be considered as outliers. They were excluded then from further analysis, which is thus based on data from 77 ICUs (with 9576 patients).

In the next step the variability of the indices (dependent variables) B20, B50 and B80 was to be explained by independent variables from the substudies (see Table 10). Apart from these variables, also the variable COUNTRY was included in the analysis as a possible confounding factor. The analysis started with univariate regression analyses, accompanied by inspection of scatter plots of

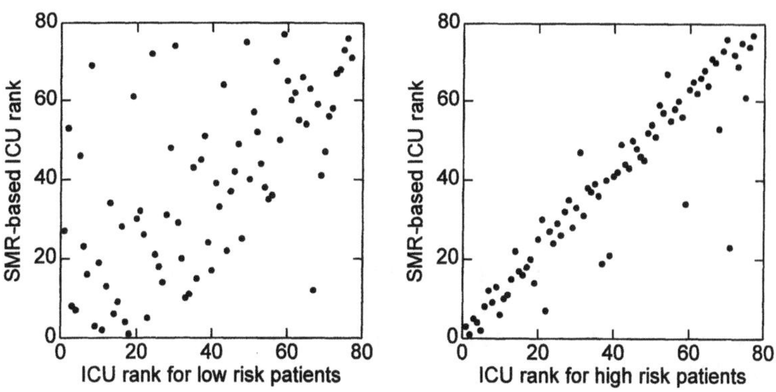

Fig. 9. Ranking of ICUs according to different indices of performance

Table 10. Summary of variables used

Substudy *Facilities*	
NoBEDS	The number of beds in the ICU
Wealth	An index of wealth of the ICU
Substudy *Personnel*	
Emothex	Emotional exhaustion
OrgCom	Organizational commitment
Substudy *Finances*	
Budget	Budget flexibility
Perceive	Perceived appropriateness of budget
Substudy *Organization*	
Central	Centralitation
EOF	Elementary organisational framework
Substudy *Culture*	
P1	Process oriented vs results-oriented
P4	Open system vs closed system

observations and residuals. On the basis of such plots it was decided to use LN = log(NOBEDS) instead of NOBEDS and to consider the quadratic regression on LN.

Table 11 summarizes the univariate analyses with and without adjustment for COUNTRY. For the model with COUNTRY the percentage of explained variability was 26%, for the other variables it was well below 10%. While this may seem a large difference, we must keep in mind that including the categorical variable COUNTRY in the model amounts to estimation of an additional 12 parameters. In the next step we examined the possibility of improving the model fit by inclu-

Table 11. Results of fitting of different regression models

Variable	df	Univariate (*p* value)			With adjustment for COUNTRY (*p* value)		
		B20	B50	B80	B20	B50	B80
LN, LN*LN	2	0.05*	0.92	0.16	0.05*	0.03*	0.22
ORGCOM	1	0.05*	0.02*	0.07	0.01*	0.00*	0.01*
CENTRAL	1	0.31	0.27	0.48	0.50	0.36	0.33
BUDGET	1	0.67	0.70	0.94	0.68	0.82	0.77
EOF	1	0.61	0.78	0.67	0.03*	0.03*	0.38
EMOEXTH	1	0.17	0.14	0.35	0.27	0.22	0.39
WEALTH	1	0.16	0.21	0.82	0.31	0.14	0.09
P1	1	0.22	0.29	0.91	0.00*	0.00*	0.04*
P4	1	0.77	0.99	0.54	0.53	0.27	0.13
PERCEIVE	1	0.22	0.13	0.17	0.42	0.17	0.07
COUNTRY	12	0.06	0.09	0.38	–	–	–

* *p* value for COUNTRY < 0.05

ding more variables in the model, starting with the significant ones from Table 11.

For B20 the best fitting model (37% explained variability) included COUNTRY (df = 12, P = 0.019), ORGCOM ($P=0.036$, $b=-0.194$, "higher ORGCOM, lower mortality") and NOBEDS ($-2.82*LN+0.657*LN^2$, "minimum mortality for NOBEDS = 9, higher mortality for smaller or larger ICUs"). The model with COUNTRY (df = 12, $P=0.013$) and EOF ($b=-0.155, P=0.025$) explained 32% of the variability. For B50 the best fitting model with COUNTRY (df = 12, $P=0.016$), ORGCOM ($P=0.08$, $b=-0.168$, "higher ORGCOM, lower mortality") and NOBEDS ($-2.11 \cdot LN + 0.488 \cdot LN^2$, "minimum mortality for NOBEDS = 9, higher mortality for smaller or larger ICUs") explained 40% of the variability. The model with COUNTRY (df = 12, $P=0.001$) and P1 ($b=-0.018, P=0.001$, "higher P1, lower mortality") explained 39% of the variability; the model with COUNTRY (df = 12, $P=0.02$) and elementary organizational framework (EOF) ($b=-0.105$, $P=0.03$, "higher EOF, lower mortality") explained 30% of the variability. For B80 no combination of variables improved significantly on models listed in Table 11. Two well fitting models thus include COUNTRY and either ORGCOM ($P=0.001$, $b=-0.15$, "higher ORGCOM, lower mortality", $R^2=25\%$) or P1 ($P=0.04$, $b=-0.0095$: "higher P1, lower mortality", $R^2=22\%$). We note that ORGCOM and LN are negatively correlated ($R=-0.31, P<0.01$) and that ORGCOM and P1 are positively correlated ($P<0.01$, $R=0.38$). Next the random effects logistic regression analysis was carried out. We used the program EGRET for fitting the "logistic-binomial models with distinguishable data", i.e. logistic models with a random intercept, and the program MIXOR for fitting models with both the random intercept and slope. The analysis is based on data from the 77 ICUs (9576 patients): as in the multiple regression analysis, two units were excluded. Table 12 gives basic information about the fit of several models. The deviances were calculated with respect to the model with separate slopes and intercepts.

The best fitting model with random intercept included variables SAPS-II ($b=0.0752$, SE = 0.0020, $P<0.001$), NOBEDS ($-1.75 \cdot LN + 0.396 \cdot LN^2$: optimal NOBEDS about 9), ORGCOM ($b=-0.129$, SE = 0.045, $P=0.004$), COUNTRY (df = 12, $P=0.075$) and a random intercept ($\delta_1=0.38$, SE = 0.045). The model

Table 12. Fit of logistic regression models (77 ICUs, 9576 patients)

I	Model	Deviance	df
1	β_0+SAPS	413.34	2
2	$\beta_0+SAPS+ICU$	148.01	78
3	$\beta_0+SAPS+ICU+SAPS*ICU$	0	154
4	$\beta_0+\delta_1+SAPS\,II$	313.64	3
5	$\beta_0+\delta_1+SAPS\,II+COUNTRY$	301.85	15
6	$\beta_0+\delta_1+SAPS\,II+EOF+COUNTRY$	298.45	16
7	$\beta_0+\delta_1+SAPS\,II+ORGCOM+LN+LN*LN+COUNTRY$	287.74	18
8	$\beta_0+\delta_1+SAPS\,II+P1+COUNTRY$	292.27	16
9	$\beta_0+\delta_1+\delta_2+SAPS\,II+LN+LN*LN$	297.92	7

with SAPS-II ($b=0.0750$, SE$=0.0020$, $P<0.001$), COUNTRY (df$=12$, $P=0.048$), P1 (b$=-0.012$, SE$=0.0037$, P<0.001) and a random intercept ($\delta_1=0.33$, SE$=0.046$) fitted slightly less well. The same can be said about the model with SAPS-II, COUNTRY and EOF ($b=0.066$, SE$=0.0035$, $P=0.06$). The best model including both random intercept and random slope was:

$$\begin{aligned}\text{logit}\,(\text{mortality}) = {} & 0.756\,(\pm 1.21) + 0.078\,(\pm 0.00295)\cdot(\text{SAPS-II}-30) - \\ & -1.213\,(\pm 1.029)\cdot \text{LN} + 0.255\,(\pm 0.213)\cdot \text{LN}^2 + \\ & +0.474\cdot U_I + 0.131\cdot U_2\cdot(\text{SAPS-II}-30)\end{aligned} \tag{6}$$

with $\text{corr}\,(U_1, U_2) = -0.58$. Inspection of the terms involving LN shows that the predicted mortality is minimal for an ICU size about ten beds. The odds ratio associated with halving this ICU size is 1.35 (95% CI: 0.86 – 1.57), the odds ratio associated with doubling it is 1.23 (95% CI: 0.89 – 1.36). Inclusion of other substudy variables to this model did not significantly increase the fit; an attempt to include COUNTRY was not successful because of numerical problems. Inclusion of random slopes significantly improved the fit. This is in accordance with the finding of nonparallel slopes under the fixed effects approach. The relatively large difference between the deviance of the model with separate slopes and intercepts and random effects models indicates that the independent variables explain only a part of the variability between ICUs. The situation is similar to that of the multiple regression approach, in which also only a relatively small part of variability among ICUs could be explained.

Conclusions

The fixed effects (multiple regression) approach and the random effects logistic regression approach lead to similar conclusions: that ICU performance (corrected for differences in SAPS-II) is significantly ($P<0.05$) related to:
- Number of beds (optimal number is about 9; smaller or larger ICUs tend to have higher mortality)
- Organizational commitment (higher commitment, lower mortality)
- Results oriented culture (higher P1, lower mortality)
- Elementary organizational framework (higher EOF, lower mortality)
- Country

An effect of the other substudy variables on the ICU performance could not be demonstrated. The analysis has also showed that relative ranking of ICUs with respect to their performance depends on the severity of the illness of a patient. In another words, ICUs that perform well on high risk patients need not do so on low risk patients, and vice versa.

References

1. Le Gall JR, Lemeshow S, Saulnier F (1993) A new Simplified Acute Physiology Score (SAPS-II) based on a European/North American multicenter study. JAMA 270:2957–2963
2. Lemeshow S, Teres D, Klar J (1993) Mortality probability models (MPM II) based on an international cohort of intensive care unit patients. JAMA 270:2478–2486
3. Hanley, McNeil (1983) A method of comparing the areas under receiver operating characteristic curves derived from the same cases. Radiology 148: 839–843
4. Lemeshow S, Klar J, Teres D (1995) Outcome predictors for individual intensive care patients: useful, misused or abused? Intensive Care Med 21:770–776
5. Miller ME, Hui SL, Tierney WM (1991) Validation techniques for logistic regression models. Stat Med 10: 1213–1226
6. Zhu BP, Lemeshow S, Hosmer DW, Klar J, Avrunin J, Teres D (1996) Factors affecting the performance of the models in the Mortality Probability Model II system and strategies of customization: a simulation study. Crit Care Med 24: 55–63
7. Rothman K (1986) Modern epidemiology. Boston, Little, Brown
8. Fidler V, Moreno R, Miranda DR (1996) Evaluation of performance of intensive care units: statistical methodology (submitted)

Part III

Part III

Participants in EURICUS-I

Steering Group

- Prof. A. Williams (Chairman)
  Centre for Health Economics, University of York, Heslington, York YO1 5DD, United Kingdom
- Dr. G. Apolone
  Instituto Mario Negri, Via Eritreia 62, 20157 Milano, Italy
- Prof. Dr. F. Lemaire
  Hôpital Henri Mondor, Service de Réanimation Médicale, 51, avenue du Maréchal de Lattre, de Tassigny, F-94010 Créteil, France
- Dr. D. Reis Miranda
  Health Services Research Unit, University Hospital Groningen, Dept. of Surgery, P.O. Box 30.001, 9700 RB Groningen, The Netherlands
- Dr. K. Rowan
  Intensive Care National Audit and Research Centre (ICNARC), Tavistock House, Tavistock Square, London WC1H 9HX, United Kingdom

Chairman EURICUS meetings

- Dr. G.J. Nooij
  OD Partner International Management Consultancy & Training, Zuiderpark 13, 9724 AG Groningen, The Netherlands

Coordination and Administrative Centre

ICU Research Group, University Hospital Groningen, Dept. of Surgery, P.O. Box 30.001, 9700 RB Groningen, The Netherlands

- Dr. D. Reis Miranda, project-leader
- Mrs. W. van Dort, project-manager
- Mr. A. van Dort, data-manager
- Dr. J. van der Veen, researcher
- Mrs. R. van der Veer, assistant

Methodology Group

- Dr. G. Apolone (Chairman)
  Instituto Mario Negri, Via Eritreia 62, 20157 Milano, Italy
- Dr. V. Fidler
  Faculty of Medicine, Section Epidemiology and Statistics,
  University of Groningen, A. Deusinglaan 1, 9713 AV Groningen, Netherlands
- Dr. R.Moreno
  Hospital St. António dos Capuchos, Intensive Care Unit, Alameda St. António Capuchos, 1150 Lisboa, Portugal
- Dr. K. Rowan
  Intensive Care National Audit and Research Centre, Tavistock House, Tavistock Square, London WC1H 9HX, United Kingdom
- Dr. V. Torri
  Instituto Mario Negri, Via Eritreia 62, 20157 Milano, Italy

Publication Advisory Board

- Prof. Dr. F. Lemaire (Chairman)
  Hôpital Henri Mondor, Service de Réanimation Médicale, 51, avenue du Maréchal de Lattre, de Tassigny, 94010 Créteil, France
- Dr. J. P. Alexander
  Middelheim General Hospital, Lindendreef 1, 2020 Antwerpen, Belgium
- Dr. D. W. Ryan
  ITU, Freeman Hospital, High Heaton, Newcastle Upon Tyne NE7 7DN, United Kingdom
- Prof. Dr. W. B. Schaufeli
  Dept. of Social and Organizational Psychology, University Utrecht, P.O. Box 80140, 3508 TC Utrecht, Netherlands

Advisors

- Miss B. L. Atkinson
  Clinical Services Manager, Intensive Care Services, Southampton General Hospital, Tremona Road, Southampton SO9 4XY, United Kingdom
- Dr. L. Dragsted
  Bispebjerg Hospital, Dept. of Intensive Care, Bispebjerg Bakke, 2400 Copenhagen NV, Denmark
- Dr. D. Edbrooke
  Consultant Anaesthetist, Intensive Care Unit, Royal Hallamshire Hospital, Sheffield, United Kingdom
- Dr. A. Granados i Navarrete
  Cap de l'Agencia d'Avaluació de Tecnologia Médica, Direcció General de Recursos Sanitaris, Travessera de les Corts, 131–159, Pavelló Ave Maria, 08028 Barcelona, Spain

- Dr. J. Pons
  l'Agencia d'Avaluació de Tecnologia Médica, Direcció General de Recursos Sanitaris, Travessera de les Corts, 131–159, Pavelló Ave Maria, 08028 Barcelona, Spain

EURICUS Substudies

Substudy Patients and Facilities

ICU Research Group, University Hospital Groningen, Dept. of Surgery, P.O. Box 30.001, 9700 RB Groningen, The Netherlands
- Dr. D. Reis Miranda
- Mrs. W. van Dort
- Mr. A. van Dort
- Dr. R. Moreno
- Dr. V. Fidler
- Dr. J. van der Veen
- Dr. K. Rowan
- Dr. G. Apolone

Substudy Finances

Centre for Financial Analysis and Policy, Free University Brussels, Pleinlaan 2, 1050 Brussels, Belgium
- Prof. Dr. M. Jegers

Substudy Organization

Dept. of Organization, Technology and Innovation, University Groningen, P.O. Box 800, 9700 AV Groningen, Netherlands (during the academic year 1996–1997 Graduate School of Business, Stanford University, Stanford, CA, USA)
- Prof. Dr. W. van Rossum

Substudy Culture

Dept. of Organization, Technology and Innovation, University Groningen, P.O. Box 800, 9700 AV Groningen, Netherlands
- Prof. Dr. G. Sanders,
- Dr. J. van der Veen

Substudy Personnel

Dept. of Social and Organizational Psychology, University Utrecht,
P.O. Box 80140, 3508 TC Utrecht, Netherlands
- Prof. Dr. W. B. Schaufeli
- Dr. P. Le Blanc

Country Coordinators

Poland

- Dr. C. Noworol, Jagiellonian University, Institute of Psychology, Department of Work Psychology and Ergonomics, 31-110 Kraków, Piłsudskiego 13
- Dr. J. Pokorski, Jagiellonian University, Collegium Medicum, Institute of Occupational Health, Department of Ergonomics, 30-969 Kraków, P.O.B. 13

Germany

- Prof. Dr. W. Kuckelt, Abt. für Anästhesiologie und Intensivtherapie, Zentralkrankenhaus „Links der Weser“, Senator-Wessling-Str. 1, 28277 Bremen, FRG

Denmark

- Dr. J. Strøm, Glostrup Hospital, 2600 Glostrup

Finland

- Dr. M. Niskanen, Department of Intensive Care, Kuopio University Hospital, SF 70210 Kuopio

Netherlands

- Dr. P. F. Hulstaert, Department of Surgery, University Hospital Utrecht, Heidelberglaan 100, 3584 CX Utrecht

Belgium

- Dr. J. P. Alexander, Middelheim General Hospital, Lindendreef 1, 2020 Antwerpen

France

- Dr. B. Guidet, Service de Réanimation Médicale, Hopital Saint-Antoine, 184 Rue du Fabourg Saint-Antoine, 75012 Paris

Luxembourg

- Dr. M. Hemmer, Director Surgical Intensive Care Unit, Centre Hospitalier, Rue Barblé 4, 1210 Luxembourg

United Kingdom

- Dr. D. W. Ryan, General ITU, Freeman Hospital, High Heaton, Newcastle Upon Tyne NE7 7DN

Italy

- Dr. G. Iapichino , Intensive Care Unit, Hospital San Paolo, Via A. di Rudini 8, 20142 Milano

Spain

- Dr. R. Abizanda, Director ICU and Dr. M. T. Rodriguez, Medicina Intensiva , Hospital General Castello, Avda. Benicassim s/n, 12004 Castello
- Dr. A. Artigas, Medicina Intensiva , Sabadell Hospital, Parc Tauli s/n, 08208 Sabadell

Portugal

- Dr. M.J. Moreira Brandão, Serviço de Cuidados Intensivos, Hospital Geral de Santo António, Largo da Escola Médica, 4000 Porto

ICUs Participating in the Study

Poland

- Intensive Care Unit, Surgical Department of Industrial Health Center, Nowa Hutu, Ujustek 3, 30–969 Kraków: Dr. M. Kostarczyk
- Intensive Care Unit, Biernacki City Hospital, Trynitarska 11, 31–061 Kraków: Dr. E. Bisaga

- Intensive Care Unit, City Hospital, Chopina 2, 35–057 Rzeszów: Dr. T. Nowosad
- Intensive Care Unit, County Hospital, Sucha Beskidzka: Dr. J. Jawor, Dr. M. Kornas
- Intensive Care Unit, Cardiology Department, Dietl City Hospital, Skarbowa 4, 31–121 Kraków: Dr. M. Kula
- Intensive Care Unit, City Hospital, Mickiewicza 25, 39–400 Tarnobrzeg: Dr. M. Sulik, Dr. K. Stolarski
- Intensive Care Unit, Cardiology Department, Rydygier City Hospital, Os. Złoa Jesie 1, 31–826 Kraków: Dr. T. /Z/elazny, Dr. T. Trybus
- Intensive Care Unit, Clinic of Toxicology, Jagiellonian University, Os. Złoa Jesle 1, 31–826 Kraków: Prof. J. Pach, Dr. L. Winnik
- Intensive Care Unit, Surgical Clinic, Jagiellonian University Hospital, Kopernika 29, 31–501 Kraków: Dr. M. Zajac P. Muller
- Intensive Care Unit, Clinic of Internal Medicine and Occupational Diseases, Institute of Occupational Health, Jagiellonian University, Ujastek 3, 30–969 Kraków: Dr. J. Pokorski, Ms. M. Dziura

Germany

- Interdisciplinary Intensive Care Unit I, Dept. of Anesthesiology, University Hospital Charité, Berlin: Dr. H. Wauer, Mrs. A. Küchenmeister
- Zentralkrankenhaus Links der Weser, Klinik für allgemeine und operative Intensivmedizin, Bremen: Prof. Dr. W. Kuckelt, Dr. C. Manhold, Dr. A. Bagdahn, Mrs. M. Pahl
- Klinik für Anästhesiologie und Intensivtherapie, Abteilung für operativ-traumatologische Intensiv-Therapie, Klinikum Schwerin, Schwerin: Dr. I. Kleit, Dr. P. Schönberger, B. Kunft

Denmark

- Intensive Care Unit, Glostrup University Hospital, Glostrup: Dr. J. Strøm, Dr. V. Bach, Mr. O. Marker, Mrs. L. Dalum, Mrs. H. Jensby
- Intensive Care Unit, Bispebjerg University Hospital, Copenhagen: Dr. A. Engqvist, Dr. L. Dragsted, Mrs. A. Bertelsen
- Intensive Care Unit, Hillerød Central Hospital: Dr. H. Blom, D. Bruun Jacobsen
- Intensive Care Unit, Frederiksberg Hospital, Frederiksberg: Dr. T. Pedersen, Dr. J. Wolf, Mrs. I. Burmeister
- Intensive Care Unit, Herlev University Hospital, Herlev: Dr. J. Bonde, Mr. P. Fosskjær
- Intensive Care Unit, Frederikssund Hospital, Frederikssund: Dr. H. Degn, Mrs. H. Magnussen

Finland

- Department of Intensive Care, Kuopio University Hospital: Dr. M. Niskanen, Mrs. P. Väisänen
- Department of Intensive Care, Jyväskylä Central Hospital: Dr. K. Hersio, Dr. R. Laru-Sompa
- Central Hospital of North Carelia: Dr. S. Karlsson, Mrs. E. Paananen
- Department of Intensive Care, Mikkeli Central Hospital Dr. M. Suistomaa, Dr. E. Loponen, H. Rintavaara
- Department of Intensive Care, Savonlinna Central Hospital: Dr. M. Suvela

Netherlands

- Surgical Intensive Care Unit, University Hospital Utrecht: Dr. P. F. Hulstaert, Mrs. F. E. van Dijk, Mr. W. H. van Haren, Mr. J. M. van den Burg
- Medical Intensive Care Unit, St. Elisabeth Hospital Amersfoort: Dr. A. K. M. Bartelink
- Intensive Care Unit, Scheperziekenhuis Emmen: Mr. A.J. Kühne
- Medical Intensive Care Unit, Diakonessenhuis, Utrecht: H. D. Eggink, P. L. Houweling, P. G. M. van der Souw
- Medical Intensive Care Unit, Beatrix Hospital, Gorinchem: Dr. M. van Berkel
- Intensive Care Unit, Onze Lieve Vrouwe Gasthuis, Amsterdam: Dr. D. F. Zandstra, Dr. H.M. Oudemans-van Straaten, R. Bosman, M. Brieko
- Medical Intensive Care Unit, Hospital Leijenburg, Den Haag: Dr. J. de Haas

Belgium

- Intensieve Zorgen, Universitair Ziekenhuis Antwerpen, Edegem: Prof. L. Bossaert, Mr. Y. Somers
- Intensieve Therapie Eenheid, Algemeen Ziekenhuis Middelheim, Antwerpen: Dr. J. P. Alexander, Mrs. L. Deckers
- Medische Intensieve Zorgen, Algemeen Ziekenhuis Middelheim, Antwerpen: Dr. J. Nagler, Mr. D. Pauwels, Dr. P. Rogiers
- Intensieve Zorgen, Algemeen Ziekenhuis Den Brandt, Boom: Dr. J. Steppé, Mrs. R. Moems
- Intensieve Zorgen, Klina Campus St Lucas, Ekeren: Dr. W. Fassin, Mrs. S. Van Belle
- Intensieve Zorgen, St. Vincentius Ziekenhuis, Antwerpen: Dr. R. Rutsaerts, H. Akkermans

France

- Service de Réanimation Médicale, Hôpital Saint Antoine, 184 rue du Faubourg Saint Antoine, 75012 Paris: Dr. B. Guidet, Mrs. S. Jacob, Mrs. A.C. Paty
- Service de Réanimation Médico-Chirurgical, Hôpital Saint-Camille, 2, rue des Peres-Camilliens, 94366 Bry sur Marne: Dr. D. Tardy, Mrs. P. Hermet, Dr. J. F. Loriferme
- Medical Intensive Care Unit, Hôpital Henri Mondor, Creteil: Prof. F. Lemaire, Dr. S. Elatrouss, A. Zeggwagh
- Réanimation chirurgicale, Hôpital Henri Mondor, Créteil: Dr. L. Beydon, Prof. Dr. F. Bonnet
- Service de Reanimation Polyvalente, HXXXpital des Diaconesses, Paris: Dr. Y. Ravaud, Dr. J. J. Jupas, Dr. F. Thomas, Dr. E. Wepierre, Dr. Armand, Dr. M. Nahon

Luxembourg

- Surgical Intensive Care Unit, Centre Hospitalier, Luxembourg: Dr. M. Hemmer

United Kingdom

- General ITU, Freeman Hospital, Newcastle upon Tyne: Mrs. R. Reach, Mrs. S.Smith, Dr. D. W. Ryan, Dr. O. Weldon, Mrs. S.Thompson
- Intensive Care Unit, South Tyneside District Hospital, Harton Lane, South Shields, Tyne and Wear NE34 OPL: Mr. P. Howe, Mrs. S. Ferguson, Dr. J. I. A. Andrews, Mrs. S. Proctor
- Intensive Therapy Unit, Wansbeck General Hospital, Ashington, Northumberland: Dr. A.G. Conn, E. Henderson
- Intensive Care Unit, Royal Hallamshire Hospital, Sheffield: Dr. D. L. Edbrooke, Mrs. S. Smith
- Intensive Care Unit, Rotherham General Hospital: Dr. D. M. Newby, Mr. D. Bainbridge, Mrs. C. White
- General Intensive Therapy Unit, Northern General Hospital NHS Trust, Sheffield: Mrs. S. M. Langan, Mrs. J. Bond, Dr. N. Appleyard
- Intensive Therapy Unit, Chesterfield Royal Hospital NHS Trust: Dr. C. Cooper, Dr. P. Rayner, Ms. L. Hutchinson, Mrs. S. Ashley, Ms. B. Clarke
- Intensive Care Unit, Doncaster Royal Infirmary, Doncaster, Dr. T. Kirkpatrick, Dr. D. Northwood, Mrs. M. Cobby

Italy

- IRCCS Ospedale Maggiore, Via Sforza 33, 20100-Milan: Dr. M. Langer, Dr. A. Sicignano, Dr. S. Rotelli, Mrs. D. Masala, Mrs. I. Adamini, Mrs. G. Trudo
- Ospedale S. Gerardo, Via Donizetti 106, 20052 Monza: Dr. R. Fumagalli, Dr. B. Marcora, Dr. L. Avalli, Dr. A. Pesenti, Mrs. E. Brina
- Ospedale di Desio, Via Mazzini 1, Azienda VSL 30, Desio: Dr. M.Peta, Dr. T. Bacchini, Dr. B. Fontana, Dr. G. Ciceri, Dr. S. Vesconi, Mrs. M. L. Casiraghi
- Ospedale di Vimercate, Via C. Battisti 23, 20059 Vimercate: Dr. F. Bassi, Dr. B. Graziano, Dr. R. Citterio, Mrs. C. Biffi
- Ospedale Predabissi, Via Pandiva 2, 20077 Vizzolo Predabissi, Melegnano: Dr. A. Guarino, Dr. A. Attanasio, Dr. G. Ronchi, Dr. S. Diterlizi, Dr. L. Della Grazia, Mrs. R. Lomi
- Ospedale de Rho, Cso. Europa 250, 20017 Rho: Dr. M. Panozzo, Dr. F. Accornero, Dr. G. M. Vaghi, Dr. P. Carmagnin, Dr. S. Bonelli, Mrs. E. Pagani
- Ospedale S. Corona, Via Forlanini 121, 20024 Garbagnate: Dr. B. Allaria, Dr. P. Ferrario, Dr. M. Dei Poli, Dr. L. de Filippi, Dr. M. Favaro, Mrs. S. Bianco

Spain

- Servicio de Medicina Intensiva, Hospital de Sabadell, Sabadell: Dr. A. Artigas, Dr. J. Mestre, C. Royo
- Servei de Medicina Intensiva, Centre Hospitalari i Cardiòlogic de Manresa, Barcelona: Dr. M. Guirado Alaiz, J. M. Alcoverro Pedrola, P. Saura Agel, J. Giladers Corominas
- Intensive Care Unit, Hospital de Terrassa: Dr. H. Bravo, Dr. M. Valdés, Dr. X. Trenchs, Mrs. C. Ramon
- Servei de Medicina Intensiva, Hospital General de Catalunya, Barcelona: Dr. M. Nolla-Salas, Dr. M.A. Leon-Regidor, Dr. J. Ibañez-Nolla, Dr. R. Diaz-Boladeras, J. Navarro-Dovenec, R. Morraja-Torras
- Servicio de Cuidados Intensivos, Hospital de Mutua de Terrassa: Dr. J. M. Nava Caballero, Dr. M. Alvares del Castillo, M. Aquilar Espinosa
- Intensive Care Unit, Hospital Universitario de Bellvitge: Dr. A. Diaz Prieto, M. Gorriz, E. Farrero, H. Torrado, M. Bello, A. Vives
- Servei de Medicina Intensiva, Hospital de la Creu Roja d'Hospitalet, Barcelona: Dr. M. Cerdà Vila, A. Rovira Plarromani, C. Cambray, A. Lopez Perez
- Servei de Medicina Intensiva, Hospital Los Camillos, Barcelona: Dr. J. Aguiló
- Servicio Medicina Intensiva, Hospital Universitario La Fé, Valencia: J. Cebrian Domeneck, B. Balerdi Perez, R. Marin Pastor, L. Gomez Salinas, J. Ruiz Ruiz, J. Botella de Maglia
- Servicio Medicina Intensiva, Hospital Clinico Universitario de Valencia: J. Cunat de la Hoz, R. Oltra Choroa, M. Blasco Cortes, J. Ferreres Franco
- Servicio Medicina Intensiva, Hospital Central de Asturias, Oviedo: F. Toboada, R. Garcia Tanjul, A. Garcia, M. Gutierrez, M.J. Espina, M. Martinez

- Servicio Medicina Intensiva, Clinico Universitario de Valladolid: Dr. J. Pino Rebolledo, J. Perez Garcia, A. Lizundia Iriondo
- Unidad de Cuidados Criticos, Servicio de Cuidados Criticos y Urgencias, Hospital Universitario Virgen de las Nieves, Granada: Dr. G. Vazquez Mata, Dr. R. M. Navarrete Navarro, Dr. E. Aguayo de Hoxos, C. Cortes Dominguez, M. Rua Bailen, P. Navarrete Navarro
- Servicio Medicina Intensiva, Hospital Arnau de Vilanova, Valencia: M. Garcia Sanz, A. Hervas Garces, M. Frances Sempere, F. Fajardo Dols, L. Cortes Tardegat, J. L. Espinos Castillo
- Servicio Medicina Intensiva, Hospital Lluis Alcanys, Xátiva: Dr. M. Rodriguez Serra, Dr. A. Cuervo Martinez, Dr. D. Garcia Lopez, Dr. A. Vinales Bernet, Dr. V. Borillo Noles
- Unidad de Medicina Critica, Servicio de Anestesiologia y Reanimación, Hospital Marina Alta, Denia, Alicante: J. Cardona Peretu, V. Madrid Rondon, F. Tarin Royo, F. Llobell Sala, J. Gonzalez Ortiz, C. Ortega Andres, A. Gimeno Infante
- Intensive Care Unit, Hospital General Castello: Dr. R. Abizanda, Dr. M. T. Rodriguez, Mrs. J. Marin
- Unidade de Cuidados Intensivos, Hospital Gran Viá, Castellon: O. Aznar Orti, H. Boix Ruiz, J. Monferrer Guardiola, M. Carbonell Uso, D. Magro Tena, T. Cortes Barcelo
- Servicio Medicina Intensiva, Hospital General Universitario de Elche: A. Mota Lopez, J. A. Rueda Cuenca
- Servicio Medicina Intensiva, Hospital Virgen de los Lirios, Alcoy: Dr. F. Guarajola Navarro, Dr. J. Marco Navarro, Dr. F. Amoros Carbonell
- Servicio Medicina Intensiva, Hospital Valle de Nalón, Sama de Langreo: J. Alfonso Megido, M. Rodriguez Junquera, B. Fernandez Gonzales, L. Velasco Alvarez, J. Gonzales Carou
- Servicio Medicina Intensiva, Hospital del Bierzo (Ponferrada): Dr. C. Ruiz Pardo, Dr. F.J. Cañizares Castellanos, Sr. L. Alvarez Viloria
- Servicio Medicina Intensiva, Hospital Rio Carrion Insalud, Palencia: Dr. A. Valverde Conde, Dr. J. Hampanera Gonzales, Dr. G. Ibañez Gallego
- Servicio Medicina Intensiva, Hospital General Universitario de Murcia: F. Felices Abad, B. Gil Rueda, J.J. Rodriguez Mondetar, T. Blanco Molina
- Intensive Care Unit, Centro de Traumatologia, Hospital Virgen de las Nieves, Granada: Dr. E. Fernandez Mondejar
- Servicio Medicina Intensiva, Hospital Arquitecto Marcide, Ferrol: I. Alvarez Dieguez, C. Botana Alba, A. Garcia Jilenez, J. Gonzales Tutor
- Servicio Medicina Intensiva, Hospital General de Galicia, Santiago de Compostela: Dr. C. Galban Rodriguez, Dr. A. Marino Rozados, Dr. A. Belmonte Sanz, Dr. T. M. Robelo Pardo, Dr. M. Sabada Acuña, Dr. E. Ferrer Vizoso

Portugal

- Serviço de Cuidados Intensivos, Hospital Geral de Santo António, Porto: Dr. M. Brandão, L. Brandão, A. Bernardino
- Unidade de Cuidados Intensivos do Serviço de Urgência, Hospital de São João, Porto: Dr. J. Duarte, Dr. F. Abelha, A. Rodrigues
- Unidade Cuidados Intensivos Polivalente, Hospital da Senhora da Oliviera, Guimarães: Dr. E. Lafuente, L. Pacheco
- Unidade de Cuidados Intensivos, Hospital de Santa Lucia, Viana do Castelo: Dr. P. Meireles, J. Correia
- Unidade de Cuidados Intensivos Polivalente, Centro Hospitalar de Vila Nova de Gaia, Vila Nova de Gaia: Dr. J. Reis, A. Rodrigues

Subject Index

Springer-Verlag and the Environment

We at Springer-Verlag firmly believe that an international science publisher has a special obligation to the environment, and our corporate policies consistently reflect this conviction.

We also expect our business partners – paper mills, printers, packaging manufacturers, etc. – to commit themselves to using environmentally friendly materials and production processes.

The paper in this book is made from low- or no-chlorine pulp and is acid free, in conformance with international standards for paper permanency.

MIX
Papier aus verantwortungsvollen Quellen
Paper from responsible sources
FSC® C105338
FSC
www.fsc.org

If you have any concerns about our products,
you can contact us on
ProductSafety@springernature.com

In case Publisher is established outside the EU,
the EU authorized representative is:
Springer Nature Customer Service Center GmbH
Europaplatz 3, 69115 Heidelberg, Germany

Printed by Libri Plureos GmbH
in Hamburg, Germany